# IMMUNOGLOBULINOPATHIES

*Publication Number 733*

AMERICAN LECTURE SERIES®


*A Monograph in*

*The* BANNERSTONE DIVISION *of*

AMERICAN LECTURES IN LIVING CHEMISTRY


*Edited by*

I. NEWTON KUGELMASS, M.D., Ph.D., Sc.D.

*Consultant to the Departments of Health and Hospitals*
*New York, New York*

# IMMUNOGLOBULINOPATHIES

### Immunoglobulins
### Immune Deficiency Syndromes
### Multiple Myeloma and Related Disorders

*By*

**RALPH L. ENGLE, Jr., B.S., M.D.**

*Associate Professor of Medicine*
*Cornell University Medical College*
*Associate Attending Physician, New York Hospital*
*New York, New York*

*and*

**LILA A. WALLIS, B.A., M.D.**

*Clinical Assistant Professor of Medicine*
*Cornell University Medical College*
*Assistant Attending Physician, New York Hospital*
*New York, New York*

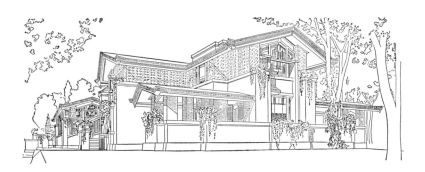

**CHARLES C THOMAS · PUBLISHER**
*SPRINGFIELD · ILLINOIS · U. S. A.*

*Published and Distributed Throughout the World by*
CHARLES C THOMAS · PUBLISHER
BANNERSTONE HOUSE
301–327 East Lawrence Avenue, Springfield, Illinois, U. S. A.
NATCHEZ PLANTATION HOUSE
735 North Atlantic Boulevard, Fort Lauderdale, Florida, U. S. A.

*With* THOMAS BOOKS *careful attention is given to all details of
manufacturing and design. It is the Publisher's desire to present books
that are satisfactory as to their physical qualities and artistic possibilities and appropriate for their particular use.* THOMAS BOOKS *will be
true to those laws of quality that assure a good name and good will.*

*Printed in the United States of America*
*K–8*

This book is dedicated to David P. Barr, M.D., outstanding clinician, teacher, investigator, and friend, whose inspiration and keen interest stimulated our work in this field.

# FOREWORD

Our Living Chemistry Series was conceived by Editor and Publisher to advance the newer knowledge of chemical medicine in the cause of clinical practice. The interdependence of chemistry and medicine is so great that physicians are turning to chemistry, and chemists to medicine in order to understand the underlying basis of life processes in health and disease. Once chemical truths, proofs and convictions become sound foundations for clinical phenomena, key hybrid investigators clarify the bewildering panorama of biochemical progress for application in everyday practice, stimulation of experimental research, and extension of postgraduate instruction. Each of our monographs thus unravels the chemical mechanisms and clinical management of many diseases that have remained relatively static in the minds of medical men for three thousand years. Our new Series is charged with the *nisus élan* of chemical wisdom, supreme in choice of international authors, optimal in standards of chemical scholarship, provocative in imagination for experimental research, comprehensive in discussions of scientific medicine, and authoritative in chemical perspective of human disorders.

Dr. Engle and Dr. Wallis of New York unravel the current concepts of immune mechanisms, of immunoglobulins, and of disease processes associated with abnormalities of immunoglobulins in a comprehensive integrated system with transcendent clarity and utter logic. It is the first unified approach to this group of heterogeneous immunologic disorders that makes penetration of physiochemical mechanisms a kind of clinical inspiration in this era. The understanding of these immune responses contributes to the study of host defense mechanisms and graft rejection phenomena, to the disciplines of classical and developmental genetics, and to the chemistry of serum proteins. The discovery of various abnormalities in immunoglobulins leads to a number of clinical conditions, the immunoglobulinopathies as a subdivision of proteinopathies, whose practical management is facilitated by the recognition of the underlying protein aberration. The newer knowledge of the physiochemical properties, molecular structure and functional activity of the immunoglobulins portrays the group of serum proteins to which antibody molecules belong. The chemical clarification of the mechanism of their production, synthesis, distribution, site of destruction, metabolism and normal levels in the serum throws new light on the esoteric heterogeneous immunoglobulinopathies: the hypoimmunoglobulinopathies associated with a deficiency of immunoglobulins; the hyperimmunoglobulinopathies associated with significant diffuse increase in immunoglobulins; and the paraimmunoglobulinopathies associated with production of unusual homogeneous immunoglobulins. This last group includes multiple myeloma and its variants, Waldenström's macroglobulinemia, heavy chain disease, essential cryoglobulinemia, paraamyloidosis, and other paraimmunoglobulinopathies.

The story of immunoglobulins in health and disease emerged from the efforts of a few architects and of many workers who changed the spirit and content of protein chemistry. The first advance in the modern era was designed by Svedberg and Tiselius, the second by E. J. Cohen and Heidelberger, and the third by Oudin and Grabar. In these lofty moments of immunochemical thoughts a tradition has arisen whereby the friendly usages of colloquial speech give way to a certain severity and formality. While this promotes precise thinking, it intimidates the neophyte. Originally, explanation signified a representation of the strange in terms of the commonplace; nowadays, it tends to be more of a description of the relatively familiar in terms of the unfamiliar. Therefore, the authors conduct the reader through the classic edifice of immunochemistry, into the workshops where construction is now in progress, to temper the customary severity of the clinical science in so far as is compatible with clarity of thought. We are led up the high hill by gentle slopes receiving chemical instruction to beguile the way. Our minds are made to move in complicated patterns in order to interpret complex biological phenomena. Once our chemical understanding is clear, clinical application is easy. To the Editor, the work has great fascination through its individualistic outlook tempered by a complete conception, correlation and criticism of immunochemical advances so crucial for clinical medicine and the life sciences.

*"Where New appearance is before the Eyes,*
*New Suppositions thereupon arise."*

I. NEWTON KUGELMASS, M.D., PH.D., SC.D., *Editor*

# PREFACE

THIS BOOK is directed primarily to physicians, both general practitioners and specialists, who want to become familiar with the many diseases in which there is an abnormality of the immunoglobulins demonstrable by electrophoresis—a group of diseases we call the immunoglobulinopathies. While this terminology may seem a bit formidable at first, its use is justified by the convenience of using compound words. Most of the book is devoted to the natural history of the diseases of the immune system; however, considerable effort has been made to present the basic science aspects of the immunoglobulins and the immune processes.

At the time we were invited to prepare this monograph, we had just completed sections on the paraimmunoglobulinopathies and on amyloidosis for the Tice-Harvey *Practice of Medicine* published by W. F. Prior Company, Inc. (Vol. I pp. 301–394, 1966). We were fortunate to get permission from Hoeber Medical Division of Harper and Row, Publishers, Inc., which has recently acquired Prior, for use of this material including some of the illustrations. Where this material has been used in the present volume, it has been expanded and brought up to date. We are also pleased to acknowledge in the appropriate captions those illustrations which we have borrowed with permission from the authors. Figures 31 to 37 and 39 to 42 are from the Tice-Harvey volume.

We would like to express our appreciation to Dr. Ralph Nachman, Dr. William Christenson, Dr. Richard Silver, and Dr. Elaine Eyster, all members of the Hematology Division of the Department of Medicine, who participated in many stimulating discussions which aided in the preparation of parts of the volume. In addition, Dr. Eyster helped to prepare some of the illustrations.

We also want to thank Mr. Milton Zisowitz for his helpful criticisms during preparation of the manuscript.

We are also grateful for the sympathetic cooperation of our respective spouses, Dr. Mary Allen Engle and Dr. Benedict Wallis.

RALPH L. ENGLE, JR.
LILA A. WALLIS

# CONTENTS

|  |  | *Page* |
| --- | --- | --- |
| *Foreword* | . . . . . . . . . . . . . . . . . . . | vii |
| *Preface* | . . . . . . . . . . . . . . . . . | ix |

*Chapter*

| 1. | INTRODUCTION . . . . . . . . . . . . | 3 |
| --- | --- | --- |
| 2. | STRUCTURE AND ACTIVITY OF THE IMMUNOGLOBULINS . . . . | 11 |
| 3. | PRODUCTION AND METABOLISM OF IMMUNOGLOBULINS . . . . | 46 |
| 4. | HYPOIMMUNOGLOBULINOPATHIES: DESCRIPTION OF SYNDROMES . . | 66 |
| 5. | HYPOIMMUNOGLOBULINOPATHIES: GENERAL ASPECTS . . . . . | 95 |
| 6. | HYPERIMMUNOGLOBULINOPATHIES . . . . . . . . | 111 |
| 7. | PARAIMMUNOGLOBULINOPATHIES: INTRODUCTION AND GENERAL ASPECTS | 126 |
| 8. | PARAIMMUNOGLOBULINOPATHIES: MULTIPLE MYELOMA . . . . . | 143 |
| 9. | OTHER PARAIMMUNOGLOBULINOPATHIES . . . . . . . . | 192 |
| *References* | . . . . . . . . . . . . . . . . . . | 218 |
| *Index* | . . . . . . . . . . . . . . . . . . . | 253 |

# IMMUNOGLOBULINOPATHIES

# Chapter 1

# INTRODUCTION

I MMUNOLOGY PLAYS an important role in almost all areas of biology and medicine and has become an essential discipline for life scientists. The antigen-antibody reaction serves as one of the major defense mechanisms of the host. At the same time it is at least partially responsible for the development of allergic and autoimmune diseases. The immune response is a manifestation of individuality and is the limiting factor in organ and tissue homotransplantation. A more complete understanding of the response may lead to successful transplantation. Studies of the many structural differences among the various immunoglobulin molecules are giving insight to mechanisms of classical genetics and, more recently, developmental genetics. Finally, the antigen-antibody reaction is a sensitive tool for characterizing and quantitating proteins and other antigens. For these and other reasons, immunology has broad applicability.

To assure a full appreciation of the present state of the science, it is important that we first review some of the highlights of its history.

## HISTORY

The phenomenon of immunity to disease, particularly to smallpox, has been known for many centuries. It was not until 1890, however, that von Behring and Kitasato demonstrated the development of a specific, transferable, neutralizing substance, later called antibody, in the blood of animals immunized by injection with tetanus toxin (von Behring and Kitasato, 1890). Before long, it was found that specific antibodies were produced to virtually all foreign proteins. In 1939, soon after the introduction of electrophoretic techniques for separating proteins, Tiselius and Kabat (1939) localized the antibody activity of the blood to the gamma globulin electrophoretic fraction of the plasma proteins. The terms *antibody* and *gamma globulin* became virtually synonymous.

By 1954 there was growing evidence that proteins related to antibodies by function and structure may be found in the beta globulin and even the alpha globulin fractions of the plasma proteins. In patients with multiple mye-

3

loma it had been shown that the serum myeloma proteins, which are related to gamma globulin, have electrophoretic mobilities ranging from the slow gamma region to the alpha region of the electrophoretic pattern. After the technique of immunoelectrophoresis was introduced by Poulik (1952) and by Grabar and Williams (1953), it was clearly demonstrated that the principal gamma globulin arc extends well over into the alpha and beta globulin regions (Williams and Grabar, 1955; Slater, 1955). This major gamma globulin arc is now called γG or immunoglobulin G, abbreviated IgG. The same technique was instrumental in defining three other major families or classes of immunoglobulins: γA or IgA, γM or IgM, and γD or IgD. Williams and Grabar (1955) discovered an arc, now called γA or IgA, which, though distinct, had immunologic determinants in common with the IgG arc. At approximately the same time, Lohss and Hillmann (1953) and Slater, Ward, and Kunkel (1955) recognized that beta serum myeloma proteins, now thought to be of this IgA class, were immunologically related to, but different from, the more frequent gamma myeloma proteins. Large molecular weight antibodies or macroglobulins, now called γM or IgM, had been identified in horse sera but their significance in human sera was not fully appreciated until after the clinical syndrome of Waldenström's macroglobulinemia had been described (Waldenström, 1944). A fourth class of immunoglobulins, called γD or IgD, was discovered by Rowe and Fahey (1965). Recently, a fifth class, called IgE, has been partially characterized, but its status is not yet clear (Ishizaka, Ishizaka, and Hornbrook, 1966).

Search for the cell responsible for antibody production led to diverse theories which are only now being integrated into a unified concept. Pfeiffer and Marx concluded in 1898 that antibodies originate in the spleen, bone marrow, lymph node, and lung, but the cell type involved was not appreciated until 1948, exactly half a century later, when Fagraeus (1948) showed the correlation between antibody formation and the development of plasma cells in the spleen. The possible role of the monocyte or macrophage as expounded by Sabin (1939) has not been entirely clarified, although it seems probable that the macrophage may prepare the antigen for its role in antibody synthesis within other cells (Fishman, Hammerstrom, and Bond, 1963). One of the major difficulties has been the confusion and disagreement concerning terminology and morphology of the cell types. Many workers, relying primarily on pathological sections in their experiments, failed to recognize plasma cells and considered them to be lymphocytes, thus adding to the confusion.

The technique of Coons (Coons, Laduc, and Connolly, 1955) in which fluorescent antibody is used to localize antigens intracellularly has made it possible to follow antibody synthesis and to identify the responsible cells as plasma cells and some lymphocytes as well as their precursors, the reticulum or reticular cells (Mellors and Korngold, 1963). There is evidence that under certain circumstances plasma cells may develop directly from lymphocytes (Nossal and Mäkelä, 1962a). All of these cells form the immunocyte system (Dameshek, 1963), since they are all thought to be involved in producing immunoglobulins.

## TERMINOLOGY AND CLASSIFICATION

The terms used in immunology and for the diseases associated with disturbances in the immune mechanism have always been confusing. We use the term *immunoglobulins* as originally proposed by Heremans (1959) and as defined by the World Health Organization Meeting on Nomenclature of Human Immunoglobulins (*Nomenclature*, 1964), since this has been generally accepted. The Meeting on Nomenclature defined the immunoglobulins as

proteins of animal origin endowed with known antibody activity, and certain proteins related to them by chemical structure and hence antigenic specificity. Related proteins for which antibody activity has not been demonstrated are included—for example, myeloma proteins, Bence Jones proteins, and naturally occurring sub-units of the immunoglobulins.

Immunoglobulins do not include complement unless one or more components of the complement system have the structure of immunoglobulins. Despite their heterogeneity, the immunoglobulins are structurally related but quite different from other protein molecules. Many immunoglobulin molecules have no known activity; however, when they do function, it is as antibodies. Immunoglobulins are formed within limited cell types, primarily plasma cells, some lymphocytes, and some reticulum cells. These are conveniently called immunocytes. The similarities in structure, function, and cell of origin justify the concept of the immunoglobulin system.

The Meeting on Nomenclature of Human Immunoglobulins (*Nomenclature*, 1964) made recommendations for terminology at the biochemical and molecular level; these terms will be used (see Table I). The clinician dealing with patients who have abnormalities of the immunoglobulins is still confronted by many different terms used to designate the various disease states. To have a proper appreciation of these terms it is essential to understand some of the manifestations of the normal and abnormal immune response.

While there is a growing recognition that some immunoglobulins may not appear in detectable quantities in the blood, nevertheless it is true that normally many immunoglobulins do circulate in the blood and are seen in the normal electrophoretic pattern of the serum proteins. These normal immunoglobulins probably result at least in part from a constant interaction between the host's immune mechanism and the many antigenic stimuli of the environment. It is possible that some of the normally circulating

## TABLE I

### NOMENCLATURE FOR HUMAN IMMUNOGLOBULINS

| | Synonyms | International Nomenclature * |
|---|---|---|
| Families or classes of immunoglobulins | $\gamma_2$, $\gamma$, $\gamma_{ss}$, $7S\gamma$ | $\gamma G$ or IgG |
| | $\gamma_{1A}$, $\beta_{2A}$ | $\gamma A$ or IgA |
| | $\gamma_{1M}$, $\beta_{2M}$, $19S\gamma$, $\gamma$-macroglobulins | $\gamma M$ or IgM |
| | | $\gamma D$ or IgD |
| | | $\gamma E$ or IgE |
| Immunoglobulin molecules identified by properties of light chains | Type I, 1, B | Type K |
| | Type II, 2, A | Type L |
| Notation for polypeptide chains | B or L chains | light chains |
| | A or H chains | heavy chains |

| | Immunoglobulin Family or Class | Notation |
|---|---|---|
| Heavy chains for each family of immunoglobulins | IgG | $\gamma$ |
| | IgA | $\alpha$ |
| | IgM | $\mu$ |
| | IgD | $\delta$ |
| | IgE | $\epsilon$ |

| | Immunoglobulin Type | Notation |
|---|---|---|
| Light chains for each type of immunoglobulins | K | $\kappa$ (kappa) |
| | L | $\lambda$ (lambda) |

* Nomenclature for human immunoglobulins. *Bull Wld Hlth Org*, 30: 447, 1964.

immunoglobulin molecules are not true antibodies in that they were not stimulated by a specific antigen but are really "blank" molecules without specific activity. Alternatively, all immunoglobulin molecules may be antibodies if only the proper antigen could be determined. In the day-to-day activities of the normal individual, there is very little fluctuation in the quantitative level of those immunoglobulins demonstrable by electrophoresis. A fairly specific stimulus to immunoglobulin synthesis, such as an acute infection, may not raise the level of immunoglobulins appreciably, even though the presence of specific antibody in high titer in the serum may be demonstrated. With special techniques, relatively profound abnormalities of the immunoglobulins can be demonstrated in association with infection, allergy, liver disease, and autoimmune phenomena without any appreciable disturbance in the electrophoretic pattern. The inability to detect these abnormalities by electrophoresis is a result of the extreme heterogeneity of the immunoglobulins, the failure of some of them to appear in appreciable quantity in the blood, and their increased catabolism under these circumstances. In other instances of the same conditions, however, quantitative changes in the immunoglobulins can be demonstrated by electrophoresis.

In those situations where a quantitative abnormality of the immunoglobulins is demonstrable by changes in the overall electrophoretic pattern we should like to suggest a new set of terms. We propose that diseases in which there are such disturbances of the immunoglobulins be called *immunoglobulinopathies,* a subdivision of the more general proteinopathies (see Table II). Three categories of immunoglobulinopathy may be recognized. Diseases associated with generalized reductions of one, two, three, or all four of the IgG, IgA, IgM, or IgD classes of immunogloublins may be called *hypoimmunoglobulinopathies* and the most common manifestation, *hypoimmunoglobulinemia*. These conditions are usually related to anatomic or functional deficiency of immunocytes.

Diseases associated with generalized elevations of one, two, three, or all four of the IgG, IgA, IgM, or IgD classes of immunoglobulins may be called *hyperimmunoglobulinopathies* and the most common manifestation, *hyperimmunoglobulinemia*. Such conditions are usually related to anatomic or functional excess of immunocytes.

Finally, in diseases such as multiple myeloma, Waldenström's macroglobulinemia, and related protein disturbances, several varieties of abnormalities may be seen. In most instances, there is an elevation in the blood of just one portion of one of the IgG, IgA, IgM, or IgD classes of immunoglobulins and suppression of all of the others. Bence Jones proteinuria may be found either with or without the serum protein abnormality. Both the serum myeloma proteins and the Bence Jones proteins are relatively homogeneous and, in a given patient, almost always of either type K or type L immunologic specificity but not both. In rare instances, two and possibly more of such homogeneous proteins appear in the same patient. Such homogeneous proteins are thought to be related to the proliferation, usually malignant, of one or rarely two or a few clones of immunocytes. For this group of diseases we suggest the term *paraimmunoglobulinopathies* and their most common manifestations, *paraimmunoglobulinemia* and *paraimmunoglobulinuria*. The prefix *para* which means beside, beyond, accessory to, or apart from, rather than the prefix *dys* which means bad or disordered (Dorland, 1940), is suggested, since present evidence favors the concept that paraimmunoglobulins are quantitatively increased amounts of proteins normally present in small amounts rather than qualitatively abnormal proteins. This problem has not been finally resolved, however. The small molecular weight fragments and subunits of the immunogloublins, such as Bence Jones proteins, heavy chain fragments, and others still unidentified, could also be called *microimmunoglobulins* and their appearance in the blood and urine, *microimmunoglobulinemia* and *microimmunoglobulinuria*.

Figure 1 illustrates starch gel electrophoretic patterns of serum proteins in hypoimmunoglobulinemia, hyperimmunoglobulinemia, three examples of paraimmunoglobulinemia, and one example of microimmunoglobulinemia as compared to a normal pattern.

# TABLE II

## CLASSIFICATION OF PROTEINOPATHIES INCLUDING THE IMMUNOGLOBULINOPATHIES

PROTEINOPATHIES

**Disturbances in Immunoglobulins**
IMMUNOGLOBULINOPATHIES

**Disturbances in all other plasma proteins** (e.g., albumin, α-mucoproteins, ceruloplasmin, fibrinogen, clotting factors)

### HYPOIMMUNOGLOBULINOPATHIES

Manifest primarily in the blood as hypoimmunoglobulinemia; deficiency of one or more of the immunoglobulin families (IgG, IgA, IgM, IgD)

A. PRIMARY HYPOIMMUNO-GLOBULINEMIAS
1. Hypoimmunoglobulinemias of early onset
   a. Reticular Dysgenesis
   b. Agammaglobulinemia with lymphopenia (Swiss type)
   c. Congenital sex-linked agammaglobulinemia
   d. Ataxia-telangiectasia
2. Hypoimmunoglobulinemias of late onset
   a. Generalized adult hypoimmunoglobulinemia
   b. Selective adult hypoimmunoglobulinemias
   c. "Familial idiopathic dysproteinemia"
B. SECONDARY HYPOIMMUNO-GLOBULINEMIAS
1. Associated with hypoalbuminemia
2. Associated with malignancies o. reticuloendothelial system
3. Associated with autoimmune diseases
4. Associated with chronic infections
5. Associated with diseases of unknown etiology
C. PHYSIOLOGIC HYPOIMMUNO-GLOBULINEMIAS
1. Of the newborn
2. Of germ-free animals

### HYPERIMMUNOGLOBULINOPATHIES

Manifest primarily in the blood as hyperimmunoglobulinemia; diffuse increase in all immunoglobulins and occasionally of just one or two of the immunoglobulin families (IgG, IgA, IgM, IgD)

A. PRIMARY HYPERIMMUNO-GLOBULINEMIAS
1. Variations related to race
2. Familial hyperimmunoglobulinemia
3. Aldrich syndrome
B. SECONDARY HYPERIMMUNO-GLOBULINEMIAS
1. Secondary to infections
2. Associated with autoimmune diseases
   a. Rheumatoid arthritis
   b. RF-Complex cryoglobulinemia and/or macroglobulinemia
   c. Systemic lupus erythematosus
   d. Other autoimmune disorders
3. Associated with malignancies
4. Associated with diseases of unknown etiology
   a. Infectious mononucleosis
   b. Sarcoidosis
   c. Benign hyperglobulinemic purpura
   d. Charrnot's syndrome
   e. Liver disease

### PARAIMMUNOGLOBULINOPATHIES

Manifest primarily in the blood as paraimmunoglobulinemia, but frequently in the urine as microimmunoglobulinuria (Bence Jones protein and other fragments of the paraimmunoglobulins), and occasionally in the tissues as paraamyloid

A. MULTIPLE MYELOMA
B. WALDENSTRÖM's MACRO-GLOBULINEMIA
C. H-CHAIN DISEASE
D. PARAIMMUNOGLOBULINOPATHIES ASSOCIATED WITH OTHER DISEASES:
1. Chronic lymphocytic leukemia, lymphosarcoma, reticulum cell sarcoma, and Hodgkin's disease
2. Other malignancies
3. Nonneoplastic conditions more often characterized by diffuse hyperimmunoglobulinemia
E. PARAIMMUNOGLOBULINOPATHIES OF UNKNOWN ETIOLOGY
1. Idiopathic paraimmunoglobulinemia
2. Idiopathic cryoglobulinemia
3. Idiopathic pyroglobulinemia
F. PARAAMYLOIDOSIS

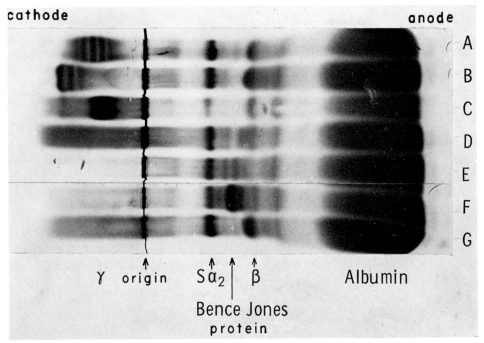

cathode

anode

A
B
C
D
E
F
G

γ    origin     Sα₂ | β              Albumin

Bence Jones
protein

FIGURE 1. Starch gel electrophoresis patterns of serum proteins illustrating patterns typical of the three kinds of immunoglobulinopathies. (A, B, and C) Paraimmunoglobulinopathy, IgG multiple myeloma, note multiple abnormal bands in gamma region. (D) Hyperimmunoglobulinopathy. (E) Hypoimmunoglobulinopathy. (F) Hypoimmunoglobulinopathy with Bence Jones proteinemia. (G) Normal.

Under certain circumstances the paraimmunoglobulinopathies are associated with tissue deposits of amyloid. We use *paraamyloid* and *paraamyloidosis* to refer to the kind of amyloid and the condition in which one of the paraimmunoglobulinopathies is associated with amyloidosis. Since physicians say "paraamyloid" and "paraamyloidosis" even though they write it "paramyloid," we suggest that the spelling conform to the pronunciation.

Those rare patients with multiple myeloma who have no demonstrable paraimmunoglobulin in the serum, urine, or tissue usually have a hypoimmunoglobulinemia and are classified in the group of hypo-immunoglobulinopathies.

All of the terms proposed come from Greek roots, a prerequisite to proper terminology among purists. Most of the terms are quite long and difficult to pronounce on first attempt. After a little practice, however, they become manageable.

This terminology removes the need for using such terms as *dysproteinemia*, which is too general and implies a distorted protein, and *monoclonal gammopathy*, which may not be monoclonal and which retains the use of gamma globulin, even though we know that many of the immunoglobulins do not migrate with gamma mobility.

## AREAS NOT COVERED

The field of immunology has grown so large that it is impossible to encompass it in a single monograph. In discussing abnormalities of the immune system, we shall confine our efforts largely to those situations in which there is an abnormality of the immunoglobulins demonstrable by electrophoresis, i.e., the hypo-, hyper-, and paraimmunoglobulinopathies. Only brief mention will be made of those conditions covered in detail in books and monographs on classical allergy (Gell and Coombs, 1963), blood bank immunology (Race and Sanger, 1962; Wiener, 1965), homo- and heterotransplantation (Woodruff, 1960), and autoimmunity (Mackay and Burnet, 1963). Likewise, we shall consider only the very general aspects of the diseases associated with hyperimmunoglobulinemia, for example, liver disease and the many acute and chronic infections, since these are covered in detail in specialized monographs and textbooks. Two publications on immunoglobulins and immune disorders have recently appeared (Samter, M., and Alexander, H. L., 1965; Schultze, H., and Heremans, J. F., 1966).

subfractions: light chains (also called L or B chains) with a molecular weight of about 22,000, and heavy chains (also called H or A chains) with a molecular weight of about 55,000 (Edelman and Poulik, 1961). A single immunoglobulin molecule of molecular weight 150,000 is thought to consist of two light chains and two heavy chains (see Fig. 3). The four immunoglobulin classes are determined by the structure of the heavy chain, which differs for each of the IgG, IgM, IgA, and IgD classes. The light chains, on the other hand, seem to be the same for each of the classes of immunoglobu-

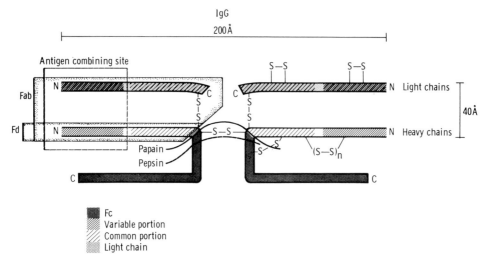

FIGURE 3. Structure of basic unit of immunoglobulin molecule. N = N-terminal end; C = C-terminal end. Each of the light chains is divided into two halves indicated by different shading. The half with N-terminal amino acid is the variable portion; the half with the C-terminal amino acid is the common portion. The intrachain S-S bonds are marked above one of the light chains, two S-S bonds per light chain. The portion of the Fd fragment with the N-terminal amino acid is the variable portion of the heavy chain; the C-terminal end of the Fd fragment is the common portion of the heavy chain. The regions where papain and pepsin act are indicated. (Reproduced [modified] with permission from OVARY, Z.: *Ann NY Acad Sci, 129*:776, 1966.)

lins. Type specificity, either type K or type L, resides in the light chains. With the four classes having specificity in the heavy chain and the two types in each class having specificity in the light chain, eight major kinds of immunoglobulins can result if light and heavy chains are combined in all possible combinations (see Fig. 4). Since there are two heavy chains and two light chains in each immunoglobulin molecule, it is theoretically possible to have pairing of identical light chains and identical heavy chains, or nonidentical pairing of either or both light and heavy chains. Present evidence indicates the natural occurrence of paired identical chains, although it is possible to construct experimentally molecules of paired nonidentical chains. Type K light chains are known as kappa ($\kappa$) chains and type L light

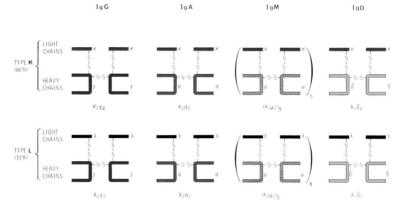

FIGURE 4. Scheme of classes and types of immunoglobulins.

chains, lambda ($\lambda$) chains. The heavy chains of IgG, IgA, IgM, IgD and IgE immunoglobulins are known as $\gamma$, $a$, $\mu$, $\delta$, and $\epsilon$ chains, respectively. Whole immunoglobulin molecules are represented by combinations of the proper peptide chains, e.g., $\gamma_2\lambda_2$.

A second method whereby biochemists have broken up the immunoglobulin molecule involves treatment with papain. While the details of this enzyme's action on human immunoglobulins still need to be clarified, it is thought that it splits the immunoglobulin molecule into three components. Two of them are probably identical, electrophoretically slow-moving Fab fragments (also called the S or A component); one is a fast-moving Fc fragment (also called the F or B component) (Edelman and Benacerraf, 1962). As the diagram (Fig. 3) shows, the Fc fragment contains portions of the heavy chains while the Fab fragments contain all of the light chains and a portion of the heavy chains. The portion of the heavy chains included in the Fab fragment is known as the Fd fragment, and it is isolated following papain digestion of heavy chains.

Not all immunoglobulins are broken down by papain in this way. Takatsuki and Osserman (1964a) found that papain in the presence of cysteine completely destroys the Fc fragments of some IgG myeloma proteins and the Fc fragments found in the urine of some patients with "heavy chain disease." Since the Fc fragments remain intact if the mixture does not contain cysteine, it has been postulated that this agent probably breaks certain crucial disulphide bonds of some immunoglobulins, thus allowing the molecule to unfold and thereby making it more susceptible to complete papain digestion (Poulik and Shuster, 1965). For a detailed review of the effects of enzymes on the immunoglobulins, the paper by Poulik (1967) should be consulted.

In contrast to papain, pepsin, when reacted with immunoglobulins, acts on the other side of the disulfide bond between the heavy chains and digests nearly all of the Fc fragment into small peptides, leaving a bivalent anti-body fragment intact (see Fig. 3). This bivalent fragment is called the F (ab′)$_2$ fragment, since it consists of the two Fab fragments and a small part of the N-terminal end of the Fc fragment containing the disulfide bond between the heavy chains (Ovary, 1966).

Even within the eight kinds of immunoglobulins already described, both the light and the heavy chains are still considerably heterogeneous. At least four different kinds of heavy chains have been described among the IgG immunoglobulins of an individual, and it has been shown that this hetero-geneity resides in the Fc fragment of the heavy chain. These subclasses within the IgG class of immunoglobulins were designated by Grey and Kunkel (1964) with the first two letters of the names of the original mye-loma patients involved, i.e., Ne, We, Vi and Ge and have been called $\gamma_{2a}$, $\gamma_{2b}$, $\gamma_{2c}$, and $\gamma_{2d}$ respectively by Fahey and coworkers (Terry and Fahey, 1964). We shall use the latter terminology in this monograph. Recently, yet another nomenclature has been recommended by a subcommittee of W.H.O. In their terminology $\gamma$G1 is $\gamma_{2b}$, $\gamma$G2 is $\gamma_{2a}$, $\gamma$G3 is $\gamma_{2c}$, and $\gamma$GA is $\gamma_{2d}$. The immunologic specificity of these subclasses was detected by several methods. Dray (1960), and later Terry and Fahey (1964), demonstrated three of the subclasses by reacting monkey antisera to human gamma globu-lin, unabsorbed and absorbed with two different myeloma proteins (para-immunoglobulins), with human gamma globulin in an immunoelectro-phoretic system. Takatsuki and Osserman (1964a) and Ballieux *et al.* (1964) found two of the subclasses by using rabbit antisera to the urinary protein of patients with heavy-chain disease. These urinary proteins are thought to be the Fc fragments of myeloma proteins. Grey and Kunkel (1964) detected at least four subclasses by using rabbit antisera to isolated paraimmunoglobulins. Evidence obtained by typing myeloma proteins shows that the $\gamma_{2b}$ subclass is the most frequent among the normal immuno-globulin molecules, about 77 per cent, while the $\gamma_{2a}$, $\gamma_{2c}$, and $\gamma_{2d}$ subclasses have frequencies of about 11 per cent, 9 per cent, and 3 per cent, respectively (from Terry, W., and Fahey, J., quoted by Fudenberg, 1965). Two un-named immunologic subclasses have been found within the heavy chains of each of the IgM (Harboe, Deverill, and Godal, 1965) and IgA classes (Vaer-man and Heremans, 1966; Terry and Roberts, 1966; Kunkel and Prender-gast, 1966).

Electrophoretic heterogeneity of both the light and heavy chains has also been demonstrated. Cohen and Porter (1964) and Cohen and Gordon (1965) using electrophoresis in urea-glycine starch gels first resolved the light chains into at least ten bands, each having molecules of type K and type L specificity. Poulik (1964) by use of tris-citrate urea starch gel electro-phoresis resolved ten to thirteen bands. Similar heterogeneity of the heavy chains has been demonstrated by other workers. Rejnek, Kostka, and Kotynek (1966) resolved ten electrophoretic subfractions of heavy chains in urea-glycine starch gels and Roholt and Pressman (1966) resolved seven subfractions within rabbit heavy chains by disc electrophoresis in acrylamide. Heavy chains from IgG have recently been resolved into fifteen to eighteen fractions by means of urea-glycine starch gel electrophoresis (Sjöquist, 1966; Sjöquist and Vaughan, 1966). Fahey showed that the electrophoretic mobility of the heavy chains approximates that of the whole immunoglobulin molecule, whereas the electrophoretic mobility of the light chain is independent of the mobility of the whole immunoglobulin molecule (Fahey, 1964). Heterogeneity of the Fc fragment of the heavy chain has been studied by Poulik and Shuster (1964), who showed ten to thirteen distinct subcomponents by starch gel electrophoresis using a discontinuous system of buffers.

The multiple discrete bands seen upon electrophoresis of light and heavy chains are thought by several workers to be due to single charge differences

TABLE IV

DISTRIBUTION OF RADIOACTIVITY IN ELECTROPHORETIC SUBFRACTIONS OF $^{131}$I-LABELLED $\kappa$- AND $\lambda$-CHAINS

Light chains were isolated from IgG of normal blood donor. Electrophoretic subfractions ($B_1 - B_{10}$) are numbered from the cathodal end of the gel. The $\kappa$-chains contain 70% of the $^{131}$I present in the original labelled light chains and $\lambda$-chains contain 30%. The values given represent percentages of total light-chain radioactivity present in each electrophoretic subfraction.

*Distribution of Radioactivity (%)*

| Light-chain subfraction | $B_1$ | $B_2$ | $B_3$ | $B_4$ | $B_5$ | $B_6$ | $B_7$ | $B_8$ | $B_9$ | $B_{10}$ |
|---|---|---|---|---|---|---|---|---|---|---|
| $\kappa + \lambda$ | 0.5 | 2.3 | 9.6 | 12.5 | 19.1 | 19.6 | 14.5 | 10.6 | 7.5 | 4.0 |
| $\kappa$ | 0.5 | 1.5 | 7.5 | 9.6 | 13.8 | 14.4 | 10.0 | 6.8 | 4.4 | 2.0 |
| $\lambda$ | 0.5 | 0.8 | 2.1 | 2.9 | 5.3 | 5.2 | 4.5 | 3.8 | 3.1 | 2.0 |
| Ratio $\kappa/\lambda$ | | 1.9 | 3.6 | 3.3 | 2.6 | 2.8 | 2.2 | 1.8 | 1.4 | 1.0 |

NOTE: Reproduced with permission from COHEN, S., and GORDON, S.: *Biochem J*, 97: 460, 1965.

in the population of molecules (Sjöquist, 1966; Roholt and Pressman, 1966) rather than to polymerization of a single subunit. The distribution by charge of the immunoglobulin molecules from a normal individual is such that there are many more molecules with relatively no charge and many fewer molecules of relatively positive or negative charge (Cohen and Gordon, 1965; Sjöquist, 1966) (see Fig. 5 and Table IV).

With immunologic as well as biochemical techniques, further heterogeneity and subgroups of light chains have been demonstrated in Bence Jones proteins which are closely related, if not identical, to the light chains of serum myeloma proteins (see discussion of Bence Jones proteins later in this chapter).

The two methods of reductive alkylation and papain digestion for dissociation of immunoglobulin molecules have permitted mapping of the molecules for sites of certain known activities. The Fab fragments, of which there are two per molecule, contain the specific antigen-combining site. It is not

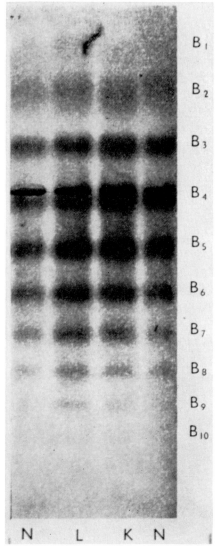

FIGURE 5. Electrophoresis in urea-glycine starch gel, pH 7, of whole light chain (N) and of preparations containing 85–90% of λ (L) or κ (K) chain. (Reproduced with permission from COHEN, S. and GORDON, S.: *Biochem J, 97*:460, 1965.)

entirely clear whether this antibody activity is related to the heavy chain or to both the heavy and light chains, though probably both chains are essential for optimal activity. If previously separated light and heavy chains of several specific antibodies are allowed to recombine in the presence of specific antigens, the light and heavy chains having antibody activity combine preferentially (Metzger and Mannik, 1964). The Fc fragment, which contains part of the heavy chain, is not required for antibody activity (Roholt, Radzimski, and Pressman, 1966) but is involved in complement fixation by $\gamma$ and $\mu$ chains as well as in precipitation with rheumatoid factor (Henney and Stanworth, 1964), in skin attachment (Porter and Press, 1962), and in placental and membrane transmission by $\gamma$ chains (Porter and Press, 1962). The carbohydrate of the immunoglobulin is attached to the Fc fragment and is an oligosaccharide containing galactose, mannose, fructose, glucosamine, and sialic acid (Rosevear and Smith, 1961).

It is possible to visualize the ultra-structure of immunoglobulin molecules by means of the electron microscope using negative staining techniques. In this technique an opaque stain such as sodium silicotungstate is dried to form a very thin layer in which the molecules are embedded. The image seen is the layer of stain and not the protein molecule itself. Valentine (1967) has reported on the electron microscopy of rabbit IgG immunoglobulins. He has described linear chains and various types of closed rings which result from polymerization of the molecules. Sometimes triangles with angles of 60° are formed resulting from trimers; sometimes squares are formed with angles of 90° resulting from tetramers; and sometimes pentagons with angles of 108° resulting from pentamers; and so on. Polymerization probably occurs between the two active sites on the Fab fragments. The various forms of polymerization visualized indicate that the juncture between the Fab and the Fc fragments must be capable of moving like a hinge in order to produce the geometrical forms seen. Svehag, Chesebro, and Bloth (1967) have made similar studies of normal rabbit and human IgM immunoglobulins and three IgM immunoglobulins from patients with Waldenström's macroglobulinemia. All of these preparations showed structures best described as five-legged spiders conforming to the proposed structure of pentamers.

Certain inherited differences in the immunoglobulins which distinguish one normal individual from another have been identified through the use of complex immunologic test systems. The genetic differences are demonstrated by an agglutination inhibition test (see Fig. 6). The reagent used is type $Rh_o$ (D) positive red blood cells coated with human anti-$Rh_o$ incomplete antibody of appropriate genetic type. These cells are agglutinated by certain normal sera (designated SNagg) or rheumatoid sera (designated Ragg) containing antibodies or rheumatoid factors directed against the isologous, genetically different, anti-$Rh_o$ antibody coated on the red blood cells.

This agglutination reaction is inhibited by sera containing antibodies of the same genetic type as the incomplete coating antibody but not by sera containing antibodies of another genetic type. Immunoglobulins in sera producing such inhibition, therefore, have immunologic determinants similar to those of the incomplete coating antibody and are said to be positive for that factor. Sera not producing such inhibition are said to be negative for that factor. The specificity of the system resides in the relationship of the

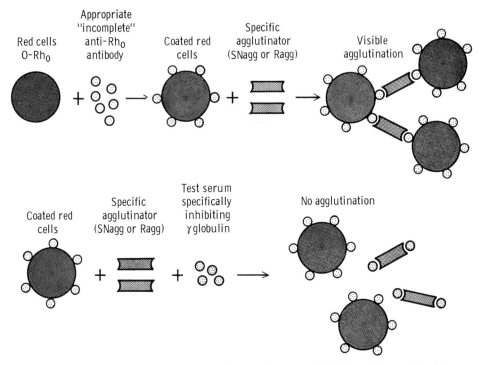

FIGURE 6. Scheme for Gm and Inv typing of immunoglobulins. (Modified with permission from Dr. James C. Allen of Johns Hopkins University.)

specific inhibiting serum to both the specific red cell coating serum and the specific rheumatoid agglutinating serum (Grubb, 1961; Steinberg, 1962; Fudenberg, 1963). Several factors have been identified in this manner and the genetics of each factor have been elucidated. These genetic variants of the immunoglobulins have been called allotypes. The major allotypic factors are Gm (a), Gm (b¹), Gm (b³), Gm (b⁴), Gm (c), Gm (f), Gm (g), Gm (n), Gm (s), Gm (t), Gm (x), Gm (y), Gm (z), Inv (a), Inv (b), and Inv (1). Gm (bʷ) is identical to Gm (b²) which is either very similar to, or identical to, Gm (f) (Steinberg, 1965). We shall use Gm (f) to designate these factors. Gm-like is now called Gm (c). Gm (b) and Gm (b¹) are the same. An international committee has suggested that numbers be used instead of letters to indicate the different Gm and Inv factors (Notation, 1966). Their recommendations are listed in Table V. They have also recommended that the phenotype be written in the form Gm (1,−2,3,4,5) to indicate both present and absent factors or Gm (1,3,4,5) to indicate just the present factors. The genotype is written with the locus in italics and superscript numbers, for example $Gm^{1,2}/Gm^1$. In his monograph we shall use the letter symbols and not the number symbols.

Gm sites are located on the heavy chains of IgG immunoglobulin molecules (see Fig. 4). Inv activity has been localized to the light chains and is

TABLE V

NOTATION FOR FACTORS AT THE GM AND INV LOCI

| | *Synonyms* | *International Nomenclature (Notation, 1966)* | |
|---|---|---|---|
| Gm locus: | a | 1 | |
| | x | 2 | |
| | $b^w$ and $b^2$ | 3 | ⎫ probably the same |
| | $f = b^2$ | 4 | ⎬ |
| | b and $b^1$ | 5 | ⎭ |
| | Gm-like and c | 6 | |
| | r | 7 | |
| | e | 8 | |
| | p | 9 | |
| | $b^\alpha$ | 10 | |
| | $b^\beta$ | 11 | |
| | $b^\gamma$ | 12 | |
| | $b^3$ | 13 | |
| | $b^4$ | 14 | |
| | s | 15 | |
| | t | 16 | |
| | z | 17 | |
| | | 18 | |
| | | 19 | |
| | fud | 20 | |
| | g | 21 | |
| | y | 22 | |
| | n | 23 | |
| Inv locus: | l | 1 | |
| | a | 2 | |
| | b | 3 | |

therefore found in all four families of the immunoglobulins. It is of interest, however, that only type K light chains have Inv activity.

At the molecular level, Meltzer *et al.* (1964) have identified a Gm (a+) peptide spot by two-dimensional electrophoresis-chromatography. (Frangione *et al.,* 1966). Analysis of Bence Jones proteins, which are closely related, if not identical, to homogeneous light chains has revealed the presence of leucine at position 189 in Inv (a+) proteins and valine at the same position in Inv (a−) and Inv (b+) proteins (Milstein, 1966b; Baglioni *et al.,* 1966; Titani, Whitley and Putnam, 1966).

The Gm ($b^1$), Gm ($b^3$), and Gm ($b^4$) antigens lose their activity upon digestion of the immunoglobulin molecule with papain while Gm (a) and Gm (f) retain activity (Steinberg and Polmar, 1965). If Gm (f+) immunoglobulins are reductively alkylated to separate heavy and light chains, Gm (f) activity is lost, but regained when the heavy and light chains are recombined. This indicates the importance of quarternary structure in such activity. The Gm (f) locus, however, can be shown to be on the heavy chain, since activity is regained only if Gm (f+) heavy chains are combined with light chains of either type K or L from either Gm (f+) or Gm (f−) immunoglobulins but not if Gm (f−) heavy chains are used (Steinberg and Polmar, 1965). The combination of heavy and light chains is also needed for full expression of the Inv (1) activity.

The Inv and Gm factors differ from one population group to another. A few typical examples are shown in Tables VI and VII. Among Caucasians 11 to 20 per cent are Inv (a+), 40 to 65 per cent are Gm (a+), and practically none are Gm (s+). Among Mongoloids 47 to 60 per cent are Inv (a+), virtually 100 per cent are Gm (a+), and 31 to 38 per cent are Gm (s+). Among Negroes 53 to 58 per cent are Inv (a) +, 100 per cent are Gm (a+), and 14 to 21 per cent are Gm (s+).

Although such incidence figures are important in determining the relationship of one racial group to another, even more important is the information on the inheritance of combinations of factors. The Inv and Gm factors are the immunologic manifestation of structural variations in immunoglobulin molecules. The immunologic techniques used to distinguish the factors must be very sensitive indicators of structure since they permit separation of Inv (a+) from Inv (a−) molecules, a difference known to result from the substitution of a single amino acid (Baglione *et al.*, 1966). Since these factors are genetically determined and have been shown to be interrelated through classical genetic mechanisms, an understanding of the inheritance of combinations of factors provides valuable information concerning allelism, linkage, and the arrangement of the responsible structural genes on the chromosomes. We shall use the term *alleles* in its narrowest sense, indicating two or more alternative protein factors (phenotypes) which are determined by one or possibly a few adjacent amino acids and which relate to a single locus on the chromosome. Although the evidence is often scanty and generalizations difficult, we shall attempt to discuss the interrelationships of these factors at the chromosomal level, realizing that our present theoretical model will probably require modifications.

There is no demonstrable genetic linkage between the Gm and Inv factors (Martensson, 1966), indicating that the loci responsible for their production are either on different chromosomes or are far apart on the same chromosome.

The Inv factors are not nearly so complicated as the Gm. Inv (1), Inv (1a), and Inv (b) act as alleles. Inv (1) is always present whenever Inv (a) is present but may also be found in the absence of Inv (a) (Lopez and Bütler, 1965) (see Table VI). There is also evidence for an as yet silent factor, Inv− (Steinberg, Wilson, and Lanset, 1962).

Gm factors are inherited in certain fixed combinations which differ from race to race. Examples of two common combinations among Caucasians, Gm (g+z+a+x+) and Gm (b$^1$+b$^3$+b$^4$+n+f+y+), are shown in Figure 7, where an attempt is made to relate the combinations to loci on chromosomes responsible for the production of $\gamma_{2a}$, $\gamma_{2b}$, and $\gamma_{2c}$ heavy chains. Since each of the two combinations is inherited as a single package, one combination is shown on one chromosome and the other on a second chromosome. From the diagram it is possible to determine which factors are present on the $\gamma_{2a}$, $\gamma_{2b}$, or $\gamma_{2c}$ heavy chains and which are on the Fc or Fd fragments. In

## TABLE VI

### INCIDENCE OF Inv DETERMINANTS IN VARIOUS POPULATION GROUPS

| Population | Reference | Number Tested | Inv(a+) | (l+) | (l+a+) | (l+a-) | (l-a-) | (l-a+) |
|---|---|---|---|---|---|---|---|---|
| | | | | | Per Cent of Population | | | |
| **Caucasian** | | | | | | | | |
| Swiss | Lopez & Bütler, 1965 | 600 | 17.7 | | | | | |
| French | Ropartz, Rousseau, et al., 1961 | 402 | 19.4 | 18.4 | 17.7 | 0.7 | 81.6 | 0 |
| German: | | | | | | | | |
| Schleswig-Holstein | Sachs, 1962 | 546 | 12.8 | | | | | |
| Rheinland-Pfalz | Ropartz et al., 1964 | 386 | 10.6 | | | | | |
| Bavaria | Ropartz et al., 1963 | 148 | 11.5 | | | | | |
| Finnish | " | 162 | 11.1 | | | | | |
| Dutch | " | 354 | 16.1 | | | | | |
| Czech | " | 190 | 12.1 | | | | | |
| Greek | " | 297 | 17.2 | | | | | |
| Yugoslavian | " | 157 | 14.7 | | | | | |
| **Mongoloid** | | | | | | | | |
| Japanese | Ropartz, Rivat, et al., 1961 | 270 | 47.8 | | | | | |
| Chinese | Steinberg, Wilson, & Lanset, 1962 | | 50–60 | | | | | |
| **Negro** | | | | | | | | |
| American | Steinberg, Wilson & Lanset, 1962 | 329 | 52.8 | | | | | |
| Dakar | Ropartz, Rivat, et al., 1961 | 399 | 53.6 | | | | | |

| Population | Reference | Number Tested | Inv(a+) | (b+) | (a+b-) | (a+b+) | (a-b+) | (a-b-) |
|---|---|---|---|---|---|---|---|---|
| | | | | | Per Cent of Population | | | |
| **Negro** | | | | | | | | |
| American | Steinberg, Wilson & Lanset, 1962 | 165 | 58.2 | 86.7 | 13.3 | 44.9 | 41.8 | 0 |
| Australian aborigines | | | | | | | | |
| Western Desert | " | 297 | 43 | 0 | | | | |
| Coastal Region | " | 268 | 37 | 31 | | | | |

## TABLE VII

### INCIDENCE OF Gm DETERMINANTS IN VARIOUS POPULATION GROUPS

| Population | Gm(a) Reference | Gm(a) Number Tested | Gm(a) % Pos. | Gm(b) Reference | Gm(b) Number Tested | Gm(b) % Pos. | Gm(s) Reference | Gm(s) Number Tested | Gm(s) % Pos. | Gm(c) Reference | Gm(c) Number Tested | Gm(c) % Pos. | Gm(x) Reference | Gm(x) Number Tested | Gm(x) % Pos. |
|---|---|---|---|---|---|---|---|---|---|---|---|---|---|---|---|
| Caucasian Swedish | Grubb by Steinberg, 1962 | 369 | 59.6 | Steinberg, 1962 | | 80–90 | Martensson & van Loghem, 1966 | 40 | 0 | | | | | | |
| Norwegian | Harboe & Lundevall, 1959 | 320 | 60.6 | | | | | | | | | | | | |
| Finnish | Grubb by Steinberg, 1962 | 477 | 65.0 | | | | | | | | | | | | |
| Danish | Linnet-Jepsen, 1958 | 1084 | 55.6 | | | | | | | | | | | | |
| Dutch | | | | | | | Martensson & van Loghem, 1966 | 870 | 1 | Steinberg, Giles & Stauffer, 1960 | 250 | 0 | Harboe and Lundevall, 1959 | 318 | 25.8 |
| Italian | Grubb by Steinberg, 1962 | 125 | 40.2 | | | | | | | | | | | | |
| French | Grubb by Steinberg, 1962 | 2659 | 52.2 | | | | | | | | | | | | |
| Negro | Ropartz by Steinberg, 1962 | | 100 | Steinberg, 1962 | | 100 | | | | Steinberg, Giles & Stauffer, 1960 | 403 | 27.5 | Steinberg, Giles & Stauffer, 1960 | 75 | 1 |
| West African | | | | | | | Martensson & van Loghem, 1966 | 110 | 14 | Ropartz by Steinberg, 1962 | | 0 | | | |
| Surinam | | | | | | | Martensson & van Loghem, 1966 | 188 | 21 | Ropartz by Steinburg, 1962 | | 0 | | | |
| Mongoloid Chinese | Ropartz by Steinberg, 1962 | | 100 | Steinberg, 1962 | | 90–95 | | | | Ropartz by Steinberg, 1962 | | 0 | Ropartz by Steinberg, 1962 | | 5–15 |
| Japanese | Ropartz by Steinberg, 1962 | | 100 | Steinberg, 1962 | | 20–25 | Martensson & van Loghem, 1966 | 176 | 38 | Ropartz by Steinberg, 1962 | | 0 | | | |
| Eskimo | Grubb & Laurell, 1956 | 74 | 94.6 | | | | Martensson & van Loghem, 1966 | 75 | 31 | Ropartz by Steinberg 1962 | | 0 | | | |
| Eskimo (U.S.) | Grubb by Steinberg, 1962 | | 100 | Steinberg, 1962 | | 20 | | | | | | | Ropartz by Steinberg, 1962 | | 6 |
| Amerinds (U.S.) | Ropartz by Steinberg, 1962 | | 100 | Steinberg, 1962 | | 2 | | | | Ropartz by Steinberg, 1962 | | 0 | Ropartz by Steinberg, 1962 | | 37 |
| Australian aborigines Western desert | Ropartz by Steinberg, 1962 | | 100 | Steinberg, 1962 | | 0 | | | | Ropartz by Steinberg, 1962 | | 0 | Ropartz by Steinberg, 1962 | | 41 |
| Coastal region | Ropartz by Steinberg, 1962 | | 100 | Steinberg, 1962 | | 31 | | | | Ropartz by Steinberg, 1962 | | 0 | Ropartz by Steinberg, 1962 | | 45 |

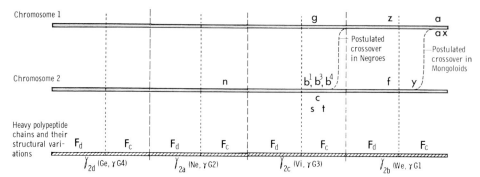

FIGURE 7. Schematic arrangement of Gm loci on two typical chromosomes from Caucasians. Racial differences in the structure of the heavy chains may be seen.

formulating this model, information has been obtained from many sources, including information on the Gm typing of the relatively homogeneous myeloma proteins and Bence Jones proteins.

Gm (g) is represented on one chromosome and Gm (b$^1$), Gm (b$^3$), and Gm (b$^4$) are represented on another chromosome; all are found on the Fc fragments of $\gamma_{2c}$ heavy chains. Gm (n) is found on the Fc fragment of $\gamma_{2a}$ heavy chains (Kunkel, Yount and Litwin, 1966). Gm (z) and Gm (f) are represented on different chromosomes and are found on the Fd fragments of $\gamma_{2b}$ heavy chains (Litwin and Kunkel, 1967). Gm (a) or (ax) and Gm (y) are represented on different chromosomes; these are found on the Fc fragment of $\gamma_{2b}$ heavy chains (Litwin and Kunkel, 1967). No Gm determinants have as yet been detected on proteins of subclass $\gamma_{2d}$.

Within a given race, combinations of factors act as units of inheritance without evidence of crossing over or recombination. The evidence that the factors within a given combination may be found on different heavy chain subclasses of the immunoglobulins favors the close linkage on the same chromosome of the loci responsible for the production of the $\gamma_{2a}$, $\gamma_{2b}$ and $\gamma_{2c}$ heavy chains (Martensson *et al.,* 1966). It is for this reason that they are shown on the same chromosome in Figure 7. The loci are arranged in the order postulated by Natvig, Kunkel, and Gedde-Dahl (1967).

Although closely linked, most of these factors are not strictly alleles so that intragenic crossover is possible. Such crossing over could explain the occurrence of racial differences. For example, many Mongoloids have the combination Gm (a+y+f+) in place of Gm (a+z+) or Gm (y+f+) found in Negroes and Caucasians. This may be explained by an intragenic crossover in common precursor chromosomes (as shown in Fig. 7). Point mutation could also account for this (Litwin and Kunkel, 1967).

The fact that Gm (f) is rare in Gm (b$^1$+) Negroes and common in Gm (b$^1$+) Caucasians and Mongoloids (Gold *et al.,* 1965; Steinberg and Goldblum, 1965) (see Table VIII) suggests that another intragenic crossover has occurred in common precursor chromosomes (as shown in Fig. 7).

TABLE VIII

INCIDENCE OF Gm(b,f) DETERMINANTS IN VARIOUS
POPULATION GROUPS

| Population | Number Tested | Gm(b+f+) | (b−f−) | (b+f−) | (b−f+) |
|---|---|---|---|---|---|
| | | | *Number Positive* | | |
| Caucasian Swedish | 620 | ( | 617 ) | 2 | 1 |
| Negro American | 10 | 3 | | 7 | |
| Senegal | 29 | 3 | | 26 | |
| Mongoloid Chinese | 27 | 25 | 2 | | |
| Eskimo (Alaskan) | 15 | 9 | 6 | | |

NOTE: Data from GOLD, E. R., *et al.: Vox Sang*, 10:299–302, 1965.

The result is a chromosome containing Gm (b¹) but lacking Gm (f). The finding that almost 100 per cent of African Negroes are Gm (a+b+) while only 50 per cent of Caucasians have this combination also favors such a model. The remaining 50 per cent of Caucasians are either Gm (a+b−) or Gm (a−b+).

Another significant racial difference is the presence of Gm (b³) when Gm (b¹) is present and its absence when Gm (b¹) is absent in Caucasians, while it may or may not be present when Gm (b¹) is present in Negroes, and may possibly exist in the absence of Gm (b¹) in Mongoloids (Steinberg and Goldblum, 1965).

Gm (a) and Gm (ax) act as alleles. Gm (x) is almost always associated with Gm (a). About 40 to 50 per cent of Gm (a+) sera from Northern Europeans are Gm (x+) while Gm (a−) sera are almost always Gm (x−) (Ropartz *et al.*, 1963; Lopez and Bütler, 1965).

Gm (c), Gm (s), and Gm (t) are found on the Fc fragments of $\gamma_{2c}$ heavy chains. Gm (c) occurs in Negroes, Gm (s) and Gm (t) in Japanese (Martensson, 1966). In Figure 7 they are shown in their approximate relationship on the chromosome to Gm (b¹) and Gm (b³).

The work on Gm (n) was done with a precipitin reaction utilizing antisera prepared in monkeys rather than with conventional agglutination inhibition techniques.

Kunkel, Yount, and Litwin (1966) demonstrated the relationship of Gm (n) to Gm (b), Gm (f) and Gm (y) as shown in Figure 7. Gm (n) closely parallels Gm (f) in various populations except among Caucasians where Gm (f+) individuals were Gm (n−) as well as Gm (n+).

For additional information on the genetic variations in the immunoglobulins the recent review by Steinberg (1967) should be consulted.

Patients who have multiple myeloma, a disease thought to result from malignant proliferation of the cells producing immunoglobulins, can produce relatively homogeneous immunoglobulins which may be present in large amounts in the blood as a myeloma protein or appear in the urine as a

Bence Jones protein. Study of these homogeneous immunoglobulin molecules has greatly enhanced our understanding of the normal immunoglobulins.

The serum myeloma proteins have essentially the same basic structure as the class of immunoglobulins to which they belong. In multiple myeloma the protein is usually of the IgG, IgA, or IgD classes while in Waldenström's macroglobulinemia the protein is usually of the IgM class. The relatively homogeneous protein, which is either of type K or type L but not both (Migita and Putnam, 1963), can be broken down into the characteristic light and heavy chains, and the Fab and Fc fragments. No two myeloma proteins from different patients have ever been found to be identical (Putnam, 1959). However, myeloma proteins are only relatively homogeneous. Individual myeloma proteins may produce multiple electrophoretic peaks (see Fig. 1). Furthermore, they have been shown to have as many as eight different light chain components and nine heavy chain components by means of disc electrophoresis in urea acrylamide gels (Terry, Small, and Reisfeld, 1966). For further information on these proteins see the chapter on the paraimmunoglobulinopathies (Chap. 7).

Bence Jones proteins are proteins of low molecular weight (22,000–44,000) which may appear in large amounts in the urine of patients with multiple myeloma and macroglobulinemia. As in the case of myeloma proteins, the Bence Jones proteins from different patients have never been found to be identical (Stein, Nachman, and Engle, 1963). Because of their small size and structural relationship to immunoglobulins, they may be called microimmunoglobulins. Bence Jones proteins have the unusual property of precipitating out of the urine between 40 to 60°C at pH 5 and dissolving at 100°C in strong acid. They are thought to be composed of single units or double polymers of light chains identical to those in the myeloma protein of the same patient and are therefore of either type K or type L specificity, but not both (Schwartz and Edelman, 1963; Gross and Epstein, 1964) (Fig. 4). Type K Bence Jones proteins also have Inv specificity. They form relatively homogeneous peaks upon electrophoresis on filter paper, in starch blocks and in agar. However, when Bence Jones proteins are studied by starch gel or acrilamide gel electrophoresis, varying degrees of heterogeneity may be found (see Fig. 8).

In general, type K proteins have four to five components and type L proteins, two components. Some, but not all, of the heterogeneity may be related to polymerization. In one patient studied in our laboratory, two electrophoretic peaks were found, one of type K and the other of type L specificity, suggesting involvement of two clones of plasma cells (Engle and Nachman, 1966). Type K Bence Jones proteins tend to appear as both dimers and monomers, while type L proteins are primarily dimers (Bernier and Putnam, 1964a). It has been suggested that the monomers of type K proteins are noncovalently bound while those of type L proteins are cova-

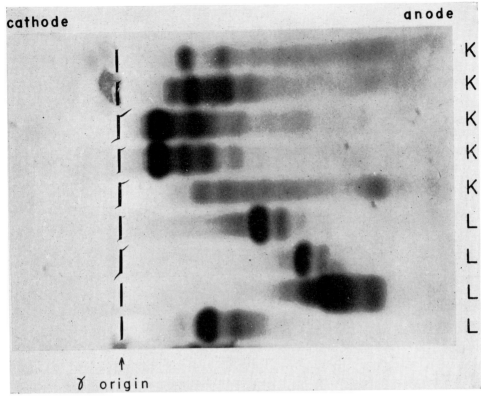

FIGURE 8. Starch gel, glycine buffer electrophoresis of Bence Jones proteins, Proteins of type K as well as type L are shown.

lently bound and therefore less likely to split into monomers (Bernier and Putnam, 1964a) .

Light chains from the normal immunoglobulins have been found in small amounts in the concentrated urine of normal individuals, in increased amounts in patients with hyperimmunoglobulinemia, and in decreased amounts in patients with hypoimmunoglobulinemia (Takatsuki and Osserman, 1964b) . These normal light chains give the Bence Jones heat test when present in sufficient concentration. Fc fragments have been found in the urine of normal individuals and of patients with hyperimmunoglobulinemia (Vaughan, Jacox, and Gray, 1967) . In rare patients with multiple myeloma or closely related diseases, there may be excreted into the urine low molecular weight proteins which do not give the Bence Jones heat test but are probably microimmunoglobulins. For example, the fast (F) fragment of heavy chains has been found in heavy chain disease (Osserman and Takatsuki, 1964) . In other instances, a protein which precipitates out and gels in the cold, and goes back into solution upon heating, has been described (Varriala, Ginsberg, and Sass, 1962) . Still other proteins of low molecular weight have been found (Weicker and Huhnstock, 1962) , some having immunologic similarities to portions of Bence Jones proteins (Solomon *et al.,* 1966; Cioli and Baglione, 1966; Williams, Pinnell, and Bratt, 1966).

Because of the relative homogeneity of these proteins found in patients with multiple myeloma and related conditions, attempts are now being made to determine the intimate structure of the molecules by means of finger-printing techniques and amino acid sequence studies. The structure of Bence Jones proteins has been a logical starting point, since these molecules are relatively small and are thought to be an integral part of the larger immunoglobulins. Analysis by two-dimensional electrophoresis-chromatography (finger-print studies) of tryptic digests of Bence Jones proteins reveals about twenty-eight peptides in the type K proteins and twenty-eight peptides in the type L. Each protein splits into nineteen to twenty-two peptides. There do not seem to be any common peptides between the type K and the type L Bence Jones proteins. This does not mean that the type K and L proteins are not closely related, since minor differences in amino acid sequence may result in different peptide spots. In fact, the two types of proteins are strikingly similar (Milstein, 1966a), suggesting that they had a common precursor. Each Bence Jones protein seems to have its own unique pattern of peptide spots. Within the type K proteins ten of the spots are common to all Bence Jones proteins of that type studied and eighteen seem to vary from protein to protein. Likewise, within the type L proteins, nine peptides are common to all and nineteen peptides vary from protein to protein. When the peptide spots are compared to the spots obtained after enzymatic hydrolysis of normal fraction II gamma globulin it is found that five of the spots common to the type K proteins and four of the spots common to type L proteins are also readily seen in the gamma globulin pattern. The remaining spots are not identified, probably because they are present in too low concentration to be seen, though it is possible that some may actually not be present in normal gamma globulin.

The amino acid sequences of three type K Bence Jones proteins and one type K light chain have now been completely elucidated. Segments of eleven other proteins have also been studied (Hilschmann, 1967a, b; Putnam, Titani, Wikler, and Shinoda, 1967; Milstein, 1966b; and Hood, Gray and Dreyer, 1966; Cunningham *et al.,* 1968). In all the proteins studied thus far, the C-terminal half of the molecule is almost identical, whereas the N-terminal half of the molecule differs remarkably at many loci. The single amino acid substitution in the C-terminal end seems to be related to the Inv locus (Milstein, 1966b; Baglioni *et al.,* 1966; Titani, Whitley, and Putnam, 1966); at position 189 leucine is present in Inv (a+) proteins and valine in Inv (b+) proteins. There are some regions of similarity, even in the variable half of the molecule. The amino acid sequences of the human type K Bence Jones proteins and light chain are shown in Table IX.

There are two intrachain disulfide linkages in each molecule, one in the variable and one in the nonvariable region. The C-terminal cystine links the light chain to the heavy chain and is responsible for complex formation. Stable monomers have the structure

$$\ldots -\text{Arg}-\text{Gly}-\text{Glu}-\text{Cys}$$
$$|$$
$$\text{Cys}$$

and stable dimers have the structure (Milstein, 1965)

$$\ldots -\text{Arg}-\text{Gly}-\text{Glu}-\text{Cys}$$
$$|$$
$$\ldots -\text{Arg}-\text{Gly}-\text{Glu}-\text{Cys}$$

Table IX also summarizes the definite sequence differences in the type K Bence Jones proteins. Substitutions of two different amino acids at fifty-one positions, three at thirteen positions, four at three positions, and five at three positions have been reported. After more proteins have been studied it may be possible to determine whether more than five different amino acids occur at a given locus but it is unlikely that all twenty may occur. There is thus a limitation on the amino acids which may occur at a single locus. If each of the well-documented amino acid substitutions occur independently it would theoretically be possible to have $2^{51} \times 3^{13} \times 4^{3} \times 5^{3} = 2,251,799,815,279,760$ different type K light chains. This degree of heterogeneity would allow for ample antibody specificity within the type K light chains alone, to say nothing of the total immunoglobulin molecule. The evidence is not yet conclusive as to whether or not the substitutions may be linked with others, and Putnam has already suggested that certain substitutions near the N-terminal end of the molecule are linked with the N-terminal amino acid. Milstein (1967) has found structural evidence of three subtypes. Such subtypes have also been postulated on the basis of immunologic evidence (Epstein and Gross, 1964; Williams, 1964; Nachman, Engle, and Copeland, 1966) and from studies of peptide maps (Nachman, Engle, and Copeland, 1966) . For each such linkage demonstrated the total number of possible molecules would be reduced by one half, one third or one quarter depending on whether it is a two, three, or four amino acid substitution point. Answers to the problem should be available after more Bence Jones proteins are subjected to sequence analysis.

As originally pointed out by Milstein and confirmed by Putnam, many of the points of substitution cluster about the two half cystine residues which are joined and therefore adjacent to each other in the three-dimensional structure. Putnam has also stressed the variability in the "switch peptide" at

# TABLE IX

## SUMMARY OF THE STRUCTURE OF SEVERAL BENCE JONES PROTEINS AND A LIGHT CHAIN OF TYPE K

| Protein | (Ref) | 0 | 1      5      10      15      20      25 |
|---|---|---|---|
| Ag | P | | Asp-Ile-Gln-Met-Thr-Gln-Ser-Pro-Ser-Leu-Ser-Ala-Ser-Val-Gly-Asp-Arg-Val-Thr-Ile-Thr-Cys-Gln-Ala- |
| Roy | H,P,M | | Asp-Ile-Gln-Met-Thr-Gln-Ser-Pro-Ser-Ser-Leu-Ser-Ala-Ser-Val-Gly-Asp-Arg-Val-Thr-Ile-Thr-Cys-Glx-Ala |
| Cum | H,P,M | Glu- | Asp-Ile-Val-Met-Thr-Gln-Thr-Pro-Leu-Ser-Leu-Pro-Val-Thr-Pro-Gly-Glu-Pro-Ala-Ser-Ile-Ser-Cys-Arg-Ser- |
| Eu | C | | Asx-Ile-Glx-Met-Thr-Glx-Ser-Pro-Ser-Thr-Leu-Ser-Ala-Ser-Val-Gly-Asx-Arg-Val-Thr-Ile-Thr-Cys-Arg-Ala- |
| B.J. | M | | Asx-Val-Glx-Met-Thr-Gln-Ser-Pro-Ser-Leu-Ser-Ala-Ser-Val-Gly-Asp-Arg-Val-Thr-Ile-Thr-Cys-Gln-Ala- |
| Ker | M | | Asx-Ile-Glx-Met-Thr-Gln-Ser-Pro-Ser-Leu-Ser-Ala-Ser-Val-Gly-Asp-Arg-Ile-Thr-Ile-Thr-Cys-Gln-Ala- |
| Day | M | | Val-Thr-Ile-Thr-Cys-Glx-Ala |
| Rad | M | Glx | Ala-Thr-Leu-Ser-Cys-Arg-Ala- |
| HBJ 3 | HO | | Asp-Ile-Val-Leu-Thr-Gln |
| HBJ 12 | HO | | Glu-Ile-Val-Val-Thr-Gln |
| HBJ 10 | HO | | Asp-Ile-Gln-Met-Thr-Gln |
| HBJ 6 | HO | | Asp-Ile-Gln-Met-Thr-Gln |
| HBJ 1 | HO | | Asp-Ile ---- Met-Thr-Gln |
| HBJ 5 | HO | | Glu-Ile-Val Leu |
| HBJ 4 | HO | | Asp-Ile-Val |
| Light chains of pooled human | | | Met / Asp Val + / + Ile + Leu Thr / Glu Gln + / Val |
| γ-globulin | HO,G | | Glu Gln + Val |

*Key to References*

P-Putnam, Titani, and Whitley, 1966
Putnam, Titani, Wikler, and Shinoda, 1967
H-Hilschmann, 1967a,b
M-Milstein, 1966c
HO-Hood, Gray, and Dreyer, 1966
G-Gray, 1966
C-Cunningham, Gottlieb, Konigsberg, and Edelman, 1968

| Protein | 26 | 27a | 27f | 30     35     40     45 |
|---|---|---|---|---|
| Ag | Ser-Gln | --- | --- | --- Asx Ile Asx Ser Phe Leu-Asn-Trp-Tyr-Gln-Gln-Gly-Pro-Lys-Ala-Pro-Lys-Ile-Leu-Ile- |
| Roy | Ser Glx | --- | --- | --- Asx Ile Ser Ile Phe-Leu-Asn-Trp-Tyr-Gln-Gln-Gly-Pro-Lys-Lys-Ala-Pro-Lys-Leu-Leu-Ile- |
| Cum | Ser-Gln-Ser-Leu-Leu-Asp-Ser-Gly-Asp-Gly-Asn-Thr-Tyr-Leu-Asn-Trp-Tyr-Leu-Gln-Lys-Gln-Gly-Gln-Pro-Ser-Leu-Leu-Ile- |
| Eu | Ser-Glx | --- | --- | --- Ser-Ile-Asx-Thr-Trp-Leu-Ala-Trp-Tyr-Glx-Lys-Pro-Gly-Lys-Ala-Pro-Lys-Leu-Leu-Met- |
| B.J. | Ser-Gln | --- | --- | --- Asp-Ile-Asn-Lys Tyr |
| Ker | Ser-Gln | --- | --- | --- Asp-Ile-Lys Asn Phe |
| Day | Ser Glx | --- | --- | --- Asx Ile Ser Asx Phe Leu Asx Trp Tyr |
| Rad | Ser Gln | --- | --- | --- Val-Ser-Ser-Asn-Ser-Tyr |

NOTES: Protein Eu is the light chain of a myeloma protein. Amino acids are listed from N-terminal to C-terminal end of molecules. Variable positions are indicated by asterisks at bottom of column. Abbreviations: Ala, alanine; Arg, arginine; Asn, asparagine; Asp, aspartic acid; Asx, undetermined whether Asp or Asn; Cys, half cystine; Gln, glutamine; Glu, glutamic acid; Glx, undetermined whether Glu or Gln; Gly, glycine; His, histidine; Ile, isoleucine; Leu, leucine; Lys, lysine; Met, methionine; Phe, phenylalanine; Pro, proline; Ser, serine; Thr, threonine; Trp, tryptophane; Tyr, tyrosine; and Val, valine.

TABLE IX (continued)

| Protein | | |
|---|---|---|

```
                  50            55            60            65            70            75
Ag   Tyr-Asp-Ala-Ser-Asn-Leu-Glu-Thr-Gly-Val-Pro-Ser-Arg-Phe-Ser-Gly-Ser-Gly-Phe-Gly-Thr-Asp-Phe-Thr-Phe-Thr-Ile-Ser-Gly-
Roy  Tyr-Asp-Ala-Ser-Lys-Leu-Glu-Ala-Gly-Val-Pro-Ser-Arg-Phe-Ser-Gly-Thr-Gly-Ser-Gly-Thr-Asp-Phe-Thr-Phe-Thr-Ile-Ser-Ser-
Cum  Tyr-Thr-Leu-Ser-Tyr-Arg-Ala-Ser-Gly-Val-Pro-Ser-Arg-Phe-Ser-Gly-Ser-Gly-Ser-Gly-Thr-Asp-Phe-Thr-Leu-Lys-Ile-Ser-Arg-
Eu   Tyr-Lys-Ala-Ser-Ser-Leu-Glx-Ser-Gly-Val-Pro-Ser-Arg-Phe-Ile-Gly-Ser-Gly-Ser-Gly-Thr-Glx-Phe-Thr-Leu-Thr-Ile-Ser-Ser-
B.J.
Ker
Day
Rad
         *   *   *   *   *   *   *       *   *   *   *   *   *   *       *   *       *   *   *   *
```

```
                  80            85            90            95            100           105
Ag   Leu-Gln-Pro-Glu-Asp-Ile-Ala-Thr-Tyr-Tyr-Cys-Gln-Gln-Tyr-Asp-Thr-Leu-Pro-Arg-Thr-Phe-Gly-Gln-Gly-Thr-Lys-Leu-Glu-Ile-
Roy  Leu-Gln-Pro-Glu-Asp-Ile-Ala-Thr-Tyr-Tyr-Cys-Gln-Gln-Phe-Asp-Asn-Leu-Pro-Leu-Thr-Phe-Gly-Gly-Gly-Thr-Lys-Val-Asp-Phe-
Cum  Val-Gln-Ala-Glu-Asp-Val-Gly-Val-Tyr-Tyr-Cys-Gln-Met-Arg-Glu-Leu-Ile-Pro-Tyr-Thr-Phe-Gly-Gln-Gly-Thr-Lys-Leu-Glu-Ile-
Eu   Leu-Glx-Pro-Asx-Asx-Phe-Ala-Thr-Tyr-Tyr-Cys-Glx-Tyr-Cys-Glx-Tyr-Asx-Ser-Asx-Ser-Lys-Met-Phe-Gly-Glx-Gly-Thr-Lys-Val-Glx-Val-
B.J.               Tyr-Tyr-Cys-Gln-Gln-Tyr-Glu-Asn-Leu-Pro-Tyr
Ker                Tyr-Tyr-Cys-Gln-Gln-Tyr-Asp-Asp-Leu-Pro-Pro-Gly-Thr-Phe-Gly-Pro-Gly-Thr-Lys
Day
Rad  Leu-Glu-Pro-Glu-Asp-Phe-Ala-Val-Tyr-Tyr-Cys-Gln-Gln-Tyr-Gly-Gln-Tyr-Gln-Gln-Tyr-Gln-Thr-Ser-Pro-Thr-Phe
         *   *   *   *       *   *   *   *   *   *   *   *   *   *   *                           *   *
```

```
                  110           115           120           125           130           135
Ag   Lys-Arg-Thr-Val-Ala-Ala-Pro-Ser-Val-Phe-Ile-Phe-Pro-Pro-Ser-Asn-Glu-Gln-Leu-Lys-Ser-Gly-Thr-Ala-Ser-Val-Val-Cys-Leu-
Roy  Lys
Cum  Arg
Eu   Lys-Gly
B.J.    *
Ker
Day
Rad

         └── Common portion starts here
```

```
                  140           145           150           155           160           190
Ag   Leu-Asn-Asn-Phe-Tyr-Pro-Arg-Glu-Ala-Lys-Val-Gln-Trp-Lys-Val-Asp-Asn-Ala-Leu-Gln-Ser-Gly-Asn-Ser-Gln-Glu-Ser-Val-Thr-

                  165           170           175           180           185           190(+)
Ag   Glu-Gln-Asp-Ser-Lys-Asp-Ser-Thr-Tyr-Ser-Leu-Ser-Ser-Thr-Leu-Thr-Leu-Ser-Lys-Ala-Asp-Tyr-Glu-Lys-His-Lys-Val-Tyr-Ala-

                  195           200           205           210
Ag   Cys-Glu-Val-Thr-His-Gln-Gly-Leu-Ser-Ser-Pro-Val-Thr-Lys-Ser-Phe-Asn-Arg-Gly-Glu-Cys
```

+ At position 191, Val is present in Inv (a+) proteins and Leu in Inv (b+) proteins.

TABLE X

AMINO ACID SEQUENCE OF TYPE L BENCE JONES PROTEIN Sh.

Italicized amino acids are those which are identical in type K Bence Jones proteins when sequences are aligned to achieve maximum homology.

10        20

Ser-Glu-Leu-*Thr-Gln*-Asp-Pro-Ala-Val-Ser-Val-*Ala*-Leu-*Gly*-Gln-Thr-*Val*-Arg-*Ile*-*Thr*-*Cys*-*Gln*-Gly-

30        40

Asp-Ser-Leu-Arg-Gly-Tyr-Asp-Ala-Ala-*Trp*-*Tyr*-*Gln*-*Gln*-Lys-Pro-Gly-Gln-*Ala*-*Pro*-Leu-Leu-Val-*Ile*-

50        60        70

*Tyr*-Gly-Arg-Asn-*Asn*-Arg-Pro-Ser-*Gly*-Ile-*Pro*-Asp-*Arg*-*Phe*-*Ser*-Gly-*Ser*-Ser-Ser-*Gly*-His-Thr-Ala-Ser-

80        90

Leu-*Thr*-*Ile*-Thr-*Gly*-Ala-*Gln*-Ala-*Glu*-*Asp*-Glu-*Ala*-Asp-*Tyr*-*Tyr*-*Cys*-Asn-Ser-Arg-*Asp*-Ser-Ser-Gly-

100        110

Lys-His-Val-Leu-*Phe*-*Gly*-Gly-*Gly*-*Thr*-*Lys*-*Leu*-Thr-Val-Leu-Gly-Gln-Pro-Lys-*Ala*-*Ala*-*Pro*-*Ser*-*Val*-

120        130

Thr-Leu-*Phe*-*Pro*-*Pro*-*Ser*-Ser-Glu-Glu-*Leu*-Gln-Ala-Asn-Lys-*Ala*-Thr-Leu-*Val*-*Cys*-*Leu*-Ile-Ser-Asp-

140        150        160

*Phe*-*Tyr*-*Pro*-Gly-Ala-Val-Thr-*Val*-Ala-*Trp*-*Lys*-Ala-*Asp*-Ser-Ser-Pro-Val-Lys-Ala-Gly-Val-Glu-Thr-

170        180

Thr-Thr-Pro-Ser-Lys-Gln-*Ser*-Asn-Asn-Lys-*Tyr*-Ala-Ala-*Ser*-*Ser*-Tyr-*Leu*-Ser-*Leu*-Thr-Pro-Gln-Glu-

190        200

Trp-Lys-Ser-*His*-Arg-Ser-*Tyr*-Ser-*Cys*-Gln-*Val*-*Thr*-*His*-Glu-*Gly*-*Ser*-Thr-*Val*-Glu-*Lys*-Thr-Val-Ala-

210

Pro-Thr-*Glu*-*Cys*-Ser

NOTE: Reproduced with permission from WIKLER, M., *et al.*: *J Biol Chem*, 242: 1668–1670, 1967.

the junction of the variable and nonvariable halves of the protein and he believes that this region is also adjacent to the disulfide linkage in the three-dimensional structure. He therefore postulates that the variable portions form a single region which functions as the specific antigen binding site.

It now seems clear that type L Bence Jones proteins have a basic structure similar to that of the type K proteins, i.e., there is a nonvariable C-terminal half and a variable N-terminal half. Wikler, Titani, Shinoda, and Putnam (1967) have reported the complete sequence of a λ Bence Jones protein and have compared its structure to that of κ Bence Jones proteins (see Table X). More recently, the same group (Putnam *et al.*, 1967) have compared the amino acid sequence of three λ Bence Jones proteins (see Table XI). Two of the proteins are three amino acids longer than protein Sh shown in table X and have PCA (pyrrolidone carboxylic acid) as the N-terminal residue. Two interchain disulfide bridges exist, as in type K proteins. In contrast to the type K proteins where Cys is the C-terminal amino acid, in the type L, a cysteine is next to the end, and this is apparently the cystine that links the light chain to the heavy chain. It is also the cystine responsible for complex formation. Stable monomers have the form

. . —Pro—Thr—Gly—Cys—Ser

|

Cys

and stable dimers,

# TABLE XI

## COMPARISON OF THE AMINO ACID SEQUENCE OF THE VARIABLE PORTION OF THREE HUMAN BENCE JONES PROTEINS (Sh, Bo, Ha) OF TYPE L

```
                                      10                                        20
Sh     Ser-Glu-Leu-Thr-Gln-Asp-Pro-Ala-Val-Ser-Val-Ala-Leu-Gly-Gln-Thr-Val-Arg-Ile-Thr-Cys-Gln-Gly-Asp-Ser-Leu-Arg-
Bo     PCA-Ser-Ala-Leu-Thr-Glx-Pro-Pro Ser Ala Ser-Gly-Ser-Pro-Gln-Ser-Val-Thr-Ile-Ser-Cys-Thr-Gly-Thr-Ser-Ser-Asp-
Ha     PCA-Ser-Val-Leu-Thr-Gln-Pro-Pro-Ser-Val-Ser-Gly-Thr-Pro-Gly-Gln-Arg-Val-Thr-Ile-Ser-Cys-Gly-Ser-Ser-Asn-
                                      10                                        20


                        30                                    40                                    50
Sh     --- --- --- Gly-Tyr-Asp-Ala-Ala-Trp-Tyr-Gln-Gln-Ala-Pro-Leu-Val-Ile-Tyr-Gly-Arg-Asn-Asn-Arg-
Bo     Val-Gly-Asx-Asx-Lys-Tyr-Val-Ser-Trp-Tyr-Gln-Gln-His-Pro-Gly-Ala-Pro-Lys-Leu-Val-Ile-Phe-Glu-Val-Ser-Glx-Arg-
Ha     Gly-Thr-Gly-Asn-Asn-Tyr-Val-Tyr-Trp-Tyr-Gln-Leu-Pro-Gly-Thr-Ala-Pro-Lys-Leu-Leu-Ile-Tyr-Arg-Asp-Asp-Lys-Arg-
                        30                                    40                                    50


                       60                                    70                                    80
Sh     Pro-Ser-Gly-Ile-Pro-Asp-Arg-Phe-Ser-Gly-Ser-Ser-Ser-Gly-His-Thr-Ala-Ser-Leu-Thr-Ile-Thr-Gly-Ala-Gln-Ala-Glu-Asp-
Bo     Pro Ser Gly Val-Pro-Asp-Arg-Phe-Ser-Gly-Ser-Lys-Ser-Asn-Asp-Thr-Val-Ser-Leu-Thr-Ile-Ser-Gly-Leu-Arg-Ala-Ala-Glx-Asx-
Ha     Pro-Ser-Gly-Val-Pro-Asp-Arg-Phe-Ser-Gly-Ser-Lys-Ser-Gly-Thr-Ser-Ala-Ser-Leu-Ala-Ile-Ser-Gly-Leu-Arg-Ser-Glu-Asp-
                       60                                    70                                    80


                       90                                   100                      108
Sh     Glu-Ala-Asp-Tyr-Tyr-Cys-Asn-Ser-Arg-Asp-Ser-Ser-Gly-Lys-His-Val-Leu-Phe-Gly-Gly-Thr-Lys-Leu-Thr-Val-Leu-Gly-
Bo     Glx-Ala-Asx-Tyr-Tyr-Cys-Ser-Ser-Tyr-Val-Asx-Asx-Asx-Phe-  ? -Val-Phe-Gly-Gly-Gly-Thr-Lys-Leu-Thr-Val-Leu-Arg-
Ha     Glu-Ala-His-Tyr-His-Cys-Ala-Ala-Trp-Asp-Tyr-Arg-Leu-Ser-Ala-Val-Val-Phe-Gly-Gly-Gly-Thr-Gln-Leu-Thr-Val-Leu-Arg-
                       90                                   100                             110    112
```

NOTE: Sequences joined by hyphens were determined by analysis. A different numbering system is employed for protein Sh (residues 1 to 108 above the sequence) and for protein Ha (1 to 112 below the sequence). The sequences of proteins Bo and Ha are aligned to achieve maximum homology with protein Sh. Thus, four amino acids are inserted in protein Bo and Ha: the NH$_2$-terminal residue PCA and three residues after Arg-27 of protein Sh. Residues which are nonidentical at the same position in the three chains are underlined. PCA = pyrrolidone carboxylic acid. Reproduced with permission from Putnam, F. W., et al.: Science, 157:1050–1053, 1967.

... —Pro—Thr—Gly—Cys—Ser

... —Pro—Thr—Gly—Cys—Ser

(Milstein, 1965).

For comparative purposes the immunologic and biochemical studies of mouse Bence Jones proteins are unusually interesting. As will be discussed in the chapter on the paraimmunoglobulinopathies, it is possible to produce a transplantable myeloma tumor in mice which forms paraimmuno-globulins and Bence Jones proteins. Mouse Bence Jones proteins are relatively homogeneous light chains of the corresponding paraimmunoglobulin, just as in man. Two immunologic types have been recognized. Each light chain is composed of a variable and nonvariable portion (Potter *et al.,* 1964). Tables XII and XIII taken from Gray, Dreyer, and Hood (1967) compare the structure of two mouse Bence Jones proteins with the human type K Bence Jones protein, Ag, studied by Titani, Whitley, and Putnam (1966). In the common portion of the molecules, residues 108–214, there are forty-five differences in a total of 107 amino acid residues between the mouse and human proteins. In the variable portion of the molecule, there are forty-two differences in 107–111 amino acid residues between one mouse protein and another mouse protein. There are about as many differences within the variable portion from mouse to man (see Table XIII). A striking similarity in the variable portion from mouse to man may also be seen (Kabat, 1967). This has led Kabat to postulate that the mechanism responsible for the variable regions of the light chains developed at an early stage in the evolution of vertebrates and was of sufficient survival value, perhaps because of its importance for antibody combining sites, to have been maintained largely unchanged.

Other studies are throwing some light on the three-dimensional tertiary or quaternary structure of the proteins. Certain immunologic determinants are blocked when the Bence Jones protein is incorporated into the whole myeloma protein (Stein, Nachman, and Engle, 1963; Nachman and Engle, 1964) or when normal light chains are incorporated into the whole immunoglobulin (Epstein, Tan, and Gross, 1964). Antisera prepared against small fragments of Bence Jones proteins, i.e., against single tryptic peptides are also capable of giving information on tertiary structure (Nachman, 1967).

Peptide maps of the Fc fragment and the closely related proteins isolated from the blood and urine of patients with H-chain disease have been studied by Putnam and coworkers (See Bernier and Putnam, 1964b). They found that about twenty tryptic peptides are shared by the Fc fragment of type K and type L 7S γ-myeloma globulins, the Fc fragment of normal 7S γ-globu-

# TABLE XII

## AMINO ACID SEQUENCES OF MOUSE AND HUMAN K-CHAINS

```
                          5                    10                   15                   20
MOUSE 41   Asp-Ile-Gln-Met-Thr-Gln-Ser-Pro-Ser-Leu-Ser-Ala-Ser-Leu-Gly-Glu-Arg-Val-Ser-Leu-Thr-Cys-
MOUSE 70   Asp-Ile-Val-Leu-Thr-Gln-Ser-Pro-Ala-Ser-Leu-Ala-Val-Ser-Leu-Gly-Gln-Arg/Ala-Thr-Ile-Ser-Cys-
HUMAN Ag   Asp-Ile-Gln-Met-Thr-Gln-Ser-Pro-Ser-Ser-Leu-Ser-Ala-Ser-Val-Gly-Asp-Arg-Val-Thr-Ile-Thr-Cys-

      25          30  a   b   c   d  31              35                   40                   45
41   Arg-Ala-Ser-Gln Asx Ile Gly --- --- --- --- Ser-Leu-Ser-Asx-Trp-Leu-Glx-Glx Gly Pro Asx Thr Glx Ile-Lys-Arg-Leu-
70   Arg/Ala-Ser-Glu-Ser-Val-Asx-Asx-Ser-Gly-Ile-Ser-Phe-Met-Asn Trp Phe Glx Glx-Lys-Pro-Gly-Glx-Pro-Lys/Leu-Leu-
Ag   Gln-Ala-Ser-Gln Asx Ile Asx --- --- --- --- Ser Phe Leu-Asn-Trp-Tyr-Gln-Gln-Lys-Pro-Gly-Lys-Ala-Pro-Lys-Ile-Leu-

          50                   55                   60                   65              70              75
41   Ile-Tyr-Ala-Thr-Ser-Ser-Leu-Asx-Ser-Gly-Val-Pro-Lys-Arg-Phe-Ser-Gly-Ser-Arg-Ser-Gly-Ser-Asp/Tyr-Ser-Leu-Thr/Ile-
70   Ile-Tyr-Ala-Ala-Ser-Asn-Gln-Gly-Ser-Gly-Val-Pro-Ala-Arg/Phe-Ser-Gly-Ser-Gly-Ser-Gly-Thr-Asp-Phe-Ser-Leu-Asn-Ile-
Ag   Ile-Tyr-Asp-Ala-Ser-Asn-Leu-Glu-Thr-Gly-Val-Pro-Ser-Arg-Phe-Ser-Gly-Ser-Gly-Ser-Gly-Thr-Asp-Phe-Thr-Phe-Thr-Ile-

        80                   85                   90                   95                  100
41   Ser-Ser-Leu/Glu-Ser-Glu-Asp-Phe-Val-Asp-Tyr/ ? Cys-Leu-Gln-Tyr-Ala-Ser-Ser-Pro-Trp-Thr-Phe-Gly-Gly-Gly-Thr-Lys-
70   His-Pro-Met-Glx-Glx-Asx-Asx-Thr-Ala-Met-Tyr-Phe-Cys-Glx-Glx/Glu-Val-Pro-Trp-Thr-Phe-Gly-Gly-Gly-Thr-Lys-
Ag   Ser-Gly-Leu-Gln-Pro-Glu-Asp-Phe-Ala-Thr-Tyr-Tyr-Cys-Gln-Gln-Tyr-Asp-Thr-Leu-Pro-Arg-Thr-Phe-Gly-Gln-Gly-Thr-Lys-

        105                  110                  115                  120                  125                  130
41   Leu-Glu-Ile-Lys-Arg-Ala-Asp-Ala-Ala-Pro-Thr-Val-Ser Ile Phe Pro Pro Ser Ser Glu-Gln-Leu-Thr-Gly Gly Ser Ala Ser
70   Leu-Glu-Ile-Lys-Arg Ala Ala Ala Pro Thr Val Ser Ile Phe Pro Pro Ser Ser Glx Leu Thr Gly Gly Ser Ala Ser
Ag   Leu-Glu-Ile-Lys-Arg-Thr-Val-Ala-Ala-Pro-Ser-Val-Phe-Ile-Phe-Pro-Pro-Ser-Asp-Glu-Gln-Leu-Lys-Ser-Gly-Thr-Ala-Ser-

        135                  140                  145                  150                  155
41   Val-Val-Cys-Phe-Leu-Asn-Asn-Phe-Tyr-Pro-Lys-Asp-Ile-Asn-Val-Lys-Trp-Lys-Ile-Asp-Gly-Ser-Glu-Arg-Gln-Asn-Gly-Val-
70   Val Val Cys-Phe Leu Asx Asx Phe Tyr Pro Lys/Asp-Ile-Asn-Val-Lys/Trp-Lys-Ile Asp Gly Ser Glu Arg Glx Asx Gly Val
Ag   Val-Val-Cys-Leu-Leu-Asn-Asn-Phe-Tyr-Pro-Arg-Glu-Ala-Lys-Val-Gln-Trp-Lys-Val-Asp-Asn-Ala-Leu-Gln-Ser-Gly-Asn-Ser-

        160                  165                  170                  175                  180                  185
41   Leu-Asx-Ser-Trp-Thr-Asx-Glx-Asp-Ser-Lys-Asp-Ser-Thr-Tyr-Ser-Met-Ser-Ser-Thr-Leu-Thr-Lys-Asp-Glu-Tyr-Glu-
70   Leu Asx Ser Trp Thr Asx Glx Asp Ser Lys/Asp Ser Thr Tyr Ser Met Ser Ser Thr Leu Thr Lys/Asx Glx Tyr Glx
Ag   Gln-Glu-Ser-Val-Thr-Glu-Gln-Asp-Ser-Lys-Asp-Ser-Thr-Tyr-Ser-Leu-Ser-Ser-Thr-Leu-Thr-Leu-Ser-Lys-Ala-Asp-Tyr-Glu-

        190                  195                  200                  205                  210
41   Arg-His-Asx-Ser-Tyr-Thr-Cys-Glx-Ala-Thr-His-Lys-Thr-Ser-Thr-Ser-Pro-Ile-Val-Lys-Ser-Phe-Asn-Arg-Asn-Glu-Cys
70   Arg/His Asx Ser Tyr-Thr-Cys-Glx Ala Thr His Lys/Thr Ser Thr Ser Pro Ile Val Lys/Ser-Phe-Asn-Arg-Asn-Glu-Cys
Ag   Lys-His-Lys-Val-Tyr-Ala-Cys-Glu-Val-Thr-His-Gln-Gly-Leu-Ser-Ser-Pro-Val-Thr-Lys-Ser-Phe-Asn-Arg-Gly-Glu-Cys
```

NOTE: The sequence of the human protein Ag is taken with permission from Putnam, F. W.; Titani, K., and Whitley, E., Jr.: *Proc Roy Soc (Biol)*, 166:124, 1966. Mouse proteins 41 and 70 are taken with permission from Gray, W.; Dreyer, W., and Hood, L.: *Science, 155*:465–467. (Copyright 1967 by the American Association for the Advancement of Science.) The sequences have been modified slightly to conform to the latest information after personal communication with authors. Diagonal bars after certain residues in the mouse proteins indicate that the alignment of peptides is derived from analogy with the other mouse protein.

TABLE XIII

CHANGES BETWEEN RELATED GENES

| | | Amino Acid Residues | Differences | Minimum Base Changes 1 2 3 | Transitions | Transversions |
|---|---|---|---|---|---|---|
| K Light Chains: | | | | | | |
| Variable | Mouse 41 | 107 | | | | |
| 1–107 | Mouse 70 | 111 | 42 (40%) | 27 12 1 | 32 | 17 |
| Common | Mouse | 107 | | | | |
| 108–214 | Human | 107 | 45 (42%) | 32 13 0 | 20 | 28 |
| Hemoglobin: | | | | | | |
| | Human | 146 | | | | |
| | Human | 146 | 37 (26%) | 28 9 0 | 28 | 16 |

NOTE: Taken with permission from GRAY, W.; DREYER, W., and HOOD, L.: *Science, 155:* 465–467, 1967. (Copyright 1967 by the American Association for the Advancement of Science.)

lin, and the two Fc fragments in subtypes Cr and Zu of the H-chain disease patients.

Frangione *et al.* (1966) have reported on the peptide maps of Fc fragments or heavy chains of 36 IgG myeloma proteins and two "heavy chain disease" proteins belonging to the $\gamma_{2a}$, $\gamma_{2b}$, $\gamma_{2c}$, and $\gamma_{2d}$ subgroups and noted striking similarities among them. The major difference was in the $\gamma_{2d}$ subgroup, which lacked three peptides found in the other three subgroups. While the Fc fragments from different proteins belonging to the same subgroup appeared very similar, differences based on currently recognized Gm factors as well as minor additional differences were noted.

The amino acid sequences of the C-terminal end of the heavy chains of two IgG myeloma proteins have been determined by Press, Piggot, and Porter (1966) and by Prahl (1966). They are shown diagrammatically in Table XIV and are compared with the amino acid sequences of comparable regions of horse and rabbit IgG. The C-terminal amino acid is glycine. This is in contrast to the C-terminal amino acid in the heavy chains of an IgM protein from a patient with Waldenström's macroglobulinemia, where cysteine has been found (Doolittle, Singer, and Metzger, 1966). Doolittle *et al.* (1966) have postulated that this cysteine accounts for polymerization of IgM subunits and that it is additional evidence that heavy chains and light chains have evolved from a common ancestral gene.

The most interesting information concerning the genetic origins of the

TABLE XIV

C-TERMINAL SEQUENCE OF THE HEAVY CHAIN OF
SEVERAL IMMUNOGLOBULINS

| | | |
|---|---|---|
| Horse IgG(T) | Weir, Porter & Givol, 1966 | (Met)-His-Glu-Ala-Val-Glu-Asn-His-Tyr-Thr-Gln-Lys-Asn-Val-Ser-His-Ser-Pro-Gly |
| Horse IgG | Weir, Porter & Givol, 1966 | (Met)-His-Glu-Ala-Leu-His-Asn-His-Tyr-Thr-Gln-Lys-Ser-Val-Ser-Lys-Ser-Pro-Gly |
| Rabbit IgG | Givol and Porter, 1965 | (Met)-His-Glu-Ala-Leu-His-Asn-His-Tyr-Thr-Gln-Lys-Ser-Ile-Ser-Arg-Ser-Pro-Gly |
| Human IgG ($\gamma_{2b}$, We) | Press, Piggot, & Porter, 1966 | (Met)-His-Glu-Ala-Leu-His-Asn-His-Tyr-Thr-Gln-Lys-Ser-Leu-Ser-Leu-Ser-Pro-Gly |
| Human IgG ($\gamma_{2c}$, Vi) | Prahl, 1966 | (Met) His-Glu-Ala-Leu-His-Asn-Arg-Phe-Thr-Gln-Lys-Ser-Leu-Ser-Leu-Ser-Pro-Gly |

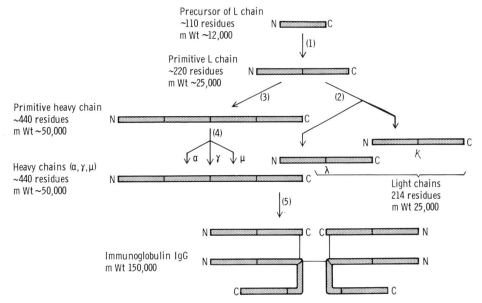

FIGURE 9. A tentative scheme for the genetic origins of the immunoglobulins. (Reproduced with permission from HILL, R. L. *et al.: Proc Nat Acad Sci, 56:*1762, 1966.)

immunoglobulin light and heavy chains has been presented by Hill *et al.* (1966). From analysis of the primary structure of human Bence Jones proteins and a large portion of the Fc fragment of a rabbit heavy chain they offer a convincing hypothesis that both chains are composed of subunits, two for light chains and four for heavy chains, which have all evolved from a common ancestor gene (see Fig. 9).

Inv and Gm types of myeloma serum proteins and Bence Jones proteins have been extensively studied. Myeloma and Bence Jones proteins are much more homogeneous than the normal immunoglobulins. IgG myeloma proteins contain either type K or type L light chains but not both (Korngold, 1961) and contain only one of the four subclasses of heavy chains (Grey and Kunkel, 1964; Terry and Fahey, 1964). Single myeloma proteins contain Gm groups which are of a single subclass and which are represented on a single chromosome (see Fig. 7). The analysis of myeloma proteins has helped to define the subclasses and the chromosomal relationships. Since the chromosomes vary from race to race, certain combinations of Gm factors may occur on the same myeloma protein from an individual of one race but not of another. The presence of Gm (a), Gm (y) and Gm (f) on the same myeloma protein of two Orientals (see Table XV) indicates that a crossover has possibly occurred during the evolution of the Caucasian and Mongoloid races, as indicated in Figure 7 (Martensson and Kunkel, 1965; Terry *et al.,* 1965; Litwin and Kunkel, 1966b).

Inv (a), Inv (1) and Inv (b) determinants have been found only on

TABLE XV

Gm FACTORS OF VARIOUS ETHNIC GROUPS

| | $a$ | $z$ | $y$ | $f$ | *Cauc.* | *Negro* | *Chin.* | *East Isl.* |
|---|---|---|---|---|---|---|---|---|
| | + | + | + | + | 42 | 2 | 17 | 23 |
| | + | + | − | − | 8 | 15 | 3 | 13 |
| Sera | − | − | + | + | 90 | 0 | 0 | 0 |
| | + | − | + | + | 0 | 0 | (30) | (12) |
| | + | + | − | − | 5 | 2 | 1 | |
| Myeloma | − | − | + | + | 11 | 0 | 0 | |
| Proteins | + | − | + | + | 0 | 0 | (2) | |

NOTE: Reprinted by permission of The Rockefeller University Press from LITWIN, S. D., and KUNKEL, H. G.: *J Exp Med, 125:* 847, 1967.

Bence Jones proteins of type K. Most $\gamma_{2b}$ and $\gamma_{2c}$ proteins associated with $\kappa$ light chains are Inv (1+) or Inv (b+) while none of 11 $\gamma_{2a}$ or $\gamma_{2d}$ proteins associated with $\kappa$ light chains contained Inv factors (Terry *et al.*, 1965). This implies selective rather than random combination of light and heavy chains. Such selective recombination of heavy and light chains has been demonstrated in the test tube (Grey and Mannik, 1965).

The question of whether or not myeloma proteins are structurally or qualitatively abnormal has not been satisfactorily answered (Harboe, 1965). While it is true that paraimmunoglobulins are antigenically deficient when compared to their normal counterparts, and while paraimmunoglobulins still react with homologous antisera even after absorption of the antisera with large quantities of normal immunoglobulins, these phenomena could be explained by the dilution of a very small amount of the paraprotein in the large amount of heterogeneous immunoglobulins. In other words, the paraimmunoglobulin in myeloma sera might be only a quantitatively increased amount of a protein normally present in small amount in that patient's immunoglobulins.

Another important observation that bears on this point is that specific antibodies have been shown to approach the same degree of relative homogeneity as can be demonstrated for serum myeloma proteins by both immunologic and chemical techniques. However, attempts to evoke antibodies to a restricted number of antigenic determinants have succeeded in producing a group of molecules that are still fairly heterogeneous upon electrophoresis. The problem of producing single species of antibody molecules is complicated by the fact that a single species of protein antigen may have many antigenic determinants, estimated to be as many as one antigenic determinant for each five amino acids in the chain. Furthermore, each antigenic determinant may call forth several different antibody molecules, each specific for a certain part or configuration of the determinant or each with a different affinity for the determinant. It seems, therefore, to be virtually impossible to select an antigen which will call forth just one species of antibody molecule. In spite of this difficulty, Nussenzweig and Benacerraf (1964) have shown that antibodies of the same specificity may have the

ing antigens. Pernis, Cohen and Thorbecke (1963) demonstrated that in rabbits specific antigenic stimulation is required to produce the specific histologic changes associated with gamma globulin formation. However they, too, found that gamma globulin synthesis was more readily demonstrable than antibody synthesis.

If there is such a thing as nonantibody gamma globulin, it might be expected that loss of gamma globulin from the blood by bleeding would stimulate gamma globulin synthesis. Thorbecke and Keuning (1956) demonstrated that loss of plasma protein was not an effective stimulus to gamma globulin production. Their studies also make it unlikely that preexistent normal gamma globulin is converted to antibody unless it is done at the time of synthesis. Many theoretical schemes of antibody production would allow for nonantibody immunoglobulin while others would not, so that this remains a very important but unanswered question.

# Chapter 3

# PRODUCTION AND METABOLISM OF
# IMMUNOGLOBULINS

## SYNTHESIS

THE IMMUNOGLOBULINS are normally produced by a number of different cell types, including the plasma cell, lymphoid plasma cell, and lymphocyte (Solomon, Fahey, and Malmgren, 1963). It is even possible that very immature cells similar to reticulum cells are involved (Mellors and Korngold, 1963). Usually only one family, either IgG, IgA, or IgM, of the immunoglobulins is found in a single cell by immunofluorescent techniques and it is not possible to distinguish the cell types responsible for each of the families (Mellors and Korngold, 1963). Recently, a positive correlation has been obtained between the number of IgA-containing intestinal plasma cells and IgA blood levels. This lends support to the thesis that the gastrointestinal tract may be a major site of IgA synthesis (Eisenstein and Spencer, 1966).

In hyperimmune rabbits it has been shown that the number of cells producing each class of immunoglobulin is roughly proportional to the percentage of each immunoglobulin class found in the blood, 5 to 8 per cent $a$ chain, 14 to 21 per cent $\mu$ chain, and 71 to 81 per cent $\gamma$ chain (Cebra, Colberg, and Dray, 1966). There is evidence that in some situations IgM and IgG immunoglobulins may be found within the same cell (Mellors and Korngold, 1963; Nossal *et al.*, 1964), suggesting that the family of immunoglobulins produced may depend, at least in part, on the degree of maturation of the cell during the immune process. Other studies indicate that macroglobulins are produced early in the process of antibody formation and are relatively rapidly catabolized, while IgG globulins are produced later and persist over a longer period of time (Barth *et al.*, 1964; Nossal *et al.*, 1964). Immunofluorescent studies indicate that individual lymphoid cells from normal lymph node or spleen contain both heavy and light chains. The light chains in an individual cell are usually of only one of the two types but not of both types (Bernier and Cebra, 1964).

Fishman has produced evidence that antigens which have been phagocytized by macrophages result in the production of a substance, presumably low- molecular-weight RNA, which is then transferred to immunocytes and can induce specific antibody synthesis in these cells (Fishman and Adler, 1963). Friedman, Stavitsky and Solomon (1965) have confirmed Fishman's findings and have shown that the RNA is bound to degraded antigen. It has been postulated that the macrophages phagocytize antigen, which is then degraded. Low-molecular-weight RNA acts as an adjuvant by combining with antigen and holding it in native, immunogenic configuration. The combination of small molecular weight antigen fragment and RNA is then transferred to immunocytes, where it induces antibody synthesis.

The possible role of eosinophils in antibody production has not been clear. Injection of an antigen stimulates a massive accumulation of eosinophils in the draining lymph nodes within the first twenty-four hours. Until recently, only antigen-antibody complexes could be demonstrated within the eosinophils. However, Roberts' (1966) report of the appearance of tritiated antigen within the eosinophils of mice within four hours after primary antigenic stimulation suggests an important function of eosinophils in the mechanisms of the primary immune response. Speirs, (Speirs and Speirs, 1964) who has long been interested in the eosinophils during the immune response, believes that they act as carriers of antigen and specific enzymes to the reacting cells.

Plasma cells have been shown by electron microscopy to have the endoplasmic reticulum which is the apparatus required for protein synthesis (see Figs. 10, 11, and 12). Lymphocytes vary greatly in appearance, and although the small ones would not be expected to be capable of producing protein (Fig. 13), it has been shown that under certain circumstances they also have the endoplasmic reticulum required for such synthesis (Zucker-Franklin, 1964) (see Fig. 16). Lymphocytes isolated from Burkitt's lymphoma have been shown to synthesize myeloma proteins *in vitro* (Fahey *et al.*, 1966). Nonetheless, the small lymphocytes surrounding lymphoid follicles seem to be devoid of antibody (Mellors and Korngold, 1963).

Recent studies have shed some light on the intracellular synthesis of the immunoglobulins. Askonas and Williamson (1966a) have shown by immunologic methods in mouse myeloma that light and heavy chains are synthesized separately on different-sized polyribosomes, the heavier polyribosomes (250 to 300S) being used in heavy chain synthesis and the lighter (150–200S) being used in light chain synthesis. They also demonstrated that free light chains were intermediate in the assembly of IgG molecules and postulated that these chains are released from the ribosomes first, forming a small pool, which is then responsible for the release of the heavy chains (Askonas and Williamson, 1966a and b).

It has been estimated from studies of plasmacytoma tissue of mice (Hum-

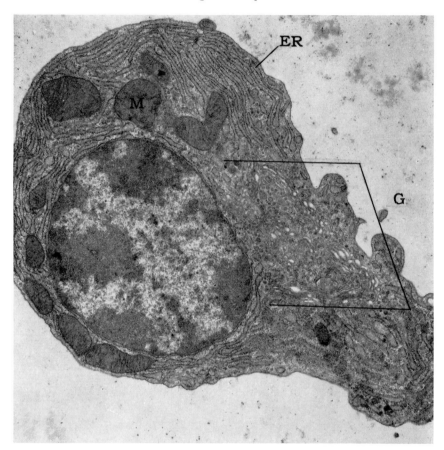

FIGURE 10. Plasma cell. Note the extensive development of rough-surfaced endoplasmic reticulum (ER) and the large area occupied by the Golgi zone (bracket). A material of homogeneous electron density is seen in the tubules of the ER—presumably representing gamma globulin. Magnification X13,000.
(Figs. 10, 11, 12, 13, 14, 15 and 16 are reproduced with permission from ZUCKER-FRANKLIN, D.: Structural features of cells associated with the paraproteinemias. *Seminars Hemat, 1*:165–198, 1964.)

phrey and Fahey, 1961) that each antibody-producing cell can form about 2,000 antibody molecules per second, so that each cell can produce $1.7 \times 10^8$ molecules per day (Nossal and Mäkelä, 1962a). Anderson (1964) has calculated that on the basis of his findings of an IgG turnover of 36 mg/kg per day, that $9.4 \times 10^{18}$ immunoglobulin molecules are produced per day in a 70 kg man, and that the number of cells involved would be $5.5 \times 10^{10}$. The volume of this number of cells would be about 10 ml, close to the estimate of the total volume of plasma cells in the body. Berenbaum (1958) estimated that single plasma cells contain between 1.25 and $7.5 \times 10^{-13}$ gm antibody per cell. This would be from one tenth to one fiftieth of the amount produced in a day per cell (Nossal and Mäkelä, 1962).

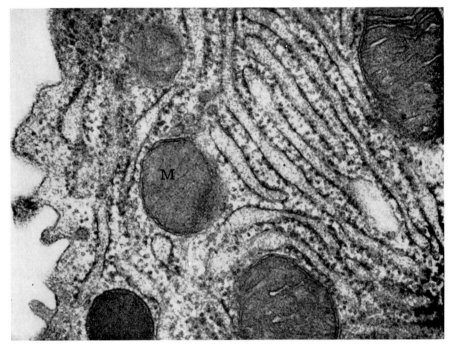

FIGURE 11. Detail of plasma cell illustrating rough-surfaced ER, mitochondrion (M). Magnification X61,500.

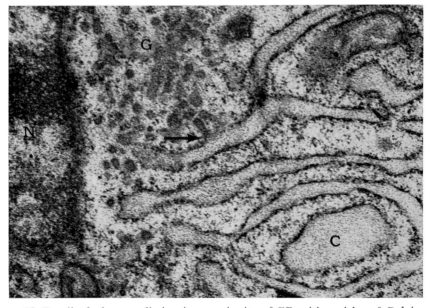

FIGURE 12. Detail of plasma cell showing continuity of ER with vesicles of Golgi apparatus (*arrow*). Nucleus (N), Golgi (G), cistern of ER (C). Magnification X49,000.

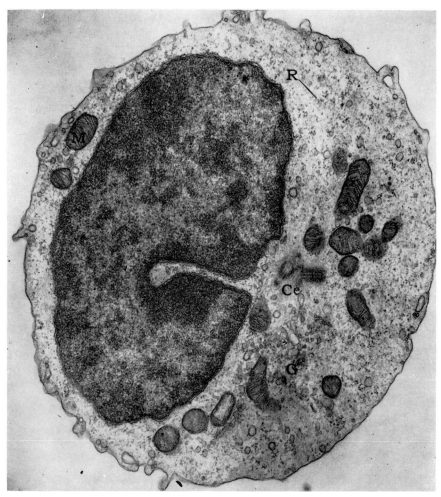

FIGURE 13. Normal lymphocyte showing the following structures: M = mitochondrion; R = ribosomes, arrow pointing at cluster of ribosomes; two centrioles (Ce), one sectioned longitudinally and the other in tangential section at right angles to each other; G = Golgi vesicles. Magnification X19,800.

In multiple myeloma and macroglobulinemia, only the relatively homogeneous, type-specific, serum protein or type-specific urinary Bence Jones protein can be found in the tumor cells. Although the morphologic appearance of the tumor cells and the character of the abnormal proteins produced vary greatly among patients (Solomon, Fahey, and Malmgren, 1963), nevertheless, in a given case, the tumor cells are characteristic for an individual patient and the proteins are of a single family, either IgG, IgA, IgD, or IgM as demonstrated by immunofluorescent techniques. Both the serum myeloma protein and the Bence Jones protein have been found in the same cell. The appearance of Bence Jones proteins in the plasma cells and lymphocytes makes it likely that they are synthesized there and fail to be incorporated into gamma globulin, rather than that they are breakdown products of gamma globulin. This is in agreement with earlier studies on the incorporation of isotopically labelled amino acids into the serum and urinary proteins of patients with multiple myeloma and the rate of appearance of the labelled proteins in the blood and urine (Putnam and Miyake, 1958; Osserman and Takatsuki, 1964). Under usual circumstances cells resem-

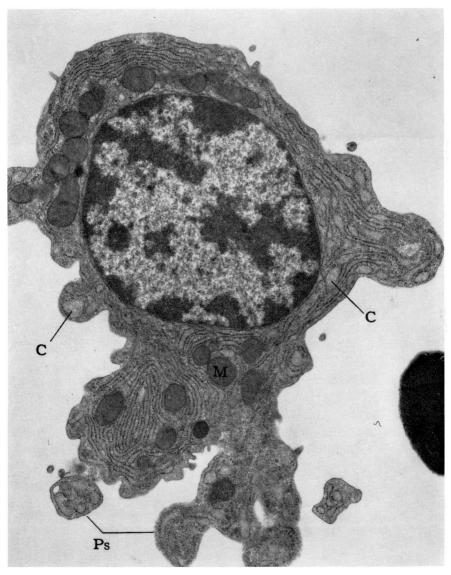

FIGURE 14. Electron micrograph of plasma cell from bone marrow of patient with 7S gamma multiple myeloma. Note deformity of cell and pseudopod formation. M = mitochondrion; C = cisternae of ER; PS = pseudopods. Magnification X15,000.

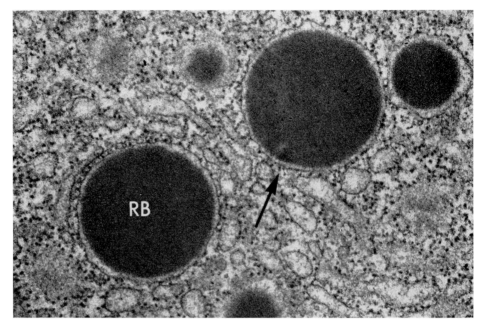

FIGURE 15. Higher power electron micrograph demonstrating relationship of Russell body to rough-surfaced endoplasmic reticulum. Arrow points to ribonucleoprotein particle attached to ER. Magnification X46,000.

bling plasma cells are seen in patients with multiple myeloma (Fig. 14) and cells resembling lymphocytes are seen in those with Waldenström's macroglobulinemia (Fig. 16). However, this is not always true; rare patients with myeloma may be found to have lymphocytes or, at least, cells indistinguishable from lymphocytes, as the predominating cell type in the marrow. Also, plasma cells are rarely the predominating cell type in macroglobulinemia.

The cells responsible for antibody production may be found in virtually any organ of the body. They seem to be concentrated, however, in the thymus, spleen, lung, lymph nodes, liver, and bone marrow. These organs have been extensively studied before and after stimulation of the animal with antigen in both the primary and secondary responses. The thymus is composed almost exclusively of lymphoid cells and occasional Hassall's bodies and normally contains neither lymphoid follicles nor plasma cells. Present evidence indicates that the thymus is not directly involved in antibody production. Thymocytes, though morphologically indistinguishable from lymphocytes, are not stimulated by phytohemagglutinin. This suggests a difference in cellular mechanism between the thymus and other lymphoid cells (Stastny and Ziff, 1966). Studies of neonatally thymectomized animals indicate that the thymus cells or thymocytes mature within the thymus under hormonal influences. These cells are released from the thymus and

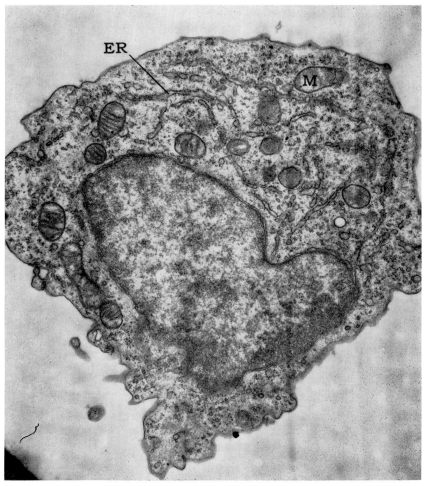

FIGURE 16. Electron micrograph of lymphoid plasma cell from the peripheral blood of a patient with macroglobulinemia of Waldenström. Note the endoplasmic reticulum (ER). Magnification X17,000.

migrate to the spleen and lymph nodes. However, the thymus continues to produce and secrete a hormone which can induce immunologic competence in other lymphoid tissues. Whether the thymus exerts its influence on cells capable of producing circulating antibodies is not clear. It is thought that the thymus is in some way involved in the recognition system in antibody production, in the effect or mechanism of delayed hypersensitivity, and in homograft rejection.

In the chicken, the bursa of Fabricius has been shown to be responsible for stimulation of circulating antibodies. The human body contains no such organ but it has been recently suggested that Peyer's patches, especially the periappendiceal lymphatic tissue, of the intestines serve this purpose in man

(Peterson, Cooper and Good, 1965). Antibody production in the spleen and lymph nodes has been localized to primitive cells located in the germinal centers and to similar cells appearing in the red pulp of the spleen and the sinusoids of the lymph nodes. These cells, which are pyrinophilic and have the characteristics of blasts, transform into more typical plasma cells. The mantle of small mature lymphocytes which characteristically surrounds the germinal center does not contain detectable quantities of immunoglobulin (Mellors and Korngold, 1963). Each germinal center has been shown to contain just one family of immunoglobulins under ordinary circumstances. There is some suggestion that the primary response reaction occurs primarily outside the lymphoid follicles, whereas during the secondary response the lymphoid follicles become involved (Fitch and Wissler, 1965).

The principal stimulus to the production of antibody is antigen, but then an antigen is defined as a substance which stimulates the development of specific antibody. If all immunoglobulin is not antibody, there must be other unknown stimulating factors. There is no evidence that removal of immunoglobulins from the blood stimulates their production. On the other hand, from the studies of Uhr and others (see review by Wigzell, 1966) it seems clear that the presence of specific antibody in the blood suppresses the formation of other immunoglobulins, probably by a feedback mechanism. Specific stimulants to antibody production include proteins, certain carbohydrates, peptides, and certain other chemical compounds provided they are combined with other antigenic substances. Certain proteins are notably unable to call forth the production of antibodies. These are the proteins which the host recognizes as being his own, the so-called self proteins. The mechanism of this antigen-specific immunologic tolerance is still not completely understood. Tolerance to proteins may be developed by several means. If the host is brought into contact with the protein early enough in life, tolerance may develop for a greater or lesser period of time. It is also possible to produce an immunologic paralysis or tolerance by administering large quantities of antigen or by frequent injections of small amounts of antigen (Gras and Dalmau, 1966). In the latter instance, antibody response occurs after a sudden increase in antigen dose.

A nonspecific stimulant to the immune system is phytohemagglutinin, an extract of the bean, *Phaseolus vulgaris*. Most, though not all, normal small lymphocytes in tissue culture are transformed into large pyrinophilic cells, many of which resemble plasma cells, following the addition of phytohemagglutinin to the medium (Robbins, 1964). At the same time there is a marked increase in the production of RNA and of the various immunoglobulins (Fudenberg and Hirshhorn, 1964). In cultures of lymphocytes from some patients with chronic lymphocytic leukemia such a transformation does not occur (Robbins, 1964). The reason for this difference has not been established. Phytohemagglutinin given *in vivo* causes suppression of antibody production if given before antigenic stimulation and enhancement if given several hours after antigenic stimulation (Elves, 1967).

Irradiation and certain drugs such as imuran, thioguanine, chlorambucil, 6-mercaptopurine, nitrogen mustards, cyclophosphamide and corticosteroids suppress the immune response, probably at the cellular level. Other agents such as aluminum salts and endotoxin, water and oil emulsions with or without mycobacteria act as adjuvants to antibody stimulation, probably by the stimulatory effect on the reticuloendothelial system.

## THEORIES OF ANTIBODY PRODUCTION

Theories of antibody production have been categorized as either instructive (Breinl and Haurowitz, 1930; Alexander, 1931; Mudd, 1932; Pauling, 1940; Haurowitz, 1965) or selective (Ehrlich, 1906; Jerne, 1955; Jerne, 1960; Talmage, 1957; Talmage and Pearlman, 1963; Burnet, 1957, 1966). Instructive and selective theories are not mutually exclusive, and there is evidence that both may need to be invoked to explain all of the facets of antibody production (Gray, 1964). Instructive theories of antibody production propose that the antigen instructs the antibody-producing cell in the production of the specific antibody. Thus, any immunoglobulin-producing cell is potentially capable of producing any antibody molecule provided it is properly instructed by the specific antigen. Instruction for the production of specific antibody may be given to the antibody-producing cell at any of several stages of protein synthesis. The direct template theories postulate that specificity is incorporated into the antibody molecule as the protein is formed on the ribosome. In some way the antigen molecule acts as a template for the three-dimensional conformation of the antibody molecule. This may occur in either of two ways. The antigen may modify the amino acid sequence of the forming antibody molecule or it may determine the folding of antibody molecules of the same amino acid sequence. In making the distinction between the two direct template theories, it is important to know whether specificity of the antibody is determined by its primary structure (amino acid sequence) or by its tertiary structure (three-dimensional conformation). This question has not been finally settled, but the work of Anfinsen (1965–66) and Freedman and Sela (1966) makes it seem likely that there is only one, or at most a few different, three-dimensional conformations for any one primary structure, since the activity of an antibody molecule may be recovered after complete reduction and unfolding of the molecule followed by oxidation and refolding. This information makes the second of the direct template theories unlikely. Indirect template theories postulate that the antigen modifies either the RNA or the DNA in a specific way, resulting in changes of the primary structure or amino acid sequence of the antibody molecule. If the DNA is modified in this way, the mechanism would be essentially a controlled somatic mutation.

Selective theories of antibody production postulate that different immu-noglobulin-producing cells produce different antibodies, and that each cell can produce a limited number of possibly only one or two antibodies. In essence, during the developmental process a clone of cells is formed for the production of each potential type of antibody molecule.

Recent evidence on the structure of the immunoglobulins raises addi-tional problems. Immunoglobulin subunits, both the type K light chains, and the type L light chains and the heavy chains, are each composed of two parts. One part, which in the case of the type K light chains is the carboxyl terminal half of the molecule, is common to all molecules of this type. The only known variation is that producing the Inv genetic determinant at position 189. The other half of the chain, the amino terminal end, has many variations in amino acid content, there being a different combination for every protein studied. It is this end which is presumed to account for the specificity of the molecule. This combination molecule with half common and half variable is unique to the immunoglobulins and is difficult to explain by any theory of antibody or protein synthesis. What is the mecha-nism which introduces these kinds of variability? Are both parts of the subunit controlled by a single gene or is each part controlled by a different gene?

Several hypotheses have been suggested to explain the unusual heteroge-neity of the immunoglobulins. However, no single theory has offered a completely satisfactory answer. An hypothesis developed by Smithies (1963) involves the production of modified genes in the developing cells either by rearrangement of the chromosomes (intrachromatid inversion) or by shifts in the coding frame of reference of the nucleic acids. These rearrangements were postulated to result from somatic crossing-over between duplicated regions of DNA in antibody genes. Additional information on the amino acid sequence of Bence Jones proteins has led Smithies to modify his origi-nal hypothesis to one in which there is crossing-over between two related but not identical genes (Smithies, 1967). Even this modification, however, does not explain all of the known substitutions, though it does offer some testable questions; e.g., are these unexplained substitutions determined by classical genetic mechanisms through the germ plasm? Milstein (1967) has recently found a third sequence in the structure of kappa light chains which would require a third structural gene using Smithies' hypothesis. Even with this addition he concludes that the number of variants that remain unexplained is in fact larger than the number explained by any hypothesis requiring crossing-over.

Burnet (1966) has suggested a more general possible mechanism produc-ing such diversity of genes, the transfer of segments of DNA from one portion of a cell to another or from one cell to another, a process equivalent to transformation in bacteria. The details of such a mechanism as applied to the immunoglobulins have not been reported. Dreyer and Bennett (1965) have proposed that the code for the variable portion comes from nucleic acid rings of varying composition which then combine with other nucleic acids of common composition to form the nucleic acid responsible for the production of the whole polypeptide chain. There would need to be as many different nucleic acid rings as there are different variable portions of the polypeptide chains.

Potter, Apella and Geisser (1965) proposed that the nucleic acid triplets coding for the regions of the antibody responsible for specificity are unusual codons. Each unusual codon is read alternatively by two or more different sRNA molecules. This ambiguous reading of the code comes about because the sRNA molecules which can interact with one unusual codon have the same anticodons for conforming to the mRNA but differ either with respect to their amino acid-activating enzyme or possibly by the structure of the sRNA molecules in the region of amino acid attachment, thus binding different amino acids to the otherwise identical sRNA. Thus, the genes involved in producing the immunoglobulins are those responsible for the structure of either the sRNAs or the amino acid-activating enzymes, rather than those responsible for the structure of the mRNAs. The principle difficulty in accepting this hypothesis concerns the nature of the unusual codons and why they are active only in certain regions of the molecule.

Brenner and Milstein (1966) suggested that an enzyme cuts the DNA and that errors are introduced at random during the repair process. With such a mechanism it would be difficult to explain the limited nature of the variability among the immunoglobulins. It has been suggested by Hood, Gray, and Dreyer (1966) that multiple germ line genes code for the variable region and that a single gene codes for the common region. Either the common and variable portions of the protein combine to make a single subunit enzymatically or the DNA or RNA responsible for each portion combines during differentiation to produce a single gene. More recently, Dreyer, Gray and Hood (1967) have postulated that this occurs at the DNA level and that there is a "copy-splice" mechanism which accomplishes the task.

In addition to Smithies, Edelman and Gally (1967) and Whitehouse (1967) have also postulated that the immunoglobulin variability results from some form of somatic recombination of duplicated genes. Edelman and Gally (1967) suggested that the somatic crossing-over occurs between tandem duplicated genes in which point mutations were assumed to have produced variations. In Whitehouse's hypothesis the somatic crossing-over is intrachromosomal between sets of gene copies which differ slightly from each other. Both of these hypotheses postulate more genes than Smithies' hypothesis and are, therefore, able to explain a greater degree of variability. At the same time, in certain situations more variability than is found might be expected.

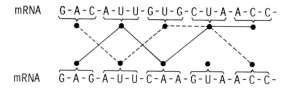

mRNA    G - A - C - A - U - U - G - U - G - C - U - A - A - C - C -

mRNA    G - A - G - A - U - U - C - A - A - G - U - A - A - C - C -

First reading (-•-)   Asp - Ilu - Val - Leu - Thr -

Second reading (-•-)  Glu - Ilu - Gln - Leu - Thr -

FIGURE 17. Reading of the code from two strands of mRNA as suggested in the hypothesis.

Many of these theories and hypotheses have been critically reviewed recently by Lennox and Cohn (1967) and by Haurowitz (1968).

While all of these hypotheses focus on very important aspects of antibody structure and synthesis, none of them is entirely satisfactory for explaining the structure of the immunoglobulins. For this reason we would like to mention yet another hypothesis, one which requires only a relatively few genes, but in which the variability is incorporated into the protein during the translation of the RNA.

Engle and Nachman (1967) have speculated that there are at least four different strands of messenger RNA which are responsible for formation of $\kappa$ light chains and which have evolved in the classical manner. Certain regions are common and certain regions are variable, depending in part upon the selective process. Prior to protein synthesis, at least two different strands line up side by side on the ribosome; the message for the synthesis is read from N-terminal to C-terminal-end between the mRNAs. At each point along the way there is a choice of at least two messages, one from each mRNA, and the choice is determined at least in part by steric relationships (see Fig. 17). In those regions of the mRNA where the strands code for the same amino acid, the message will be the same, but in those regions where the strands code for different amino acids, there will be a distribution of the allowed amino acid substitutions.

They proposed that there are at least four different strands of mRNA, because only four different amino acids have been found at a single point in the Bence Jones protein molecules. In the future, more than four different mRNA strands may be needed to explain the protein structure. However, under any circumstances, it would be a reasonably small number. It is possible that each kind of mRNA strand is present in a different amount, thus affecting the odds with which any particular amino acid is incorporated.

Antigen is known to enhance the general as well as the specific immune response. In this model they proposed that antigen stimulates the synthesis of the messenger mRNAs which in turn produce nonspecific immunoglobulin. In addition antigen modifies antibody synthesis either directly or indirectly during the sequential insertion of amino acids into the growing polypeptide chain by affecting the selection between the two possible codons offered by the aligned mRNAs. Thus, antigen-specific light chains are synthesized. Similarly, in the malignant disease, multiple myeloma, and related conditions, where a relatively homogeneous immunoglobulin such as Bence Jones protein is produced, it is postulated that the synthetic mechanism is locked in one conformation. Such locking might also explain the continued production of specific antibody in the absence of antigen.

The mechanism for lining up the different mRNA molecules side by side may be active at the ribosome level. Alternatively, the message pairing might occur at the DNA level and be inherited, or it might occur during mRNA synthesis. In any case, the information would be transferred in side-by-side arrangement to the point of protein synthesis on the ribosome. This mechanism could act anywhere in the DNA → mRNA → protein process. However, because of the structure of the genetic code, it is difficult to construct a suitable model except at the mRNA → protein level. Except at the RNA to protein step where the code is read as triplets, such mechanisms would allow the appearance of more amino acids than are found in some single positions where substitutions are known to occur.

This model could explain the synthesis of both the common and variable portions of the immunoglobulin light chains. It does not exclude the possibility that the variable and common portions are produced by different genes (Hood, Gray, and Dreyer, 1966) or that light chains may vary in length (Gray, Dreyer, and Hood, 1967). The model might also apply to immunoglobulin heavy chains which are thought to have a structure similar to light chains.

While on the surface this would appear to be strictly an instructive theory, it is possible that it may work together with a selective mechanism. There may be clonal differences in DNA activation. For example, there are probably also four different mRNAs responsible for the synthesis of λ light chains. These are also under classical genetic control. The fact that κ and λ chains are usually not found in the same cell, suggests that the same mechanisms are occurring in at least two different strains of cells and that selection may occur between them. It is also possible that there is selection of as yet unrecognized subtypes. Such subtypes might result from selection of a particular combination of two of the four possible mRNAs responsible for the synthesis of the protein.

The major problem in accepting the proposed model is that no mechanism of the type proposed is known to exist. Present evidence favors the concept of a single strand of mRNA on the ribosome at the time of protein synthesis (Watson, 1965b). However, we believe that not enough is known about protein synthesis in mammalian systems and particularly within immuno-globulin-forming cells to exclude the proposed theory (Watson, 1965b; Singer and Leder, 1966; Schweet and Heintz, 1966).

The proposed model is more consistent with one form of instructive theory, namely, the template theory of antibody production as proposed and recently elaborated upon by Haurowitz (1965, 1968), than with other theories. However, as mentioned before, it does not exclude the possibility of certain selective aspects. It is true that many of the objections raised to a template theory alone still exist in the presently proposed model. These include the difficulty in explaining the anamnestic response and the phenomenon of tolerance or "self-recognition." These have been discussed in detail by Haurowitz (1965), who does not feel that they stand in the way of a primarily template-oriented theory. As in any template theory which acts at cytoplasmic level, it is somewhat more difficult to explain the continued synthesis of antibody in the absence of antigen and the ability to transplant multiple myeloma serially from one mouse to another. It becomes necessary to assume not only that the immune response or malignancy in some way freezes the synthesizing mechanism, but also that the frozen mechanism (mRNA) is capable directly, or indirectly through the DNA, of replicating and of being transmitted to daughter cells during mitosis. Since there is still so much that is not known about cytoplasmic genetics (Brachet, 1967), further speculation is unwarranted.

A mechanism of the type proposed might be expected to have other biological applicability. The phylogenetic development of an enzyme with optimum specificity bears some resemblance to the synthesis of a specific antibody in somatic cells. The mechanism of synthesis proposed here for antibody molecules allows for the production of large numbers of different molecules, only one of which has the desired specificity. Is it not possible that during the phylogenesis of an enzyme, a similar mechanism might have produced a spectrum of molecules, one of which had the desired enzyme activity? Over a long period of time, selection has favored the optimum nucleic acid codons which are responsible for producing the ideal enzyme. The postulated multi-track process of antibody production could represent a vestigial mechanism which is retained because of the continual stimulus of many highly specific but diverse molecules, the antigens.

It has been suggested that nerve cells store information in much the same way as plasma cells (Schmitt and Davison, 1965; Katchalsky and Oplatka, 1966). The proposed process could form the basis for an intracellular storage mechanism which allows encoding of much more information through the many more combinations than would be possible by classical genetic process. It is, however, difficult to explain the long held view of an all or none response of nerve cells with an intracellular information storage mechanism.

## DISTRIBUTION

Once antibodies have been formed in the cells, theoretically the antibodies might be stored there for future use. Since plasma cells are not long-lived, however, it is very likely that the antibodies quickly find their way into the tissues and blood. The mechanism of release of antibody from the plasma cell is not entirely clear. It seems likely, however, that the plasma cell breaks up and that the cytoplasm containing the antibody distributes itself into the blood and tissues. In patients with multiple myeloma it is possible to see fragmentation of plasma cells with small bits of cytoplasm appearing in the blood. It is also possible that there is an excretory mechanism in the plasma cell. The Golgi apparatus is thought by some to function in this way (see Fig. 12).

Some antibodies are considered to remain closely attached to cells. These are the antibodies that may be particularly involved in the delayed immunologic response and in homograft rejection. Virtually all of the antibodies that have been studied quantitatively appear in the blood and are known to occur in the extracellular tissue spaces. A dynamic equilibrium exists between the immunoglobulins present in the intravascular and in the extravascular spaces. Turnover studies indicate that about 45 per cent of the IgG molecules are in the intravascular space and 55 per cent in the extravascular space at any one time (see Table XVI). On the other hand, the distribution of IgM molecules is primarily intravascular, probably because of their large molecular weight. IgA is found predominantly in the parotid saliva, colostrum, tears, gastrointestinal secretions, tracheobronchial washings, nasal secretions and, to a lesser extent, in the blood (Tomasi *et al.*, 1965). The IgG molecules are known to cross the placenta while virtually no such transfer of the IgM, IgA, or IgD molecules occurs. There is some evidence

TABLE XVI

METABOLIC FEATURES OF THE IMMUNOGLOBULINS *

|  | IgG | IgA | IgM | IgD |
|---|---|---|---|---|
| Serum level (mg/ml) | 10.7 | 2.5 | 0.77 | 0.023 |
|  | (6.0–15.6) | (0.19–4.95) | (0.57–1.98) | (0.003–.141) |
| Synthetic rate (mg/kg/day) | 42 | 21.1 | 4.13 | 0.396 |
|  | (16–51) | (2.67–55.0) | (3.16–16.9) | (0.028–1.49) |
| Fractional Catabolic Rate | 0.068 | 0.237, 0.37 § | 0.179 | 0.37 |
| (Fraction of intravascular pool catabolized per day) | (0.058–0.078) | (0.144–0.338) | (0.141–0.251) | (0.18–0.60) |
| Intravascular distribution | 44 | 40 § | 70 | 73 |
| (% total body pool intravascular) | (32–53) | — | (65–100) | (63–86) |
| Biological half-life (days) | 23 † | | 5*‡ | |
|  | (17–32) | | | |

* Median value is presented with the range of values in parentheses below
§ Values obtained by Solomon and Tomasi, 1964
† Solomon, Waldmann, and Fahey, 1963
‡ Cohen and Freeman, 1960; Barth *et al.*, 1964
NOTE: Reprinted with permission from ROGENTINE, G. N.; ROSE, D. S.; BRADLEY, J.; WALDMANN, T. A., and FAHEY, J.: *J Clin Invest; 45:* 1467, 1966.

for an active placental IgG transport mechanism (Kohler and Farr, 1966). The question of whether some amyloid deposits in the tissue are immunoglobulins has not been completely resolved. Some workers find that amyloid is stainable with fluorescent antibodies to gamma globulin, but others do not agree.

## SITE OF DESTRUCTION

Very little is known about the destruction of the immunoglobulins. The combination of antibody with specific antigen predisposes the complex to phagocytosis by phagocytic cells, which then presumably break down the proteins (Benacerraf, Sebestyen, and Cooper, 1959). It is also possible that some antibodies are removed by a less specific means. Removal would be expected to occur in any organ containing large numbers of reticuloendothelial elements. The liver in particular has been implicated. Some immunoglobulin is lost through the gastrointestinal tract, and it has been estimated that as much as 40 per cent of immunoglobulin is broken down in the intestinal lumen. There is, however, considerable difference of opinion concerning whether or not the gastrointestinal tract is a site of loss in normal individuals (Andersen, 1964). In certain kidney diseases considerable quantities of immunoglobulins are lost in the urine.

## METABOLISM

Most studies of the metabolism of the immunoglobulins depend on the use of radioactively labelled molecules. Such techniques have been limited by a number of problems, the most important of which has been the difficulty of obtaining isolated immunoglobulins in undenatured form. Denatured isotopically labelled immunoglobulins are removed from the blood more rapidly than normal. Some classes of immunoglobulins are normally present in such low concentration that they cannot be adequately studied. Therefore, most of the work has been done with the IgG class. The other classes have been studied for the most part in patients who have pathologic elevations. The metabolic features of the immunoglobulins are summarized in Table XVI.

Normal IgG molecules labelled with iodine 131 have a biologic half-life of seventeen to thirty-two days with a mean of twenty-three days in normal individuals (Solomon, Waldmann, and Fahey, 1963). There is no difference in the rate of removal of autologous and homologous protein, at least among individuals of the same Gm group (Freeman, 1965). Normal IgM molecules have a half-life of five days in normal individuals, which is appreciably shorter than that of the IgG. (Barth *et al.*, 1964; Cohen and Freeman, 1960). Barth *et al.* (1964) have reported that approximately 18 per cent of the circulating normal macroglobulin is catabolized daily as compared to only 3 per cent of the 7S gamma globulin. The synthetic rate of macroglobulin is only 7 mg/kg per day, 15 to 20 per cent of the synthetic rate of 7S gamma globulin.

The serum level of immunoglobulins depends on a balance between the rate of synthesis and the rate of catabolism. Observations of Fahey and Robinson (1963) in mice indicate that the rate of immunoglobulin synthesis is the primary factor determining the serum immunoglobulin level, and that the fractional catabolic rate depends on the serum concentration. The fractional catabolic rate is the fraction of the body pool degraded per day. At the same time the catabolism is apparently regulated so as to maintain a steady concentration irrespective of synthesis (Freeman, 1965).

The homeostatic mechanism of IgG catabolism is quite specific and selective. Fahey and Robinson's (1963) studies on plasma cell tumor-bearing mice indicate that marked serum increases of IgA, IgM, or albumin do not accelerate the IgG catabolism. Similarly, injections of the slow fragment of the IgG papain digest have no effect on IgG catabolism. On the other hand, IgG from a variety of sources including antibodies obtained through normal antigenic stimulation, proteins from plasma cell tumors, and proteins obtained from exogenous sources as well as the fast fragment of the IgG papain digest, all accelerated IgG catabolism. Immunoglobulin catabolism is also increased with an increased metabolic rate and with fever.

Increases in fractional catabolic rate are limited to two to three times the normal (Fahey and Robinson, 1963) while absolute catabolic rates are unlimited. When the maximal fractional catabolic rate is reached, it becomes independent of the blood level or the rate of synthesis.

While the catabolism of the immunoglobulins might be expected to be related to their function as antibodies, strangely enough this is not the case. Specific antibody is not eliminated more rapidly in the presence of its antigen (Humphrey and McFarlane, 1954), since the fractional disappearance rate of specific antibody in hyperimmunized rabbits was the same as that of normal gamma globulin. Likewise, gamma globulin from monkeys (Smithies, 1964) or patients (Cohen and McGregor, 1963) with malaria has the same fractional catabolic rate as normal gamma globulin in monkeys or patients with malaria. It has, therefore, been postulated that only a small percentage of the increased gamma globulin associated with malaria has antibody activity, and that there must be two stimuli to immunoglobulin production; one, specific antigen, and the other, something nonspecifically stimulating all immunoglobulin production (Freeman, 1965).

The mechanisms involved in the metabolism of IgM must be quite different from those in IgG, since similar fractional catabolic rates were found in subjects with a wide range of serum levels (Fahey and Robinson, 1963).

## NORMAL LEVELS OF IMMUNOGLOBULINS IN SERUM

Stiehm and Fudenberg (1966a) have reported the levels of immunoglobulins in the serum of normal subjects at different ages (see Table XVII

## TABLE XVII

### LEVELS OF IMMUNE GLOBULINS IN SERUM OF NORMAL SUBJECTS AT DIFFERENT AGES

| Age | No. of Subjects | Level of γG* | | Level of γM* | | Level of γA* | | Level of Total γ-Globulin* | |
|---|---|---|---|---|---|---|---|---|---|
| | | mg/100 ml (range) | % of Adult Level | mg/100 ml (range) | % of Adult Level | mg/100 ml (range) | % of Adult Level | mg/100 ml (range) | % of Adult Level |
| Newborn | 22 | 1,031 ± 200 (645–1,244) | 89 ± 17 | 11 ± 5 (5–30) | 11 ± 5 | 2 ± 3 (0–11) | 1 ± 2 | 1,044 ± 201 (660–1,439) | 67 ± 13 |
| 1– 3 mo | 29 | 430 ± 119 (272–762) | 37 ± 10 | 30 ± 11 (16–67) | 30 ± 11 | 21 ± 13 (6–56) | 11 ± 7 | 481 ± 127 (324–699) | 31 ± 9 |
| 4– 6 mo | 33 | 427 ± 186 (206–1,125) | 37 ± 16 | 43 ± 17 (10–83) | 43 ± 17 | 28 ± 18 (8–93) | 14 ± 9 | 498 ± 204 (228–1,232) | 32 ± 13 |
| 7–12 mo | 56 | 661 ± 219 (279–1,533) | 58 ± 19 | 54 ± 23 (22–147) | 55 ± 23 | 37 ± 18 (16–98) | 19 ± 9 | 752 ± 242 (327–1,687) | 48 ± 15 |
| 13–24 mo | 59 | 762 ± 209 (258–1,393) | 66 ± 18 | 58 ± 23 (14–114) | 59 ± 23 | 50 ± 24 (19–119) | 25 ± 12 | 870 ± 258 (398–1,586) | 56 ± 16 |
| 25–36 mo | 33 | 892 ± 183 (419–1,274) | 77 ± 16 | 61 ± 19 (28–113) | 62 ± 19 | 71 ± 37 (19–235) | 36 ± 19 | 1,024 ± 205 (499–1,418) | 65 ± 14 |
| 3– 5 yr | 28 | 929 ± 228 (569–1,597) | 80 ± 20 | 56 ± 18 (22–100) | 57 ± 18 | 93 ± 27 (55–152) | 47 ± 14 | 1,078 ± 245 (730–1,771) | 69 ± 17 |
| 6– 8 yr | 18 | 923 ± 256 (559–1,492) | 80 ± 22 | 65 ± 25 (27–118) | 66 ± 25 | 124 ± 45 (54–221) | 62 ± 23 | 1,112 ± 293 (640–1,725) | 71 ± 20 |
| 9–11 yr | 9 | 1,124 ± 235 (779–1,456) | 97 ± 20 | 79 ± 33 (35–132) | 80 ± 33 | 131 ± 60 (12–208) | 66 ± 30 | 1,334 ± 254 (966–1,639) | 85 ± 17 |
| 12–16 yr | 9 | 946 ± 124 (726–1,085) | 82 ± 11 | 59 ± 20 (35–72) | 60 ± 20 | 148 ± 63 (70–229) | 74 ± 32 | 1,153 ± 169 (833–1,284) | 74 ± 12 |
| Adults | 30 | 1,158 ± 305 (569–1,919) | 100 ± 26 | 99 ± 27 (47–147) | 100 ± 27 | 200 ± 61 (61–330) | 100 ± 31 | 1,457 ± 353 (730–2,365) | 100 ± 24 |

* Mean is ± 1 S.D

NOTE: Reproduced with permission from Stiehm, E. R., and FUDENBERG, H. H.: *Pediatrics*, 37:715, 1966.

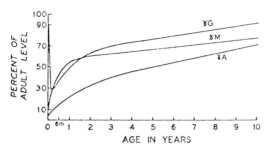

FIGURE 18. Alterations in levels of serum immune globulins in the first ten years of life, expressed as percent of normal adult values. (Reproduced with permission from STIEHM, E. R., and FUDENBERG, H. H.: *Pediatrics, 37:*715, 1966.)

and Fig. 18). No variations were noted by sex during the first year of life. The level of IgG decreased rapidly after birth to a low level at three to six months of age. Most of the IgG at birth is maternal in origin and there is very little synthesis of the infant's own IgG during this period. The level of IgG then increases rapidly for two years and at a slower rate until adult levels are reached by age nine to sixteen. The level of IgM increases rapidly after birth for the first year and than at a slower rate until age sixteen when adult levels are reached. IgM is the chief immunoglobulin synthesized by the neonate. The IgA level increases slowly during the first year and thereafter at a faster rate, continuing to rise into early adulthood.

*Chapter 4*

# HYPOIMMUNOGLOBULINOPATHIES:
# DESCRIPTION OF SYNDROMES

HYPOIMMUNOGLOBULINOPATHIES are conditions presumably associated with a defective body immune system and characterized by deficiency, total lack, or relative decrease in serum level or body content of one or more of all of the immunoglobulins. Some of these conditions are distinct clinical entities, frequently genetic, sometimes acquired, associated with specific symptomatology and laboratory findings. Others are less well defined, perhaps a continuum of similar and overlapping syndromes. Some conditions described here are probably two or more distinct syndromes considered together because each is rare and because of our present inability to define their distinctness and classify them properly. We shall first describe the clinical syndromes, postponing considerations of etiology, common aspects of symptomatology, diagnosis and treatment until Chapter 5. Familiarity with the syndromes is essential for an understanding of general considerations.

The first of these that was described is what we now call congenital sex-linked agammaglobulinemia. Bruton in 1952 reported lack of gamma globulin in a male infant who was overwhelmingly susceptible to infections. Since then, many more cases have been reported and this classically distinct, well-defined syndrome is the best recognized entity among the hypoimmunoglobulinopathies. Later, other related entities were described.

***Classification.*** Our classification of these conditions does not adhere to the historical order. We have separated the hypoimmunoglobulinopathies into primary and secondary hypoimmunoglobulinemias (see Table XVIII). Within the primary group we first consider the most severe deficiencies, least compatible with life, manifesting themselves at an early age and resulting in early death. The subsequent entities are discussed in the order of decreasing severity and of appearance at a later age.

TABLE XVIII

HYPOIMMUNOGLOBULINOPATHIES

A. Primary Hypoimmunoglobulinemias
  1. Hypoimmunoglobulinemias of early onset
    a. Reticular Dysgenesis—congenital alymphoplasia with aleukocytosis
    b. Agammaglobulinemia with lymphopenia (Swiss type)—congenital alymphoplasmacytic agammaglobulinemia with thymic dysplasia
    c. Congenital sex-linked agammaglobulinemia
    d. Ataxia-telangiectasia
  2. Hypoimmunoglobulinemias of late onset, also called primary adult hypogammaglobulinemias or primary "acquired" hypogammaglobulinemias
    a. Generalized adult hypoimmunoglobulinemia
    b. Selective adult hypoimmunoglobulinemia
      (1) Selective hypo IgA-globulinemia
      (2) Selective hypo IgG-globulinemia
      (3) Selective hypo IgA and G-globulinemia with increased IgM and IgD also called "dysglobulinemia"
      (4) Selective hypo IgA and M-globulinemia with normal IgG, Giedion-Scheidegger syndrome
      (5) Selective hypo IgA and M-globulinemia with slight decrease in IgG
      (6) No selective hypo IgM-globulinemia described
      (7) No selective hypo IgD-globulinemia described
  3. "Familial idiopathic dysproteinemia" of Homburger and Petermann
B. Secondary Hypoimmunoglobulinemias (also called secondary acquired hypoimmunoglobulinemias)
  1. Associated with hypoalbuminemia
    a. Nephrotic syndrome
    b. Amyloidosis (some cases)
    c. Protein-losing enteropathies of various causes
    d. Malnutrition and cachexia
  2. Associated with malignancies of the reticuloendothelial system
    a. Multiple myeloma
    b. Waldenström's macroglobulinemia
    c. H-chain disease
    d. Lymphoma
    e. Chronic lymphocytic leukemia
  3. Associated with autoimmune diseases
    a. Rheumatoid arthritis
    b. Lupus erythematosus
    c. Idiopathic thrombocytopenic purpura
    d. Rheumatic fever
  4. Associated with pernicious anemia
  5. Associated with chronic infections
  6. Associated with diseases of unknown etiology (e.g., sarcoidosis)
C. Physiologic Hypoimmunoglobulinemias
  1. Transient physiologic hypoimmunoglobulinemia of the newborn
  2. Hypoimmunoglobulinemia of germ free animals

## PRIMARY HYPOIMMUNOGLOBULINEMIAS

### Hypoimmunoglobulinemias of Early Onset

### *Reticular Dysgenesis*

This is also called *congenital thymic alymphoplasia with aleukocytosis and agammaglobulinemia.* The distinctive feature of this entity is that all white blood cells, lymphocytes and granulocytes are markedly decreased with total white count of 200 to 600 per cu mm, 15 to 20 per cent polys, the rest of the white cells in the blood being monocytes. This very rare and profound alteration in the body immune system was described (de Vaal and Seynhaeve, 1959; Gitlin, Vawter, and Craig, 1964) in three patients, twin boys and one girl. All these succumbed to overwhelming infections during the newborn period (5 days, 8 days, and 15 days of age), after a violent course of diarrhea, omphalitis, conjunctivitis, and sepsis. The smears of nasal, oral, and rectal discharges revealed gram-positive cocci, but no leukocytes.

At autopsy, the thymus was small and atrophic. Small numbers of primitive lobules were separated by relatively thick fibrous septa and surrounded by a broad zone of fibrous connective tissue. No small lymphocytes were seen. The cells making up the lobules were the so-called large thymocytes (reticulum cells with elongated or round vesicular nuclei containing a distinct chromatin pattern and rather indefinite cytoplasmic boundaries). There was no differentiation into cortex and medulla. Hassall's bodies were completely missing. *Lymph nodes* were few but slightly enlarged and consisted almost entirely of reticulum cells resembling those seen in the thymus. Only *stromal* differentiation into cortex and medulla was seen. No primary follicles and no germinal centers were found (these structures are not ordinarily found in a newborn infant). A small number of cells with ovoid nuclei and eosinophilic or slightly basophilic cytoplasm were seen, somewhat similar to plasma cells. In the spleen, Malpighian follicles were replaced by reticulum cells. The bone marrow showed no myeloid precursors; megakaryocytes and erythroid precursors were present in normal numbers.

There was extensive necrosis in the bone marrow, liver, and pancreas. No immunologic studies were performed because of the early deaths but these infants almost certainly would have been found to be immunologically deficient.

This defect may be either directly or humorally conveyed. It selectively affects the development of the lymphocyte and granulocyte but not that of the megakaryocyte, proerythroblast, and monocyte. It manifests itself at or before the tenth week of gestation. De Vaal and Seynhaeve (1959) postulated that the reticular anlage of the lymphocytes and other white cells failed to develop, and hence suggested the term *reticular dysgenesis*. The disease may be due to a congenital blockage in the development of bone marrow stem cells, a blockage occurring before the cells have differentiated into lymphocyte and neutrophile precursors.

The mode of inheritance of this rare entity is not clear. The first two patients were twins. In the family of the third patient, some members died from infection in infancy in the third generation (40 to 50 years ago, before antibiotics), but they did survive beyond the first few weeks of life.

### Swiss-Type Agammaglobulinemia with Lymphopenia

This is also called *congenital alymphoplasmocytic agammaglobulinemia with thymic dysplasia* and *lymphopenic hypogammaglobulinemia*.

In this entity, failure of normal development leads to absence of all immunocytes (lymphocytes and plasma cells) so that all immunoglobulins are absent. Granulocytes are not affected. About fifty cases have been reported (Gitlin and Craig, 1963; Gitlin, Vawter and Craig, 1964; Hitzig, Kay, and Cottier, 1965; Rosen, Gitlin, and Janeway, 1962; Sacrez *et al.,* 1963; Allibone, Goldie, and Marmion, 1964; Delta *et al.,* 1965; Schaller, Davis, and Wedgwood, 1966).

These infants with lymphopenic hypoimmunoglobulinemia incur serious infections in the first weeks of life, while patients with the congenital sex-linked agammaglobulinemia do not manifest infections until the fifth or sixth month of life. Severe thrush, chronic diarrhea with malabsorption, occasional ulcerative colitis (Sacrez *et al.,* 1963), recurrent pulmonary infections, and a rapidly deteriorating course almost always lead to death within the first eighteen months of life. Pneumocystis carinii pneumonia, systemic moniliasis, and progressive vaccinia are frequent causes of death. These infants do not respond to gamma globulin therapy. Growth is stunted. They have less than 25 mg% of gamma globulin in the serum, and less than 1,000 lymphocytes per cu mm of blood, and usually no lymphocytes in the bone marrow. They do not produce antibodies when challenged with a monilia antigen, nor do they show the expected contact allergy reaction to a second exposure to dinitrofluorobenzene (DNFB), a highly sensitizing skin irritant. They show no evidence of skin homograft rejection.

At postmortem examination the thymus is atrophic and contains neither Hassall's corpuscles nor lymphocytes (see Fig. 19). The lymph nodes and spleen as well as the gastrointestinal tract are without germinal centers, small lymphocytes, or mature plasma cells (Rosen, Gitlin, and Janeway, 1962) (see Fig. 20).

Agammaglobulinemia and lymphopenia, Swiss type, in many respects resembles the wasting disease of mice thymectomized at birth. Miller (1961, 1963) noted that mice thymectomized in the immediate neonatal period suffered from a severe depletion in the lymphocyte population and serious immunological defects, including tolerance to skin grafts up to two months, compared to ten to twelve days in control animals. Mortality was high, owing to increased susceptibility to common laboratory infections. Lymph nodes and spleens of thymectomized animals revealed a conspicuous deficiency of germinal centers and only a few plasma cells. This wasting disease can be prevented by grafting thymus into the animal (Levey, Trainin, and Law, 1963). Miller (1963) postulated that the thymus, particularly in early life, regulates lymphocyte production, not only by being the main producer of such cells, but also by secreting a factor, such as Metcalf's lymphocytosis-stimulating factor, which after birth stimulates lymphopoiesis in other lymphoid organs. Perhaps thymus provides an environment which allows lymphoid cells to acquire immunologic competence (Ford and Micklem, 1963). Another hypothesis is that the thymus produces the precursors of immunologically competent cells, many of which migrate to other sites at about the time of birth (Miller, 1963). In either case, thymectomy would

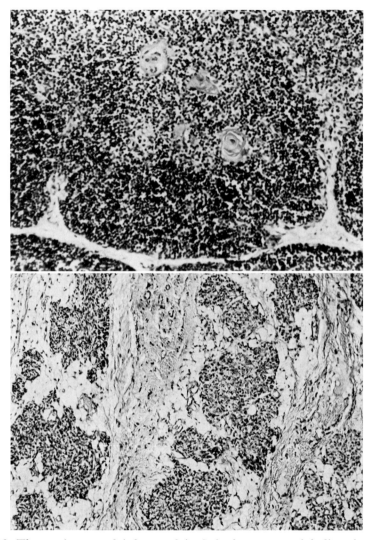

Figure 19. Thymus in normal infant and in Swiss hypogammaglobulinemia. (*Upper*) Normal thymus from a nine month old infant showing lobular structure with cortex and medulla, numerous lymphocytes, and Hassall's corpuscles. Original magnification x100. (*Lower*) Thymus tissue from the patient with lymphopenic hypogammaglobulinemia (Swiss) showing small islands of cells without cortical or medullary structure, lymphocytes, or Hassall's corpuscles. Original magnification X96. (Reproduced with permission from Schaller, J.; Davis, S. D., and Wedgwood, R. J.: *Amer J Med, 41:*462, 1966.)

interfere with immune processes. Schaller, Davis, and Wedgwood (1966) feel that in some cases of lymphopenic hypogammaglobulinemia (Swiss type) there is a lack of lymphoreticular stem cells, a more basic defect than neonatal thymectomy.

It is of interest that in rats thymectomized at birth, plasma cells appear in

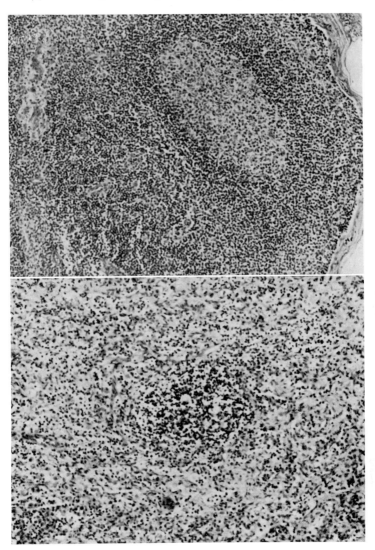

FIGURE 20. Lymph node in normal control and Swiss hypogammaglobulinemia. (*Upper*) Normal lymph node showing germinal center formation after antigenic stimulation. Original magnification X125. (*Lower*) Mediastinal node from the patient with lymphopenic hypogammaglobulinemia (Swiss) showing paucity of lymphocytes and absence of germinal centers. Original magnification X125. (Reproduced with permission from SCHALLER, J.; DAVIS, S. R., and WEDGWOOD, R. J.: *Amer J Med, 41:*462, 1966.)

relatively normal numbers in the tissues and these animals synthesize normal amounts of 7S ($\gamma_2$) globulin (Waksman *et al.*, 1962).

Agammaglobulinemia and lymphopenia of Swiss type is a familial disorder; consanguinity is frequently found in affected families. Both boys and girls can be affected, in contrast to congenital sex-linked agammaglobulinemia without lymphopenia which affects male infants only. Delta *et al.* (1965) described the Swiss-type disorder in two brothers who had several asymptomatic family members of both sexes exhibiting immunoglobulin defects. This finding suggests an autosomal recessive transmission. This is supported by Hitzig's genealogical work on the disease. Family studies by Gitlin and Craig (1963) suggest a sex-linked transmission for their patients.

There is no known successful treatment. Because of the analogy with the wasting disease of thymectomized mice, thymus grafting has been suggested. Thymus grafts, fetal bone marrow transplants, combination of thymus grafts and fetal bone marrow, and combination of thymus grafts and fetal liver cells as a source of competent stem cells have been tried with variable but generally unsatisfactory results (Hitzig, Kay, and Cottier, 1965). Of course, antibiotics and other forms of supportive therapy are indicated, though these too are usually unsuccessful. Prompt diagnosis, especially in children from affected families, would permit trial of experimental tissue grafting well before the onset of symptoms. Early study of antibody-synthesizing capacity, by immunization with bacteriophage and typhoid antigens, is a reasonable screening test for the disease. In view of extremely decreased resistance to infections, these infants should not be immunized with preparations of live virus (vaccinia, measles, orally administered polio) or BCG vaccine (Schaller, Davis, and Wedgwood, 1966).

### Congenital Sex-Linked Agammaglobulinemia

This classical disorder, the best defined syndrome in the entire group, was first described by Colonel Ogden Bruton in 1952. Congenital agammaglobulinemia is an hereditary disorder affecting the male infant and is transmitted as a sex-linked recessive characteristic. The role of paternal factors may be important in the development of the clinical disorder in some families (Kirkpatrick and Schimke, 1967).

The first severe infection heralding the disease usually occurs around six months of age, when transplacentally acquired maternal antibodies disappear from the circulation (Gitlin, Gross, and Janeway, 1959). Occasionally, the onset is delayed until the third year of life. The pattern and severity of infections are quite variable. Repeated attacks of pneumonia, recurrent meningitis, and repeated septicemia may occur either alone or in combination. Suppurative otitis media and sinusitis are frequent. Severe pyoderma may be the initial infection. Slow-healing leg ulcers have been reported (Firkin and Blackburn, 1958). Death ensues unless antibiotic therapy is given in adequate amounts.

The infecting microorganisms are primarily of the pyogenic group: *Staphylococcus aureus, pneumococcus, meningococcus* and *Haemophilus influenzae*. Infections with gram-negative enteric bacilli are not common.

Fungal infections such as candidiasis are frequent and are probably provoked, in part, by intensive antibiotic therapy.

Children with congenital hypogammaglobulinemia have a peculiar susceptibility to succumb to pneumonia caused by *Pneumocystis carinii* (Blattner, 1965). This organism has not been classified with certainty. Some regard it as a protozoan, others as a yeast-like fungus. It attacks premature infants as well as older children and adults with impaired defense mechanisms (UCLA Interdepartmental Conference, 1966). *Pneumocystis carinii* cysts, $10\mu$ in diameter, have been observed in the tissues of many small mammals, including domestic animals. Subclinical infection in man may be common, and the agent may be acquired by the newborn infant from a clinically inapparent infection in the mother's genital tract. A chain of indirect contacts is also suggested in the epidemiologic pattern in institutional outbreaks. The mortality rate is high. Recently, successful treatment has been reported with pentamidine isothionate supplemented with gamma globulin (Blattner, 1965).

The resistance of these children to viral infections such as rubeola, varicella, mumps, poliomyelitis, herpes simplex, and vaccinia is normal. Second exposure to a viral disease which ordinarily produces a lasting immunity does not result in a second attack. Usually revaccination produces an immune response despite failure to form detectable antibodies in the serum. However, unusual responses to varicella, progressive vaccinia after vaccination, three attacks of mumps in one patient, and fatal viral hepatitis have been reported in these patients (Gitlin, Gross, and Janeway, 1959; Peterson, Cooper, and Good, 1965).

The defect in this condition is due to an almost complete failure to synthesize all classes of immunoglobulins and specific antibodies after infection or antigenic stimulation. The patients have gamma globulin concentrations below 50 mg% and usually below 25 mg%. All immunoglobulins (A, G, and M) are absent or low. Only 15 per cent of patients with this syndrome had detectable isohemagglutinins (Gitlin, Gross, and Janeway, 1959). Antigenic stimulation with vaccination does not usually result in antibody response, although a minimal response is sometimes observed. Half-life of infused gamma globulin is normal, indicating that the defect is that of synthesis and not breakdown.

Despite the immunoglobulin deficiency, hypersensitivity reactions of delayed type are not infrequent and can be induced: delayed hypersensitivity to penicillin, adhesive tape, poison ivy, *Candida,* tuberculin, histoplasmin, and reactivity to DNFB. This hypersensitivity is mediated by leucocytes and can be transferred from one person to another with these cells.

Contrary to earlier reports (Good and Mazzitello, 1956) skin homografts in children with congenital agammaglobulinemia are eventually rejected as a result of delayed hypersensitivity (West, Hong, and Holland, 1962). Presence of this limited response to antigens is in contrast to the complete immunologic impairment presented by patients with alymphocytosis and agammaglobulinemia (Swiss type).

These children die early of overwhelming infections. The incidence of lymphocyte malignancies, especially of acute lymphatic leukemia, is increased. About half of the children have manifestations of collagen disease, especially symptoms like those of rheumatoid arthritis. Rarely, there are gastrointestinal symptoms.

Lymph nodes of patients with congenital agammaglobulinemia have a thinner cortex than normal, fewer lymphocytes, practically no primary follicles, and quite prominent reticuloendothelial cells of the sinusoids (see Fig. 21). On antigenic stimulation the nodes in patients with congenital agammaglobulinemia fail to form secondary germinal centers and plasma cells. Plasma cells are absent and lymphoid elements are deficient in the spleen, thymus, gastrointestinal tract, and even the bone marrow. Lymphoid pharyngeal tissue is conspicuously absent, as may be observed on the lateral roentgenograms of the nasopharynx. The appendiceal lymphoid tissue is quite defective. The thymus is usually normal. Lymphocytes in the periph-

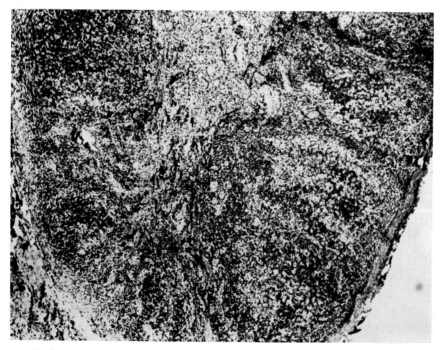

FIGURE 21. Lymph node from patient with congenital sex-linked agammaglobulinemia. The lymphoid tissue is not organized, and germinal follicles and plasma cells are absent. (Reproduced with permission from PETERSON, R. D. A.; COOPER, M. D., and GOOD, R. A.: *Amer J. Med, 38*:579, 1965.)

eral blood are normal. Neutropenia occurs frequently, especially with severe infections (Firkin and Blackburn, 1958). Cyclic neutropenia has been observed, but in most cases neutropenia disappears once the infection has been controlled. Aplastic anemia, thrombocytopenia, and lymphopenia have also been noted.

Treatment consists of antibiotic therapy given according to specific needs of each patient, and administration of human gamma globulin. These modes of treatment as well as the rarely indicated steroid therapy are discussed in Chapter 5.

## Ataxia-Telangiectasia

This disease, first described in 1941, consists of progressive cerebellar ataxia, oculocutaneous telangiectasia, and frequent severe sinopulmonary infections. The ataxia usually begins in infancy or early childhood and progresses to complete incapacitation by early adolescence. The telangiectasia becomes apparent at about three years of age and involves the bulbar conjunctivae, malar eminences, ears, antecubital fossae, and occasionally other body areas. Sinopulmonary infections are present in 85 per cent of cases and frequently are the principal cause of death. The disease is familial,

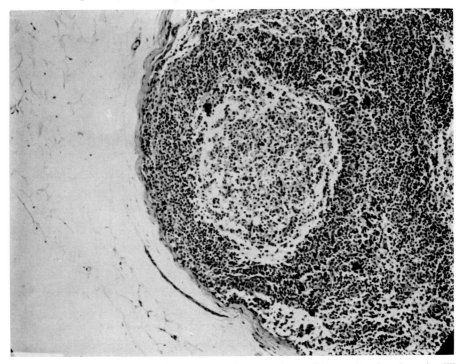

FIGURE 22. Germinal center in lymph node from patient with ataxia-telangiectasia. The usual cuff of small lymphocytes is not seen and reticular stromal cells are the major elements bordering the follicle. (Figs. 22, 23, and 24 reproduced with permission from PETERSON, R. D. A.; COOPER, M. D., and GOOD, R. A.: *Amer J Med, 41*:342, 1966.)

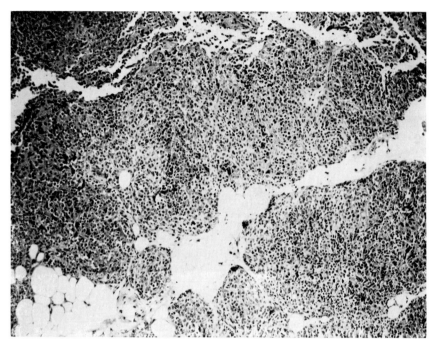

FIGURE 23. Thymus from patient with ataxia-telangiectasia. Although the normal lobular structure is seen, the lobules are composed almost entirely of epithelial-stromal cells. The small and darkly stained thymocytes are few in number and Hassall's corpuscles are conspicuously absent.

apparently being inherited as a simple autosomal recessive. It is associated with an abnormal thymus, immunological deficiency, and increased susceptibility to lymphoreticular malignancy (Peterson, Cooper and Good, 1966).

Plasma cells are usually rare or absent in the bone marrow but are sometimes normal. Some of these patients have grossly deficient lymphocytic collars around normal medullary centers in the lymph nodes (see Fig. 22). Plasma cells may be even missing from the imprints of antigenically stimulated lymph nodes (Peterson, Kelly, and Good, 1964). Thymic tissue is usually atrophic. There are no Hassall's corpuscles; only stromal cells are seen suggestive of the epithelial anlage (see Fig. 23). The thymus in these patients resembles an embryonic thymus before the lymphoid induction.

A number of patients with ataxia-telangiectasia develop malignancies of the reticuloendothelial system such as reticulum cell sarcoma, Hodgkin's disease, "round cell sarcoma," and lymphosarcoma (see Fig. 24).

Upon immunoelectrophoresis the sera show either absent or very low levels of IgA (0 to ½ normal) (Fireman, Boesman, and Gitlin, 1964; Peterson, Kelly, and Good, 1964) while IgG is normal and IgM is either normal or increased by two to three times. Serum isohemagglutinins are low in some of these patients. There is also failure to produce any detectable

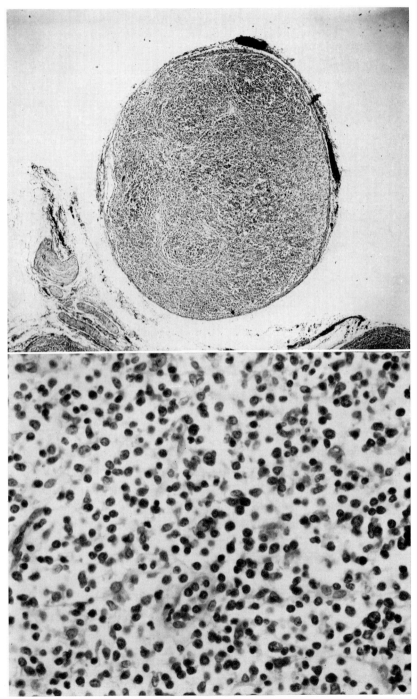

FIGURE 24. Lymphosarcoma involving a lymph node from a patient with ataxia-telangiectasia. (*Upper*) Note destruction of the normal architecture of the node. (*Lower*) Higher magnification of the same specimen showing the predominance of small lymphocytes.

antibody to bacteriophage. diphtheria toxoid, and typhoid and paratyphoid antigens. There is frequently a difficulty in sensitization to DNFB. Skin homografts have prolonged survivals and the usual rapid rejection of the second grafts does not occur. The defect is that of synthesis. The gamma globulin half-life was definitely prolonged in one case (Peterson, Kelly, and Good, 1964).

The relationship of the IgA deficiency to the characteristic sinopulmonary infectious in these patients is of interest, since IgA is the serum immunoglobulin that normally predominates in respiratory tract secretions (Tomasi and Zigelbaum, 1963). While the defect of serum IgA synthesis is severe, it is incomplete; IgA production in the salivary gland seems to be unaffected (McFarlin *et al.*, 1965).

Some of the relatives of the patients studied by Peterson, Kelly, and Good (1964) lacked IgA globulin and had early clinical stigmata of ataxia-telangiectasia. This was not true of families studied by Fireman, Boesman, and Gitlin (1964).

## Hypoimmunoglobulinemias of Late Onset

Hypoimmunoglobulinemias of late onset are also called *primary adult hypogammaglobulinemias* or *primary acquired hypogammaglobulinemias*.

This is a group of syndromes which is being recognized more frequently, and the literature on it is growing rapidly. With the realization that immunoglobulin deficiency may lead to recurrent infections and enteritis, sera of individuals with chronic suppurative diseases, with bronchiectasis, and with chronic diarrhea are being screened by immunoelectrophoresis for immunoglobulin abnormality. New cases of hypoimmunoglobulinopathy previously missed are being uncovered (Hermans *et al.*, 1966). In the majority of these patients, first symptoms can be traced to early childhood. However, the bulk of symptomatology becomes apparent in adult life—in the thirties, forties, and fifties. This group is sometimes called acquired type. However, family studies have uncovered the presence of various immunologic deficiencies, not necessarily of the type found in the propositus, in the asymptomatic family members. A genetic defect is suggested by some, a somatic mutation by others. It is possible that some of the syndromes described below are genetic and some are acquired. Of those that are genetic, the transmission of the defect seems to be ill-defined, with the type and degree of deficiency varying from one member of the family to the other. What seems to be heritable is a vague "weakness" of the immune body system, an "immunoparetic diathesis." The environmental factors seem to dictate the direction and degree of the deviation.

Primary adult hypoimmunoglobulinemia can be generalized, involving all classes of immunoglobulins, or selective. Either IgA, IgG, IgA and IgG, or IgA and IgM are decreased, with the remaining classes of immunoglobu-

globulins with an increase in IgM, as well as high isohemagglutinin and Forssman antibody titers without any unusual clinical manifestations. Bone marrow aspirate was deficient in plasma cells.

Huntley, Lafferty, and Lyerly (1963) described a nine-year-old boy with draining ears and neck and an acutely inflamed appendix. The IgA and IgG were markedly decreased. The IgM-globulins were increased, as were the titers of isohemagglutinins (1:512) and of heterophile agglutinins of Forssman type (1:224). A positive Schick test persisted after immunization; there was absence of a rise in the titer of polio neutralizing antibodies after a booster injection. The patient's symptoms responded to treatment with pooled gamma globulin. A steady drop in the IgM concentration after initiation of gamma globulin replacement suggested that the overproduction of IgM-globulins was related to the low IgG level.

Rosen and Bougas (1963) reported the case of a thirty-seven-year-old-woman with chronic progressive bronchiectasis with what they called "acquired dysgammaglobulinemia" characterized by a marked elevation in the serum concentration of macroglobulin and high titers of the antibodies associated with this group of immunoglobulins (antibodies against the somatic or 0 antigen of the gram-negative bacteria), but the virtual absence of 7S gamma globulins from the serum. On lung biopsy well developed primary lymphoid follicles were found in the peribronchiolar exudate. The periodic acid-Schiff (PAS) positive "plasmacytoid" cells that have been associated with the synthesis of 19S globulins in Waldenström's disease (Dutcher and Fahey, 1960) and in congenital dysgammaglobulinemia (Cruchaud *et al.,* 1962) were abundantly present in the periphery of the lymphoid follicles. These cells are distinguished from plasma cells by a high nuclear-cytoplasmic ratio and positive PAS staining. A maturation arrest with failure to form plasma cells but increased formation of functioning "plasmacytoid" cells seemed to be present. The patient did well on massive periodic injections of gamma globulin (22cc every 2 weeks).

Hinz and Boyer (1963) reported a case of a sixty-two-year-old woman, not unusually susceptible to infections, who had a severe hemolytic anemia brought on by the presence of an autoantibody directed against her group MM red cells. The antibody was an IgM and there was an increase of IgM in the patient's serum as well as a decrease in all of her 7S gamma globulins. The patient improved with prednisone. The authors felt that the patient's anemia was merely an incidental result of her basic dysproteinemic state and due to an "accidental fit" of the elevated protein for an existing erythrocyte antigen. They believed that macroglobulin elevation represented one part of a widespread disorder of altered immunoglobulin synthesis rather than being a result of specific sensitization.

A variant of this condition was reported by Barth and coworkers (1965) in a fifteen-year-old Navajo girl who had repeated respiratory infections since infancy, with generalized adenopathy, hepatosplenomegaly, cardiomegaly and retarded growth. She had persistent *Giardia lamblia* infestation and recurrent Salmonella infections. Serum paper electrophoresis failed to reveal any abnormality, while immunoelectrophoresis showed marked reduction of the IgA and IgG globulins, both less than one hundredth of normal, and increased IgM, ten to fifteen times greater than normal, and increased IgD, 0.6 to 3.6%, twelve to one hundred and twenty times the normal level. The macroglobulins appeared to be normal in physicochemical and immunochemical properties except for a low antibody content. Lymphocytes as well as plasma cells were present in normal amounts in the bone marrow and lymph nodes and had a normal appearance both with Giemsa stain and under the electron microscope. Immunofluorescent studies suggested that the plasma cells were synthesizing the heavy $\mu$ chains (IgM) and the $\kappa$ and $\lambda$ light chains and only a few contained the IgG globulin. Immune response was impaired in these patients but not absent. The family study in this case failed to reveal immunoglobulin deficiencies or clinical history of susceptibility to infection, but was limited by unavailability of close relatives.

Stiehm and Fudenberg (1966b) reported a case of this syndrome in an infant followed from the age of seven months to his death at nineteen months. The child exhibited recurrent respiratory infections, hepatosplenomegaly, adenopathy, hemolytic anemia, and pancytopenia.

Mongan, Kern, and Terry (1966) reported a sixty-one-year-old white woman with a normal IgM but markedly decreased IgG and IgA with multiple bacterial infections, an episode of autoimmune hemolytic anemia as well as a thymoma and evidence of cytomegalovirus pulmonary infection on autopsy. This patient produced two abnormal autoantibodies, an antinuclear antibody and an antibody directed against her own red cells.

The cases first reported occurred in young boys (Rosen *et al.*, 1961; Hong *et al.*, 1962; Huntley, Lafferty, and Lyerly, 1963), and Huntley and coworkers suggested that the disease affected boys only and is inherited through the mother. In his family study the disease affected two sons of the same mother with different fathers; the mother had increased serum albumin and increased globulins. However, subsequent papers recorded the disease in a girl (Barth *et al.*, 1965) and in three older women (Hinz and Boyer, 1963; Rosen and Bougas, 1963; Mongan, Kern, and Terry, 1966).

Incidence of this condition is probably greater than realized. Paper electrophoresis may be normal, as increased IgM may mask the hypo-IgG and hypo-IgA-globulinemia. Soothill (1962) studied serum IgM levels in seventy patients with hypogammaglobulinemia. In seven the IgM levels were two to five times greater than normal.

It is of diagnostic and etiologic significance that the clinical onset of the condition can be traced to the patient's childhood, five to ten years of age, and occasionally to infancy (Stiehm and Fudenberg, 1966b). There is usually an increased susceptibility to infections, manifested to a minor degree in childhood, but to an increasing degree later in life; respiratory tract infections, otitis media, adenitis, chronic progressive bronchiectasis, *Giardia lamblia* and salmonellosis have been reported. Hepatomegaly, splenomegaly and lymphadenopathy may be present. Gastrointestinal symptoms, especially diarrhea, are sometimes prominent. Several of these patients have symptoms suggestive of rheumatoid arthritis.

Plasma cells in this syndrome may be either absent (Hinz and Boyer, 1963), decreased (Hong *et al.*, 1962), or normal (Barth *et al.*, 1965; Huntley, Lafferty, and Lyerly, 1963). The IgM-immunoglobulins appear to be produced in the spleen in the "transitional cells," or "plasmocytoid cells" as Cruchaud and coworkers (1962) demonstrated by the fluorescent antibody technique.

While IgG and IgA immunoglobulins are decreased, and may be absent even after immunization, the IgM and IgD immunoglobulins are normal or increased. Rosen found that his patient with this condition responded to an antigenic challenge with an increase in IgM but not IgG antibodies. Barth's patient, however, had a poor response or none to almost all antigens tested despite a high IgM level and lack of any cellular deficiency. Studies in animals have shown that IgM antibody formation does not lead to persisting immunologic memory. However, patients with hypo-IgG and IgA-globulinemia and increased IgM-globulinemia (type I dysgammaglobulinemia) when repeatedly immunized with bacteriophage exhibited anamnestic response in the IgM (Gleich *et al.*, 1966). The bulk of antibody formed in these patients in response to bacteriophage administration is of 19S type even after five injections. Previous failures to demonstrate an IgM anamnestic response to viral antigens in guinea pigs and rabbits may be related to the inhibitory effects of IgG antibody on IgM antibody synthesis.

Isoagglutinins may be either very low or very high. Whereas early symptoms in this condition are related to susceptibility to infections, with progression of compensatory hyper-IgM-globulinemia, the patients also show the consequences of the elevated macroglobulins. Autoimmune hemolytic anemia and thrombocytopenia may be associated with this condition (Hinz and Boyer, 1963; Rosen *et al.*, 1961). Splenectomy in two such cases resulted in cessation of 19S gamma globulin synthesis, reversion to agammaglobulinemia, and remission of hemolytic anemia and thrombocytopenia. The spleen is probably the site of manufacture of IgM-globulins in these patients.

The basic defect in this entity probably is in the controller (or operator) gene for various chains, with a relative decrease in synthesis of $\gamma$ and $a$ chains, and superabundance of $\mu$ and $\delta$ chains (Barth *et al.*, 1965; Stiehm and Fudenberg, 1966b). In addition, the excess of IgM and IgD may represent a physiologic as well as a genetic compensatory mechanism. With gamma globulin therapy, the serum IgM level fell. IgG may regulate the synthesis of IgM molecules by a homeostatic mechanism, as specific antibody may reduce the stimulus to immunoglobulin formation. Alternatively, the exogenous IgG may effect the controller genes of the immunoglobulin synthetic process.

In addition to the defect in synthesis, the patient studied by Barth also had an accelerated catabolism of [131]I-labelled normal IgG. This was probably due to a mild, transient and reversible protein-losing enteropathy secondary to salmonella enteritis and giardial infestation. Serum albumin, low prior to treatment for these conditions rose to normal after therapy, lending further credence to this possibility.

*4. Selective Hypo-IgA and M-Globulinemia with Normal IgG (Giedion-Scheidegger Syndrome).* Giedion and Scheidegger (1957) described a patient subject to recurrent bacterial infections who had a normal level of 7S gamma globulins but who demonstrated a severe deficiency of 19S gamma globulin and of IgA-globulin.

No detectable isohemagglutinins were present even after stimulation. The patient was unable to shift the antibody response from one type (IgM) to another (IgG). A few similar patients have since been described (Barandun, Cottier, and Hassig, 1958).

All patients reported were boys. The mode of inheritance is unknown. Parents of one patient were first cousins. There is increased susceptibility to infection. One or more patients had splenomegaly, cerebral palsy, glaucoma, eczema, bronchiectasis, and enterocolitis. Plasma cells were present in the bone marrow and lymph nodes (Barandun, Cottier, and Hassig, 1958).

*5. Selective Hypo-IgA and M-Globulinemia with Slight Decrease in IgG.* Gilbert and Hong (1964) reported a twenty-nine-year-old Negro housewife with a three-year history of pulmonary infections, a genitourinary tract infection, almost total absence of IgA and IgM, and slight decrease in IgG to half the usual value. Other features included a rheumatoid-like arthritis, diarrhea with xylose malabsorption, hypokalemia and hypocalcemia. A muscle biopsy showed necrosis and was consistent with myositis. A jejunal biopsy showed "nonspecific enteritis" with only slight flattening of the villi. A bone marrow study showed a marked decrease in plasma cells, but in peripheral blood there was a mild leukocytosis and a normal number of lymphocytes.

Immunologic investigation revealed a remarkable inability to form measurable humoral antibodies to bacterial and viral antigens despite only a small decrease in IgG level. The authors felt that the patient's IgG was qualitatively inadequate. However, cellular reactivity was normal as measured by PPD, histoplasmin and other skin tests as well as by homograft rejection. Properdin was absent from this patient's serum while the levels of this euglobulin have been normal in patients with various antibody deficiency syndromes. Natural isohemagglutinins were present in the patient but no increase was detectable after stimulation. In congenital agammaglobulinemia, isohemagglutinins are usually absent or low. In the acquired form, about half of the patients demonstrate normal isohemagglutinin titers. In Giedion-Scheidegger syndrome no isohemagglutinins were found even after stimulation. Normal isohemagglutinins have been observed in patients with deficiency in IgG and IgA with normal or elevated IgM.

Several family members of the reported patient, although asymptomatic, revealed various quantitative immunoglobulin abnormalities, either diminution in IgM or elevation in IgG or IgA.

A similar constellation of immunoglobulin deficiency (decreased A and M, slightly decreased G) was described as a distinct syndrome by Hermans and coworkers (1966) in nine patients studied at the Mayo Clinic. In addition to increased susceptibility to infections of the upper and lower respiratory tract, and intermittent or chronic diarrhea of moderate severity which was steatorrheic at times, these patients had alterations of the small intestine consisting of little or no villus atrophy, absence of plasma cell infiltration and presence of a considerable degree of lymphocytic infiltration associated with a nodular lymphocytic hyperplasia in which large germinal centers could be discerned. The striking nodular character of the infiltration was apparent on the small bowel roentgenograms. *Giardia lamblia* was almost invariably found in the feces and did not disappear after several courses of quinocrine. In some of the patients diarrhea responded to treatment with tetracycline. A carcinomatous lesion of the gastrointestinal tract was present in three out of nine (adenocarcinoma of stomach in two, and carcinoma of rectosigmoid in one) and pernicious anemia with achlorhydria in one, all at a relatively young age.

Conn and Quintiliani (1966) reported a case of hypoimmunoglobulinemia, with greatly decreased IgM and IgA and mild decrease in IgG in a seventy-four-year-old laborer with recurrent respiratory infections, and severe diarrhea controlled by gamma globulin administration. This patient had pneumococcal pneumonia, salmonella enteritis, a normal jejunal biopsy and small bowel x-rays, no malabsorption, and a spindle cell thymoma as well as amyloidosis of the gastrointestinal tract, spleen, adrenal and thyroid.

6. No selective hypo-IgM-globulinemia has been described so far.

7. No selective hypo-IgD-globulinemia has been described.

### "Familial Idiopathic Dysproteinemia" of Homburger and Petermann

In 1949, Homburger and Petermann (1949) reported a family in which members of three generations had hypoalbuminemia, hypogammaglobulinemia and edema with leg ulcers in the male and peripheral vascular changes in the female patients. Some cases were associated with malforma-tion of the thoracic cage and an anomalous distribution of occipital hair. Approximately half of the members of three generations of both sexes were affected. Failure to produce antibodies to injected pneumococcal polysac-charides was demonstrated in one of these patients. The mechanism of this aberration and its relationship to other hypoimmunoglobulinemias is pres-ently unknown.

### SECONDARY HYPOIMMUNOGLOBULINEMIAS
#### (Secondary Acquired Hypoimmunoglobulinemias)

### Secondary Hypoimmunoglobulinemias Associated with Hypoalbuminemia

Hypoimmunoglobulinemia may be part of generalized hypoproteinemia. In this situation, hypoalbuminemia is usually the most striking protein abnormality.

By far the commonest of the conditions associated with hypoimmuno-globulinemias and hypoalbuminemia is the nephrotic syndrome. Loss in the urine and increased catabolism may be the principal causes of the decrease in the plasma immunoglobulins in this condition, as the rate of synthesis is normal (Gitlin, Gross, and Janeway, 1959). Gamma globulin in children with the nephrotic syndrome frequently drops to 200 mg%; this decrease may contribute to the well-known susceptibility to severe septic infections in these children. Blainey and coworkers (1960) found that it is primarily the IgG and IgA that are decreased while IgM is frequently normal; this may be due to the character and degree of the renal defect which permits preferen-tial urinary loss of the smaller immunoglobulins.

In some cases of amyloidosis, hypogammaglobulinemia occurs along with hypoalbuminemia and may be due to a combination of an increased cata-bolism (renal loss) as well as decreased synthesis secondary to the immuno-cyte disorder.

That a variety of gastrointestinal diseases can be associated with a loss of protein through the gastrointestinal tract (protein-losing enteropathy) has become well known over the last decade (Holman, Nickel, and Sleisenger, 1959; Barth *et al.*, 1964).

Hypoimmunoglobulinemia may be part of the syndrome of hypoproteine-mia in Menetrier's disease, carcinoma of the stomach, gastric polyps, regional enteritis, acute enteritis, nontropical sprue, lymphangiectasia of the small intestine (Strober *et al.*, 1966; McGuigan *et al.*, 1968) and chronic ulcera-tive colitis (Hermans *et al.*, 1966). In some of these entities, intestinal pro-tein leak is coupled with malabsorption.

Nutritional hypogammaglobulinemia was reported in one patient (Git-lin, Gross, and Janeway, 1959); as a rule, however, protein starvation leads to hypoalbuminemia but not to hypogammaglobulinemia. In the so-called nutritional-recovery syndrome after kwashiorkor, hypergammaglobulinemia may be observed.

### Secondary Hypoimmunoglobulinemias Associated with Malignancies of the Reticuloendothelial System

In various malignancies of the reticuloendothelial system there is marked decrease in one or two or all classes of immunoglobulins.

This situation occurs classically in paraimmunoglobulinopathies such as multiple myeloma (Snapper, Turner, and Moscovitz, 1953; Fahey *et al.,* 1963), Waldenström's macroglobulinemia, and H-chain disease where the pathologically altered immunocyte produces large amounts of a paraimmunoglobulin (such as myeloma protein, Bence Jones protein, macroglobulin) and fails to produce the normal immunoglobulins. In the deranged immunocyte the synthesis of immunoglobulins may be blocked at an early stage with a resultant hypoimmunoglobulinemia and no paraimmunoglobulinemia. Hypoimmunoglobulinemia associated with various paraimmunoglobulinopathies is discussed in greater detail in the chapters on the paraimmunoglobulinopathies.

Hypoimmunoglobulinemia has also been noted in various lymphomas (Arends, Coonrad, and Rundles, 1954; Poe, Gable, and Jarrold, 1966), chronic lymphatic leukemia (Jim and Reinhard, 1956), as well as in amyloidosis (Engle and Wallis, 1966). In the last condition it is frequently associated with hypoalbuminemia and could possibly reflect renal loss of those proteins. The predisposition of these patients to bacterial infections is well known.

Chronic lymphocytic leukemia and lymphosarcoma are commonly associated with hypogammaglobulinemia at some time during the course of the disease. While chronic myelocytic leukemia and acute lymphoblastic leukemia are associated primarily with low IgA levels, in chronic lymphocytic leukemia all immunoglobulins are low, and especially the macroglobulins. Using the bacterial adherence test Brody and Beizer (1966) demonstrated a remarkable difference between a normal lymphocyte and the lymphocytes from patients with chronic lymphocytic leukemia. Since the test depends on the manufacture of 19S antibody by the lymphocyte from an individual previously immunized to salmonella, they concluded that the leukemic lymphocyte demonstrated a failure of this specific 19S production. This immunological indolence may bear a fundamental responsibility for the poor resistance to infections seen in patients with chronic lymphocytic leukemia. The fall in the serum immunoglobulins usually occurs late in chronic lymphocytic leukemia and lymphosarcoma and has been postulated to be the consequence of an interference with normal lymphopoiesis and plasma cell production. Radiation therapy, alkylating agents and other cytotoxic agents have been implicated as contributors to hypoimmunoglobulinemia.

Hodgkin's disease, on the other hand, is rarely associated with low gamma globulin. Poe, Gable, and Jarrold (1966) reported a well documented case of Hodgkin's disease with liver involvement, generalized hypoimmunoglobulinemia and lack of plasma cells in the bone marrow. With nitrogen mustard treatment, the serum electrophoresis pattern returned to almost normal; IgG and IgA globulins rose and normal plasma cells appeared in the bone marrow. There was no parallel improvement in the liver involvement.

## Secondary Hypoimmunoglobulinemia Associated with Autoimmune Diseases

A number of diseases characterized by evidence of immune derangement may be associated with hypoimmunoglobulinemia. The electrophoretic protein pattern in rheumatoid arthritis, lupus erythematosus, idiopathic thrombocytopenic purpura, rheumatic fever and sarcoidosis is usually completely normal but sometimes shows hyperimmunoglobulinemia or even hypoimmunoglobulinemia.

The high incidence of a syndrome resembling rheumatoid arthritis in the patients with congenital and adult type hypoimmunoglobulinemia, and the high incidence of rheumatoid factor, positive LE (lupus) preparations and collagen diseases in relatives of patients with adult hypoimmunoglobulinemia will be discussed in the next chapter.

## Secondary Hypoimmunoglobulinemia Associated with Pernicious Anemia

Several patients have been reported with hypoimmunoglobulinemia associated with pernicious anemia. Clark and associates (1967) studied two such patients and reviewed four other documented cases. The relationship of the immunoglobulin deficiency and resulting susceptibility to infections and gastric atrophy and intrinsic factor deficiency is not clear. Impaired antibody responsiveness was associated with a failure to demonstrate serum antibodies against parietal cell, intrinsic factor, or thyroid antigens. Herbert (1967) found that about a half of patients with pernicious anemia had varying degrees of hypoimmunoglobulinemia and postulated that vitamin $B_{12}$ deficiency led to an impairment in immunoglobulin synthesis through its nonspecific effect on the synthesis of all proteins. Recently, Conn, Binder, and Burns (1968) have also reported on this association.

## Secondary Acquired Hypoimmunoglobulinemias Associated with Chronic Infections

A significant number of patients with chronic progressive bronchiectasis are found to have acquired hypoimmunoglobulinemia (Rosen and Bougas, 1963), involving all three classes of immunoglobulins. It is sometimes impossible to tell if the hypoimmunoglobulinemia preceded or followed the onset of the pulmonary infection. Was this hypoimmunoglobulinemia a heritable disorder manifesting late in life with resulting susceptibility to infection culminating in chronic progressive bronchiectasis? Or was the infectious disorder responsible for exhausting the immune response and causing a truly acquired hypoimmunoglobulinemia? For the time being we assume that some cases fall into one and some into the other category.

## Secondary Acquired Hypoimmunoglobulinemia Associated with Diseases of Unknown Etiology

An interesting case with manifestations of hypoimmunoglobulinemia (pneumonia, sinusitis, and furunculosis) preceding the classical symptoms of sarcoidosis was reported by Bronsky and Dunn (1965). The patient, a thirty-seven-year-old Negro, had a markedly reduced IgG, and no IgM or IgA globulins.

## PHYSIOLOGIC HYPOIMMUNOGLOBULINEMIAS

### Transient Physiologic Hypogammaglobulinemia of Infants

The IgG-globulins pass the placental barrier and are present in high concentration in the serum of the umbilical cord and newborn. Thereafter the level of IgG drops rapidly and is lowest at three months, even though the infant begins to synthesize his own IgG at four weeks. Thereafter the level increases rapidly. At two years there is a nearly normal adult concentration (see Fig. 18). The rate of increase diminishes; by age sixteen, adult level IgG is attained (Stiehm and Fudenberg, 1966a).

If the development of the ability to synthesize IgG is abnormally delayed in the infant, the plasma concentration will continue to fall to dangerously low levels. Between four and twelve weeks of age, gamma globulin is between 300 and 600 mg per 100 ml and in certain infants the level may fall to 150 mg or less. Serious infections may occur. However, this state is temporary, and as the infant begins to synthesize his own immunoglobulins, the plasma level begins to rise, usually by the fifth month.

The IgA and IgM do not play a significant role in the hypoimmunoglobulinemia of infancy (Fig. 18). IgM globulins are present in small amounts ($\frac{1}{10}$ of adult) in the newborn and are the chief immunoglobulins synthesized in the neonatal period (Stiehm and Fudenberg, 1966a). Their concentration increases rapidly; at four months they are at 50 per cent of the adult level; at nine months almost at the normal adult level (Huntley, Lafferty, and Lyerly, 1963), and at sixteen years are at the normal adult level (Stiehm and Fudenberg, 1966a).

IgA globulins are usually absent in the newborn, but have been found in trace quantities in one third of the samples of umbilical cord serum (Stiehm and Fudenberg, 1966a). The concentration increases slowly and is at a normal adult level at four years (Huntley, Lafferty, and Lyerly, 1963). According to Stiehm and Fudenberg (1966a) the concentration of IgA's continues to rise throughout early adulthood.

There is no difference in levels of immunoglobulins between the male and the female, whether in infants, children, or adults.

### Normal Hypoimmunoglobulinemia of Germ-Free Animals

Germ-free animals exhibit a generalized hypoimmunoglobulinemia, suggesting that bombardment with antigenic stimuli is responsible for the "normally" encountered levels of gamma globulin. The germ-free guinea pigs have serum levels one half to one sixth of those of nongerm-free guinea pigs. Studies of the gamma globulin metabolism in these animals, employing $^{131}$I-labelled gamma globulin, indicate that the rate of catabolism of gamma globulin is the same in the germ-free and nongerm-free guinea pigs, suggesting that the low serum levels of gamma globulins in the germ-free animals are due to lower rates of synthesis. The calculated rates of synthesis are two-to-five times slower (Sell, 1964).

Germ-free chickens injected with bovine serum albumin exhibit a delayed and a lower initial response in antibody production, reflecting a state of "inexperience" in the reticuloendothelial system. However, antibody production in the germ-free birds is more prolonged than that in the conventional chickens (Wostmann and Olson, 1964). If a cell usually produces one antibody at one given time (Nossal *et al.*, 1964), a competitive interaction of different antigenic stimuli may foreshorten the response in the conventional system (Wostmann and Olson, 1964).

# Chapter 5

# HYPOIMMUNOGLOBULINOPATHIES: GENERAL ASPECTS

## ETIOLOGY

THE ETIOLOGY of hypoimmunoglobulinemias cannot be explained by a single mechanism. The causes of various entities are probably separate but more generally interrelated. The most comprehensive concept of the pathogenesis of various immunologic deficiency states has been proposed by Peterson, Cooper, and Good (1965) (see Fig. 29). They recognize two components of the immune system in the higher vertebrates including man: they are (1) the thymus-dependent lymphoid tissue, consisting primarily of small lymphocytes and responsible for the recognition of antigenicity, initiation of specific immune response, and the mechanism of cellular immunity; and (2) the "bursa-appendix-Peyer's patches-and possibly tonsil"-dependent lymphoid tissue which they call "immunoglobulin producing system" consisting mainly of large pyroninophilic lymphocytes and plasma cells and responsible for the major production of immunoglobulins. Both of these cell systems populate the "peripheral" lymphoid organs (lymph nodes, spleen, liver, etc.); however, both are derived from "central," gut-wall associated lymphoid tissue.

Embryologic studies suggest that thymus is formed in the region of the third and fourth pharyngeal pouches as a result of a proliferation of gut epithelial cells. This epithelial anlage is transformed into a lymphoid thymus, mesenchyme being necessary for the maturation (see Fig. 29). The thymic lymphocytes differentiate further and become the smaller cells recognizable as lymphocytes elsewhere in the body. Thymic lymphocytes actually leave the thymus and populate the peripheral lymphatic tissue. In addition, the thymus appears to influence the peripheral lymphoid tissue by secreting a humoral substance. In animals deprived of the thymus and thymus-dependent peripheral lymphoid tissue, the immunoglobulin-producing system is intact or even hypertrophied with generalized hyperimmunoglobulinemia; these animals, however, lack the ability to develop specific

95

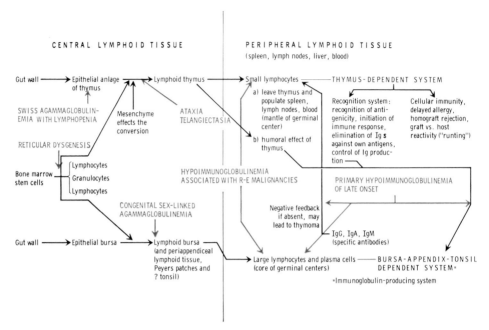

FIGURE 29. Schematic presentation: development of the immune system and hypoimmunoglobulinemias. (Modified with permission from PETERSON, R. D. A.; COOPER, M. D., and GOOD, R. A.: *Amer J Med, 38:*579, 1965.)

antibodies to various specific antigens. Rabbits, if newborn and thymectomized, may develop autoimmune hemolytic anemia, lupus-like lesions in the kidneys and later amyloid disease. This association suggests a defect in self-recognition.

The immunoglobulin-producing system also originates in the gut wall. In the chicken the place of origin seems to be the epithelial cells lining the bursa of Fabricius in the hindgut. The mammalian organs that most closely resemble the chicken bursa are the periappendiceal lymphoid tissue, sacculus rotundus, and Peyers patches and probably the palatine tonsil. The epithelial cells from these areas are transformed into bursal lymphocytes; these are the precursors of the large pyroninophilic lymphocytes present in follicles in the spleen and of plasma cells scattered throughout the white pulp of the spleen. These cells are the main immunoglobulin producers. Bursal ablation of a newly-hatched chicken will cause quantitative lowering of serum levels of 7S immunoglobulins; 7S-19S immunoglobulins can be further decreased by radiation of bursectomized chickens. However, since cellular immunity is a function of the thymus-dependent lymphoid tissue, it remains intact in these animals.

The thymus-dependent system and the bursa and appendix-dependent (immunoglobulin-producing) system are interdependent. The thymus and/

or the thymus dependent system recognizes the antigenic stimulus as not self, initiates the specific immune response and directs and controls the immunoglobulin-producing system toward a specific immune response. The immunoglobulin-producing system may serve as a negative feedback, the increased immunoglobulin level inhibiting the thymus-dependent tissue, the decreased immunoglobulin level stimulating the thymus-dependent system.

According to the scheme of Peterson, Cooper and Good (see Fig. 29), Swiss agammaglobulinemia with lymphopenia is due to failure of development of the normal epithelial anlage of the thymus and probably other lymphoid tissue from the gut endoderm. Reticular dysgenesis is attributed to failure of development of the lymphocytes and other white blood cells from the stem cells. In ataxia-telangiectasia the thymus resembles embryonic thymus before lymphoid induction. Normal mesenchyme is known to be necessary for the lymphoid maturation of the thymus. An abnormality in the mesenchyme of these patients, perhaps reflected in their vascular lesions, could cause failure to induce normal lymphoid development of the thymus. The progressive degeneration of the central nervous system may also be secondary to a vascular abnormality. A primary mesenchymal abnormality may thus account for all the facets of ataxia-telangiectasia.

Congenital sex-linked agammaglobulinemia with its striking absence of pharyngeal lymphoid tissue is akin to the condition of chickens bursectomized at birth or in which bursal development has been prevented by treatment with 19-nortestosterone. The defect is probably in the formation of the bursa-appendix type tissue. Primary hypogammaglobulinemias of late onset and "acquired" hypogammaglobulinemias associated with diseases characterized by immune derangement (rheumatoid arthritis, lupus erythematosus, idiopathic thrombocytopenic purpura, rheumatic fever, regional enteritis) but not associated with lymphomas, are attributed to failure either of one of the components of the immune system or of a homeostatic mechanism that presumably regulates the intercommunication of these systems. When this homeostatic control is disturbed, absence of normal immunoglobulins may result in abnormalities in the thymus such as the thymomas observed in these patients. On the other hand, thymic abnormality may result in autoimmune disease, possibly reflecting overcompensation of the immunoglobulin producing system.

The pathogenesis of hypoimmunoglobulinemia associated with malignancies of the reticuloendothelial system has been assumed to be the crowding out of immunologically competent cells by invasive malignant cells. Peterson, Cooper and Good (1965) propose, however, that in these patients a defect in differentiation of the lymphoid system underlies both the immunologic deficiency and the lymphoreticular malignancy. The abnormality of the lymphoid tissue which is reflected in hypoimmunoglobulinemia predis-

TABLE XIX

RELATIONSHIP BETWEEN IMMUNOLOGIC DEFICIENCY
AND MALIGNANCIES

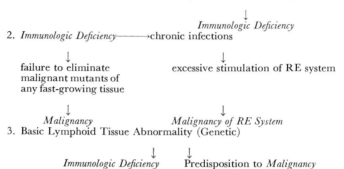

1. *Lymphoreticular Malignancy*→crowding out of immunocompetent cells

↓

*Immunologic Deficiency*

2. *Immunologic Deficiency*————→chronic infections

↓                                    ↓

failure to eliminate            excessive stimulation of RE system
malignant mutants of
any fast-growing tissue

↓                                    ↓

*Malignancy*                    *Malignancy of RE System*

3. Basic Lymphoid Tissue Abnormality (Genetic)

↓        ↓

*Immunologic Deficiency*    Predisposition to *Malignancy*

poses to subsequent malignancies. Furthermore, an immunologic deficiency
may facilitate development of a malignancy by permitting mutant cells to
proliferate (see Table XIX).

The general outline of the developmental schema described above has
been accepted by most workers. However, many specific points need confirmation from further studies and clarification.

The etiology of hypoimmunoglobulinemia has also been considered on a
cellular and molecular level. Rieke (1966) demonstrated that thoracic duct
lymphocytes from neonatally thymectomized rats failed to produce runt
disease in newborn allogeneic rats injected with up to ten times the number
of normal lymphocytes needed to cause runting. This suggested that the
immunologic deficiency caused by thymectomy does not arise solely from a
failure of central immune mechanism which may be dependent upon
thymic action *in vivo;* the lymphocytes themselves become immunologically
deficient.

Furthermore, studies of *in vitro* cultures of lymphocytes suggest that the
defect in antibody production may result from a failure of protein synthesis
rather than from a failure of plasma cell maturation. Peripheral lymphocytes taken from patients with congenital sex-linked agammaglobulinemia
when cultured in the presence of phytohemagglutinins and streptolysin were
able to differentiate into plasma cells (Fudenberg and Hirschhorn, 1964)
but failed to produce or contain certain immunoglobulins, when exposed to
specific antigens, as demonstrated by negative specific fluorescence, in contrast to normal human lymphocytes (Hirschhorn and Ripps, 1966). This
points to a genetic deficiency in gamma globulin synthesis as the basic defect
of congenital sex-linked agammaglobulinemia. Differentiation of lymphocytes into plasma cells seems to be concomitant with, rather than a prerequisite for, antibody formation. The defect in synthesis may be attributable to
mutations resulting in formation of either insufficient or altered and faulty

messenger RNA either incapable of coding for normal immunoglobulin or capable of binding to and blocking the ribosomes responsible for synthesis of the various polypeptide chains of immunoglobulins. Indeed, RNA synthesis has been found defective in lymphocytes from patients with congenital agammaglobulinemia (Cline and Fudenberg, 1965).

This observation of intrinsic defect of synthesis in agammaglobulinemic lymphocytes was not borne out by studies of Cooperband and coworkers (1966), who used leucine $C^{14}$ incorporation into immunoglobulins and $P^{32}$ incorporation into DNA by human lymphocytes cultured in the presence of an antigen. In their studies they observed no difference between lymphocytes taken from normal and from agammaglobulinemic subjects.

Fudenberg, Heremans, and Franklin (1963) drew an analogy between the immunologic deficiency syndromes and thalassemia, suggesting that a genetically determined inability to synthesize one or more of the gamma globulin chains is similar to the failure of synthesis of the various chains of hemoglobin in thalassemia. Defects produced by mutations at the Gm locus, which controls the synthesis of heavy chains of 7S gamma globulin, would result in inhibition of synthesis of 7S alone. Similarly, defects in other postulated not yet discovered Gm loci would specifically suppress the synthesis of IgA or IgM. Decreases in two of the three immunoglobulins would result in double heterozygosity involving two of three gene loci and a most serious clinical disorder. A mutation at the Inv locus leads to impaired synthesis of light chains, and as these are common to all of the immunoglobulins, there would result deficiency in all three immunoglobulins such as is seen in classical congenital agammaglobulinemia. As this disorder is sex-linked, the authors postulate involvement of a regulator gene on the X chromosome, since the structural Inv gene is located on the autosome.

Primary hypogammaglobulinemias of late onset and acquired hypogammaglobulinemias associated with disease characterized by immune derangement (rheumatoid arthritis, lupus erythematosus, idiopathic thrombocytopenic purpura, rheumatic fever, regional enteritis) have been thought to be acquired in nature and secondary to the underlying disease. However, Fudenberg, German, and Kunkel (1962) found a high incidence of rheumatoid factor, serum globulin abnormalities and clinical collagen disease in the families of patients with such "acquired" hypogammaglobulinemia. This suggested a genetically determined disorder which may have certain similarities to other genetic disorders which do not express themselves until adult life, e.g., Huntington's chorea, pseudoxanthoma elasticum, and some cases of the adult Fanconi syndrome.

The question as to whether agammaglobulinemia manifesting later in life represents an acquired or a heritable disorder is well discussed by Cruchaud and coworkers (1966). They reported agammaglobulinemia in one of two monozygous twins with symptoms appearing at five years of age.

The other twin, studied at thirty-four, another brother, and the parents of the patient were studied and found normal. The authors thought that a genetic abnormality in this case, such as a chromosomal accident or a spontaneous point mutation involving the gene responsible for gamma globulin synthesis in one of the twins is a highly improbable possibility. They felt that this was a true acquired idiopathic agammaglobulinemia. Clinical and biological facts lend consistency to Good's hypothesis that during embryonic life or immediately after birth, a deleterious factor may alter a part of the "central lymphoid system" equivalent to the bursa of Fabricius in the chicken, which is responsible for development of peripheral immunologically competent organs (a somatic mutation).

## COMMON ASPECTS OF SYMPTOMATOLOGY
### Susceptibility to Infections

With rare exceptions, generalized and discrete immunoglobulin deficiencies are associated with increased incidence of infections. This susceptibility to infections may vary in onset, degree and prognosis. Patients with reticular dysgenesis die of overwhelming infection in the newborn period. Patients with Swiss-type agammaglobulinemia incur serious infections in the first weeks of life; recurrent pulmonary infections including *Pneumocystis carinii* pneumonia, severe thrush, systemic moniliasis and progressive vaccinia are frequent causes of death within the first eighteen months of life. In congenital sex-linked agammaglobulinemia, severe infections occur between nine months and two years of age and consist of recurrent episodes of pneumonia, meningitis, septicemia, otitis media, sinusitis, and pyoderma, alone, in combination or in succession. The responsible microorganisms are *Staphylococcus aureus, pneumococcus, meningococcus, Haemophilus influenzae,* and fungi. Although viral infections usually run a normal course, occasional unusual response to varicella and mumps as well as progressive vaccinia have been recorded. Sinopulmonary infections are present in 85 per cent of cases of ataxia-telangiectasia and frequently are the principal cause of death.

In primary adult hypogammaglobulinemia, generalized and selective, the propensity to recurrent infections may manifest itself in childhood, with unexplained febrile episodes, recurrent respiratory tract infections, and recurrent otitis media. More often, however, the infections are ascribed to the usual high incidence of respiratory infections in children and the basic disorder does not come to the attention of physicians until later in life in the young adult or, more frequently, in middle age. At that time bronchiectasis may become apparent, and chronic diarrhea, malabsorption, acute Salmonella infections and rheumatoid-like arthritis may appear, thus raising the possibility of immune deficiency.

While selective deficiencies of IgG, IgA and IgG, and IgA and IgM are associated with increased susceptibility to infections, an isolated IgA deficiency may be present without any detectable clinical manifestations. On the other hand, isolated increase in IgA level (Aldrich syndrome) may indeed be associated with heightened susceptibility to infection.

In various secondary acquired hypoimmunoglobulinemias (nephrotic syndrome, reticuloendothelial malignancy, autoimmune disease) incidence of recurrent infections varies and is probably related to the degree of depletion of the immunoglobulins, as well as to other factors.

## Intestinal Lesions

The association of gastrointestinal symptoms and lesions with immuno-globulin deficiency is a fascinating problem. Approximately 20 per cent of patients with hypogammaglobulinemia have diarrhea (Conn and Quintiliani, 1966). While gastrointestinal pathology is rare in sex-linked congenital agammaglobulinemia and ataxia-telangiectasia, occasional ulcerative colitis is seen in the Swiss type of agammaglobulinemia.

However, in the primary hypoimmunoglobulinemias of late onset, both of the generalized and selective type, gastrointestinal symptoms are a characteristic, frequently presenting and overwhelming complaint. They consist of chronic or intermittent, often debilitating diarrhea, sometimes bloody, associated with malabsorption, recurrent acute salmonella infection, and refractory *Giardia lamblia* infections. Malabsorption can frequently be documented with low serum carotenoids, low xylose excretion, hypokalemia, hypoferremia, hypocalcemia, and hypophosphatemia. X-rays may permit demonstration of a deficiency pattern of small intestine and generalized osteomalacia. Small intestinal biopsy may be normal, or it may reveal absence of villi, dense lymphocytic infiltration into the lamina propria either diffuse (Pelkonen, Siurala, and Vuopio, 1963) or nodular (Hermans *et al.*, 1966), or a vasculitis (Holman, Nickel, and Sleisenger, 1959).

The relationship between the hypoimmunoglobulinemia and the gastrointestinal disorder is not clear, but there are several possibilities.

1. Hypoimmunoglobulinemia is the result of exudative protein-losing enteropathy in Menetrier's disease (giant rugae of the stomach) (Citrin, Sterling, and Halsted, 1957), carcinoma of the stomach (Jarnum and Schwartz, 1960), gastric polyps (Dich, Paaby, and Schwartz, 1961), regional enteritis (Steinfeld *et al.*, 1960), acute enteritis (Jeffries, Holman, and Sleisenger, 1962; Waldmann *et al.*, 1961), nontropical sprue (Parkins, 1960; Vesin *et al.*, 1960), lymphangiectasia of the small intestine (Holman, Nickel, and Sleisenger, 1959; Schwartz and Jarnum, 1959), and chronic ulcerative colitis (Steinfeld *et al.*, 1960); some of these entities are also associated with malabsorption. The above conditions are classified among the secondary acquired hypoimmunoglobulinemias.

In the primary hypoimmunoglobulinemias, however, protein loss in the gastrointestinal tract, even if it occurs, is not a major cause of the hypoimmunoglobulinemia. Studies of the hypo IgA-M-immunoglobulinopathy patients (Hermans *et al.*, 1966) and of the generalized hypoimmunoglobulinemia patients (Collins and Ellis, 1965) with [131]I labelled PVP reveal no abnormal gastrointestinal loss. Many of these patients failed to respond to a strict gluten-free diet. The lymphocytic infiltration of the lamina propria of the small intestine of patients with generalized hypoimmunoglobulinemia was described as more dense than that seen in the usual celiac disease specimens (Collins and Ellis, 1965), and the nodular lymphocytic infiltration of the small intestine was described as quite specific for the group of patients with hypo IgA-M-immunoglobulinopathy (Hermans *et al.*, 1966). The low levels of intestinal mucosal enzymes probably indicate a severe degree of mucosal damage per se rather than the existence of an underlying celiac disease (Collins and Ellis, 1965).

Furthermore, when hypogammaglobulinemia occurs as a consequence of generalized gastrointestinal protein loss, it is almost always associated with more marked hypoalbuminemia. In their patients with hypoimmunoglobulinemia, Hermans and coworkers (1966) and Collins and Ellis (1965) found normal or only slightly decreased serum albumin levels.

2. The supposition that intestinal malabsorption could conceivably lead to impaired absorption of globulin-building blocks is unlikely in view of the studies of patients with nontropical sprue (Huizenga *et al.*, 1961) which demonstrated that the serum gamma globulin was only rarely depleted to a critical level.

3. Another possibility is that the hypoimmunoglobulinemia, in one way or another, is responsible for the gastrointestinal disorder. Clinical evidence suggests that gamma globulin deficiency precedes the development of malabsorption in these patients (Collins and Ellis, 1965; Hermans *et al.*, 1966; Huizenga *et al.*, 1961; Green and Sperber, 1962; Sanford, Favour, and Tribeman, 1954; Holman, Nickel, and Sleisenger, 1959). However, diarrhea is a rare occurrence in patients with a congenital type of agammaglobulinemia. Gamma globulin injections failed to decrease the diarrhea significantly in some patients (Collins and Ellis, 1965); in others there was an excellent response of diarrhea to gamma globulin (Conn and Quintiliani, 1966).

According to the concept of Peterson, Cooper, and Good (1965) the central lymphoid tissues developing in close association with the epithelium of the gut influence immunoglobulin development. The lymphoid tissue abnormalities found in the patients with hypo-IgA-M-immunoglobulinemia (the diffuse and the nodular lymphocytic infiltration of the small intestine) may be a *compensatory hyperplasia* of functionally inadequate central lymphoid tissue.

It is possible that the *integrity* of the gut, normally exposed to a variety of bacterial and other pathogens, depends on the presence of immunoglobulins in the serum which may exercise a trophic influence on the gastrointestinal mucosa and submucosa. When these are lacking, nonspecific atrophic changes may occur leading to a nonspecific lymphoid infiltration and functional abnormalities.

Finally, the gastrointestinal tract may respond to the hypoimmunoglobulinemia in a manner similar to that of the respiratory tract, namely by permitting a variety of pathogens to infest it. The diffuse and the nodular lymphoid infiltration of the gut may be the body response to bacterial overgrowth or to infection. The presence of intractable *Giardia lamblia* infestation in an overwhelming majority of Hermans' patients is very thought-provoking. These patients are particularly susceptible to pathogenic bacteria known to cause diarrhea, such as shigella, salmonella (Conn and Quintiliani, 1966), and staphylococci. The response of diarrhea to tetracycline (Hermans *et al.*, 1966) is interesting but not predictably universal in this syndrome (Collins and Ellis, 1965).

4. Whether hypoimmunoglobulinemia and the gastrointestinal disorder are both secondary to some other primary underlying defect must also be considered. However, no such defect is apparent.

## Association of Hypoimmunoglobulinemia with Arthritis and Collagen Disorders

From one third to one half of patients with either congenital or acquired hypoimmunoglobulinemia develop a disease state clinically indistinguishable from rheumatoid arthritis (Gitlin, Gross, and Janeway, 1959; Rotstein and Good, 1961; Collins and Ellis, 1965; Neustadt, 1965).

Other collagen disorders such as dermatomyositis, scleroderma, lupus-like syndrome, diffuse "fibrinoid" disease, and atypical forms of arthritis have appeared in a relatively high percentage of patients with agammaglobulinemia. The frequency is too high to be coincidental (Rotstein and Good, 1961).

In half of sixteen patients with congenital agammaglobulinemia who survived beyond two years of age, Gitlin, Gross and Janeway (1959) observed a chronic arthritis clinically resembling rheumatoid arthritis. Several of these conditions were diagnosed as rheumatoid arthritis before the diagnosis of agammaglobulinemia was suspected. The process starts in the knees and in some patients later involves the ankles, wrists and even the fingers; the systemic manifestations are mild. The clinical spectrum of articular involvement varies from nonspecific tendovaginitis and atypical joint manifestations to classical rheumatoid arthritis with characteristic subcutaneous (rheumatoid) nodules. However, erythema and tenderness are typically absent. Pathological examinations reveal changes consistent with rheumatoid arthritis (edema, villous hyperplasia, fibrin deposition, lymphocytic accumulation and "fibrinoid degeneration"). Histologic sections of the subcutaneous nodules reveal the classic features of a rheumatoid nodule except for the absence of plasma cells. The sera of these patients do not contain a rheumatoid factor and do not exhibit the expected inhibition of the rheumatoid agglutinating reactions (Collins and Ellis, 1965).

Interestingly, there is no increase in the frequency of rheumatoid arthritis in the families of patients with the congenital form of agammaglobulinemia, while there is a definite increase in rheumatoid factor, serum globulin abnormalities and clinical collagen disease in the families of patients with acquired hypoimmunoglobulinemia of late onset. The noted increase in incidence of chronic rheumatoid arthritis in patients with agammaglobulinemia has led to much reconsideration of the widely held concept of rheumatoid arthritis as a consequence of an altered immunologic process related to excessive amounts of certain gamma globulins. Absence of immunoglobulins could be considered a deterrent to such an immunoarthritic process. However, a selective increase of certain immunoglobulins in the face of a total decrease may still be consistent with this concept. Some investigators refuse to accept the arthritis accompanying agammaglobulinemia as definite rheumatoid arthritis but consider it a "toxic phenomenon" due to repeated subclinical bacterial infections. Thus, Rotstein and Good (1961) and Good and coworkers (1960) feel that connective tissue disease in this setting may result from an infection—either as a direct response of the host to the infecting agent, a hypersensitivity reaction in which mechanisms of delayed allergy are operative, or a response of another type of cellular hypersensitivity, similar but not identical to delayed allergy. During long-term treatment with large doses of gamma globulin, the associated rheumatoid arthritis may ameliorate or even disappear completely.

## Association of Hypogammaglobulinemia with Thymoma

This association has been reported in seventeen patients with hypogammaglobulinemia of late onset (Conn and Quintiliani, 1966; Mongan, Kern and Terry, 1966; teVelde, Huber, and van der Slikke, 1966; Gabrielsen and Good, 1966; Rogers, Manaligold and Blazek, 1968). Most of these patients had splenomegaly, anemia, and leukopenia. Some had thrombocytopenia as well. Thymectomy performed in eight patients brought about no decrease in susceptibility to infection and no hematologic improvement. In twelve patients the tissues were examined histologically; in ten they were of spindle cell type and very similar to each other; in one (Mongan, Kern and Terry, 1966) tissues were of lymphocytic cell type, and in one (teVelde, Huber, and van der Slikke, 1966) epithelial cell type (see Fig. 30). Transient symptoms suggestive of myasthenia gravis were reported in two patients: in one, 15 years prior to the discovery of thymoma, and in the other

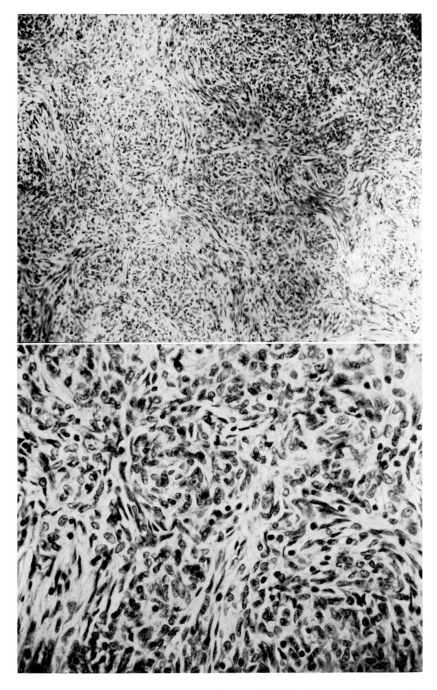

FIGURE 30. Thymoma in a patient with primary adult hypoimmunoglobulinemia. Low power (*Upper*) and high power (*Lower*) views demonstrate spindle cells in this tumor. Cystic and epithelial tumors are also seen in this syndrome. (Reproduced with permission from PETERSON, R. D. A.; COOPER, M. D., and GOOD, R. A.: *Amer J Med, 38:*579, 1965.)

at the time of the discovery (teVelde, Huber, and van der Slikke, 1966). In one third of the cases the thymomas have preceded the onset of infections by as long as twelve years. In one third, both conditions were diagnosed simultaneously. Two of the patients with thymoma and hypoimmunoglobuline-mia had evidence of cytomegalovirus infection.

The frequent concurrence of these two relatively rare conditions excludes coincidence. It is not clear whether the thymomas cause hypogamma-globulinemia by replacing normal thymus tissue or by suppressing other antibody-producing tissues or whether they represent compensatory changes secondary to antibody deficiency.

## Association of Hypogammaglobulinemia with Malignancies of the Reticuloendothelial System

Increased susceptibility to lymphoreticular malignancy has been observed in ataxia-telangiectasia (Peterson, Cooper, and Good, 1966) and in several cases of various forms of adult hypoimmunoglobulinemia (Green *et al.,* 1966). In adult cases the simplest explanation for this association is that the lymphosarcoma was really present all the time in a clinically undetected form and that it had produced hypoimmunoglobulinemia. However, this explanation is clinically untenable in most cases. The second possibility is that the hypoimmunoglobulinemia predisposes to the development of lymphoma. The mechanism could be excessive stimulation of the reticuloendothelial system by the various infections, persistence and growth of aberrant cell lines permitted by lack of immunological response.

The third possibility, that both conditions are produced by a common cause, possibly a genetic predisposition, is difficult to refute. The fourth possibility, that they are coincidental, is unlikely (see Table XIX).

### DIAGNOSIS

Early diagnosis of agammaglobulinemia, congenital or of delayed onset, is extremely important to avoid such sequelae of severe and recurrent infections as bronchiectasis, deafness and impaired cerebral function.

Absent or low isohemagglutinins in the serum of any patient except one with AB blood, or failure to develop antibodies after standard immunizations as indicated by a positive Schick test, should alert the physician.

The full immunologic investigation should ascertain humoral antibody function such as level of antibodies to naturally occurring antigens (isohem-agglutinins, antithyroid antibodies), effect of stimulation with pork A substance, humoral antibody formation to administered antigens (Salk vaccine, mumps vaccine, typhoid and paratyphoid vaccine and diphtheria vaccine). Reagin formation is studied by scratch and intradermal testing with allergenic extracts (Gilbert and Hong, 1964).

Cellular reactivity, including delayed hypersensitivity (PPD, histoplasmin test, smallpox immunity), is intact in patients with congenital and acquired hypoimmunoglobulinemia. Other aspects of cellular reactivity such as homograft rejection are deficient in patients with Swiss agammaglobulinemia and in those with ataxia-telangiectasia. Homograft rejection is delayed in patients with congenital agammaglobulinemia and usually normal or almost normal in hypoimmunoglobulinemia of late onset. A contact allergy response to a second exposure to dinitrofluorobenzene (DNFB), a highly sensitizing skin irritant, parallels the skin homograft rejection in these entities.

Complement was usually normal when determined. Marked decrease in properdin was reported in a variant of hypo-IgA-M-immunoglobulinemia (Gilbert and Hong, 1964).

Plasma cells are usually diminished in the bone marrow of patients with hypoimmunoglobulinemia: 3/5,000 nucleated cells (Gilbert and Hong, 1964).

Serum paper electrophoresis is a good screening test for diffuse hypoimmunoglobulinemia but may be normal in selective hypoimmunoglobulinemia. Immunoelectrophoresis should help establish the diagnosis.

Since the newborn infants' plasma contains gamma globulins passively transferred from the mother, a definite diagnosis is difficult before five or six months of age.

Thymic alymphoplasia with agammaglobulinemia, Swiss type, may be diagnosed with a rectal or lymph node biopsy because the lymphocyte deficiency is especially striking in these tissues, while the peripheral lymphocytes may be nearly normal. Study of antibody-synthesizing capacity after immunizations with bacteriophage and typhoid antigens in the neonatal period is a good screening test for these children. Early diagnosis of this entity is of utmost importance to permit experimental therapeutic trial of transplantation of thymus, bone marrow or other immunocyte-containing organs.

## TREATMENT

The treatment of hypoimmunoglobulinopathies consists of four modes: antibiotics, gamma globulins, steroids and immuno-organ transplants.

1. Antibiotics are given according to the specific needs of each patient. In some patients, intermittent broad spectrum prophylaxis is recommended. Pentamidine isothionate has been reported successful in *Pneumocystis carinii* infections in children with congenital agammaglobulinemia (Blattner, 1965).

2. Human gamma globulin administration is required in all patients with agammaglobulinemia. It must be given periodically, regularly, in adequate dosage and over a long period. Dosage levels of 0.6 to 0.8 cc/kg of body weight are administered intramuscularly, usually every twenty-one to thirty days (Domz and Dickson, 1957). The tolerance to this heroic regimen exhibited by patients with congenital agammaglobulinemia and the protection

afforded are both remarkable. Five-year courses have been followed without any known untoward effect (Neustadt, 1965).

Gamma globulin is a very useful form of treatment in a variety of patients other than those with hypoimmunoglobulinemia and other forms of defective immune mechanism. Gamma globulin preparations are also used in passive immunizations to prevent or modify measles in susceptible contacts, to modify symptoms induced by vaccination with an attenuated live measles vaccine, to prevent rubella (German measles) in susceptible persons, to modify chicken pox in selected contacts, to attenuate infectious hepatitis in contact cases or in individuals entering endemic areas, and to attenuate serum hepatitis resulting from transfusion of blood and other blood products.

The few reactions reported have occurred mostly in the patients with hypoimmunoglobulinemia of late onset. All in all, eleven reports of anaphylactoid reactions to intramuscular gamma globulin have been recorded (Richerson and Seebohm, 1966; Baybutt, 1959; Owings, 1953; Glaser and Wyss-Souffrant, 1961; Kamme *et al.*, 1966). The reaction was demonstrated to be due to aggregate formation in the well-studied case of Richerson, and it is likely that this was responsible in some or all of the other ten cases as well. In the others, the cause postulated was "hypersensitivity," including severe allergic past history, but not well documented, of recipients and their families. The reactions have consisted of hives, nausea, cough, flushing, stiffness of face and neck, lumbar pain, chest pain, cold sweat, cyanosis, syncope, and, in two patients, loss of consciousness and transient apnea. After an hour or so, chills and fever may occur and last a few hours. Use of antihistamines and epinephrine was very effective and all patients recovered.

Commercial human gamma globulin consists of IgG; on standing it forms aggregates spontaneously with sedimentation coefficients from 9.5S to 40S and becomes increasingly anticomplementary. *In vitro* it may cause inactivation of complement, agglutination of human erythrocytes and rabbit platelets and release of histamine and 5-hydroxytryptamine from rabbit blood. When given intravenously, even in small amounts, or when absorbed rapidly from a large intramuscular depot, the IgG aggregates become biologically active and may lead to increased permeability of skin capillaries, Arthus-like reactions and erythema-wheal formation.

For safe use of human gamma globulin in patients with immune derangement, care should be taken to avoid intravenous administration and large intramuscular depots of the preparation. Divided, small doses at more frequent intervals are recommended by Richerson—2.5 cc injections not exceeding eight injections at one round. If a reaction occurs, it is not necessary to stop future use of human gamma globulin in that patient, but extra care should be taken in administration of the drug, the batch may have to be changed and the size of each injection decreased.

True antigen-antibody (true anaphylactic) reactions have not been reported to human gamma globulin. The patients who exhibited reactions to intramuscular gamma globulin when tested did not demonstrate any antigammaglobulin in their sera (Kamme *et al.*, 1966). However, there is evidence that the administration of gamma globulin to man at times results in an antibody response because of genetic variation. This is especially true with reference to the Gm factors, as Inv factors are not very antigenic. Thus, Allen and Kunkel (1963) found that seventeen of twenty-four sera from children who had received multiple blood transfusions contained agglutinating antibodies against a Gm factor absent from their own serum immunoglobulin. Also, Stiehm and Fudenberg (1965) reported the presence of antibodies against human gamma globulin in six of eighteen children receiving prophylactic gamma globulin; these antibodies were found in hypoimmunoglobulinemic children but not in the agammaglobulinemic children, who were obviously unable to synthesize any immunoglobulin. The clinical significance of such antibodies is unknown.

Serum hepatitis has not been reported as resulting from administration of human gamma globulin, probably because the virus is not present in this fraction.

What ill effects the long-term, ten years and longer, administration of human gamma globulin might have is unknown.

Although the widely accepted method of gamma globulin administration to patients with immunoglobulin deficiency has been massive doses 0.6–0.7 cc/kg of body weight (40–60 cc to a 60 kg man) every three to four weeks, it seems that this method should be revised. Guided both by the recommendations of Richerson and Seebohm (1966) who warn against IgG aggregates, and by studies of immunoglobulin catabolism by Fahey and Robinson (1963) and Waldmann and Schwab (1965), new guidelines should be constructed, especially in adult patients with hypogammaglobulinemia, since this is the group which seems to be most sensitive to the side effects. Metabolic studies demonstrate that the fractional catabolic rate of IgG is directly correlated with, and controlled by, the serum concentration or total body pool of the IgG. Thus, sudden massive influx of IgG would only result in a more rapid than usual catabolism of the IgG and only minimal benefit to the patient. It would seem reasonable to expect that, whenever possible, intramuscular injection of 4 to 12 cc, in divided doses, once or twice weekly might be more beneficial than the massive monthly dosage.

Patients with severe hypogammaglobulinemia should be kept under close observation for a few hours after the injection. Adverse effects are more apt to occur if the dose is divided into two portions given at an interval of some hours. Untoward reactions are sporadic, and the occurrence of one on a single occasion does not contraindicate continued treatment with gamma globulin.

Persons injected intravenously with human gamma globulin may develop flushing of the face, a constricting feeling in the chest, muscle pain in the trunk or thighs, nausea, vomiting, fever, and rarely, shock. Pepsin-treated gamma globulin, however, given slowly at a rate less than 2 cc of five per cent protein per minute was administered repeatedly and to a patient with hypoimmunoglobulinemia without causing a reaction. Furthermore, there was a striking response in the immunoglobulin level. (Jager, 1967). It is thought that treatment with pepsin averts aggregate formation.

3. Steroids are not contraindicated in patients with immunoglobulin deficiency. Indeed it is sometimes necessary to administer steroids to patients with a concomitant arthritis. The possibility of obscuring symptoms and signs of infection must be considered. Sanford, Favour, and Tribeman, (1954) gave an account of an impressive clinical remission in gastrointestinal symptomatology in an adult agammaglobulinemic patient with cortisone. This offers encouragement despite the obvious hazards of steroids in the presence of immunoglobulin deficiency. Cautious use of steroids has been suggested for treatment of selected patients with agammaglobulinemia (Fudenberg, German, and Kunkel, 1962). The rationale for this therapy has been the observation that there is a definite association between this entity and the presence of the rheumatoid factor, lupus erythematosus, periarteritis nodosa in the family studies as well as an association between congenital agammaglobulinemia and incidence of rheumatoid-like arthritis. Small doses of prednisolone 10 mg/d were reported to produce moderate improvement in control of recurrent upper respiratory infection and in chronic fatigue associated with a striking increase in gamma globulin levels in two patients (Fudenberg, German and Kunkel, 1962).

4. Recent advances in organ transplantation offer more hope in the management of patients with the more severe derangement of the immune mechanism. Patients with thymic alymphoplasia (Swiss) do not respond to human gamma globulin administration. Thymic transplants, although reportedly of no benefit to a few of these patients, may, when modified be more successful. Normal bone marrow transplants have been reported helpful in this entity (Gitlin, Vawter, and Craig, 1964). Transplantation of spleen (Marchioro *et al.*, 1964) may also be of benefit. Any of these procedures when performed on patients with various forms of hypoimmunoglobulinopathies would provide the means of producing all three or four immunoglobulins, while the gammaglobulin preparations available for replacement therapy contain only IgG and not the IgA or IgM fractions. It is not known, however, whether replacement of all immunoglobulin would result in a basic cure of the condition, and particularly if it would reverse the processes of malabsorption and arthritis. Splenectomy has been successful in patients who have hypo-IgG-A-immunoglobulinemia with increased IgM and resulting hemolytic anemia and thrombocytopenia.

*Chapter 6*

# HYPERIMMUNOGLOBULINOPATHIES

T<small>HIS</small> <small>CHAPTER</small> does not dwell on conditions of normal immunological response elicited in individuals by various antigens. These responses usually consist of an increase in specific antibodies to antigen, rarely if ever resulting in a detectable overall increase of immunoglobulins. Specifically, there will be no discussion here of immunological responses to *environmental* allergens such as inhaled dust and pollens, bacteria, fungi, ingested food, and parenterally injected protein particles. Neither will there be any consideration of *heteroimmunologic* responses to protein of another species such as insulin resistance, dog and horse allergy, and heterotransplants. Nor will much time be devoted to *homo-* or *isoimmunological* responses such as ABO and Rh incompatibility (erythroblastosis fetalis, transfusion reactions) and homotransplants.

Significant alterations in immunoglobulin pattern with diffuse or isolated hyperimmunoglobulinemia are seen, however, in certain populations, as well as in certain chronic infections, some autoimmune diseases with over-

TABLE XX

HYPERIMMUNOGLOBULINOPATHIES

I. P<small>RIMARY</small> H<small>YPERIMMUNOGLOBULINEMIAS</small>
   a. Variations related to race
   b. Familial hyperglobulinemia
   c. Familial hyper-IgA-globulinemia (Aldrich syndrome)
II. S<small>ECONDARY</small> H<small>YPERIMMUNOGLOBULINEMIAS</small>
   a. Secondary to infections
   b. Associated with autoimmune diseases
      (1) Rheumatoid arthritis
      (2) Rheumatoid factor complex cryoglobulinemia and macroglobulinemia
      (3) Systemic lupus erythematosus
      (4) Other autoimmune disorders (Rheumatic fever, Sjögren's syndrome, thyroiditis, periarteritis nodosa, scleroderma, dermatomyositis, erythema nodosum, autoimmune hemolytic anemia, cold agglutinin disease)
   c. Associated with malignancies
   d. Associated with diseases of unknown etiology
      (1) Infectious mononucleosis
      (2) Sarcoidosis
      (3) Benign hyperglobulinemic purpura
      (4) Charmot's syndrome
      (5) Liver diseases

111

TABLE XXI

SERUM IMMUNOGLOBULIN CONCENTRATIONS IN VARIOUS
CLINICAL DISORDERS

| Disease | No. Cases | IgG | (Average mg/cc) IgA | IgM | IgG/IgA |
|---|---|---|---|---|---|
| Systemic lupus erythematosus | 22 | 17.6 | 2.6 | 1.3 | 10.3 |
| Pulmonary fibrosis | 7 | 19.7 | 2.4 | 1.5 | 9.0 |
| Ulcerative colitis | 6 | 12.4 | 1.8 | 0.85 | 6.9 |
| Boeck's sarcoid | 11 | 39.9 | 4.6 | — | 8.9 |
| Sjögren's syndrome | 17 | 33.2 | 3.0 | 1.8 | 14.4 |
| Low titer rheumatoid arthritis | 11 | 44.4 | 2.1 | 1.2 | 8.1 |
| High titer rheumatoid arthritis | 15 | 11.3 | 4.0 | 2.1 | 3.3 |
| Infectious hepatitis | 6 | 18.3 | 1.5 | 1.9 | 13.2 |
| Lupoid hepatitis | 10 | 49.4 | 1.9 | 1.3 | 26.3 |
| Laennec's cirrhosis | 8 | 18.3 | 6.6 | 1.7 | 2.8 |
| Normal | 24 | 10.0 | 1.6 | 1.1 | 6.4 |

NOTE: Reprinted with permission from Tomasi, T. B., Jr.: *Blood, 25:* 382–403, 1965.

whelming immunoglobulin response, certain malignancies and in a number of diseases of unknown etiology (see Table XX).

For reasons that have not yet been determined, rate of synthesis of the immunoglobulins is frequently increased in cirrhosis of the liver, collagen disease, infections, and myeloid leukemia (Andersen, 1964). The fractional turnover rate is usually normal but may be increased in infectious disease, stress or other hypercatabolic states.

Table XXI demonstrates the immunoglobulin alterations in various clinical disorders.

## PRIMARY HYPERIMMUNOGLOBULINEMIAS

### Variations in Globulins Related to Race

It has been known for the last ten years that sera from the African Negroes are characterized by diffuse hyperimmunoglobulinemia. This increase was considered secondary to frequent and intensive exposure of the African Negro to parasitic and bacterial antigens. Recently a study was made comparing healthy Negroes to Puerto Rican and other Caucasian populations in New York City. The average gamma globulin level was highest among Negroes, next, in Puerto Ricans, and lowest in other Caucasians. Because of careful matching of the series these differences were supposedly independent of socioeconomic condition and duration of residence in New York City (Siegel *et al.,* 1965). This study supports existence of physiological quantitative variations in immunoglobulins related to race.

### Familial Hyperglobulinemia

This poorly defined entity has been observed by many authors, usually in families of patients suffering from systemic lupus erythematosus, discoid lupus, rheumatoid arthritis, scleroderma, and dermatomyositis. Often asymptomatic diffuse hyperimmunoglobulinemia occurs in the unaffected members of the family (Larsson and Leonhardt, 1959; Waldenström, 1961). Wilson, Williams, and Tobian (1967) described three families with diffuse increase in serum IgA, IgG and IgM; in each of the families one individual exhibited renal tubular acidosis, anemia, hepatosplenomegaly, xerostomia, and high latex fixation titers.

## Familial Hyper-IgA-Globulinemia (*Aldrich Syndrome*)

A familial syndrome of eczema, thrombocytopenia and recurrent infection was described by Wiskott in 1937 and defined as a sex-linked recessive disease by Aldrich and his coworkers in 1954. Since then several reports have documented this disorder in seventeen families (Lanzkowsky and Levy, 1965). The distribution is worldwide, mostly in Caucasians, but also in Negroes. Average age at onset of symptoms in these male children is six years. Patients usually die early either from infection or hemorrhage, although there have been records of survival to seven years and $10\frac{1}{2}$ years. One patient with mild disease was alive at forty (Lanzkowsky and Levy, 1965). The majority of children afflicted died from an overwhelming bacterial infection. Visceral invasion by measles virus and cytomegalovirus, and progressive herpes simplex infection, sometimes fatal, were encountered. Infections varied from otitis media to pyoderma, septicemia, meningitis and pneumonia. Other features included bloody diarrhea, purpura, splenomegaly, anemia and eosinophilia. Intensive gamma globulin therapy, repeated transfusions, administration of immune-donor leukocytes, and antibiotics did not alter the course of infection. Steroids do not affect platelets but improve eczema. These children are uniformly lymphopenic and have an increase in IgA in serum (West, Hong and Holland, 1962). They have absent or low titre of isoagglutinins and possess circulating antibodies to whole cow's milk. The expression of delayed cutaneous hypersensitivity is defective. This is probably a manifestation of altered cellular resistance, perhaps secondary to a genetic deficit in synthesis of interferon.

The etiology of thrombocytopenia is not clear. No platelet agglutinating antibodies were found (Krivit and Good, 1959). There is most likely a defect in production of platelets (Krivit, 1966). Splenectomy is contraindicated as overwhelming infection develops promptly. The only acceptable treatment at present is supportive therapy, blood transfusions, antibiotics and prevention of suppuration. There is increased frequency of reticulum cell sarcomatous proliferation in the lymph nodes and other organs (Hastrup and Grahl-Madsen, 1965; St. Geme *et al.*, 1965).

Cooper *et al.* (1968) studied eighteen patients with this syndrome. They were impressed by the reduction in lymphocytes, particularly the small cell type, and by a depletion of small lymphocytes in the thymus-dependent paracortical areas of the lymph nodes. They found that these patients were unable to form antibodies to several antigens which depend on polysaccharide configurations for their antigenicity. This class of antigens is widely distributed in bacteria, viruses, fungi, and even metazoan parasites. Cooper and coworkers postulated that the genetic fault in Wiskott-Aldrich syndrome consists of inability to recognize or process these polysaccharide antigens as required for normal induction of an immune response. This defect involving the afferent limb of immunity results in susceptibility of the patients to all infections (bacterial, viral, fungal, and metazoan). The increase in IgA, to a certain extent also in IgG, may represent compensatory hyperplasia of the lymphoreticular system due to frequent antigenic stimulation.

Harzheim, Stechele, and Kunzer (1965) described a form of Aldrich syndrome where skin manifestations were missing from the triad. This disymptomatic form, consisting of thrombocytopenia and susceptibility to infection with increased IgA, seems to carry a somewhat better prognosis. The two traits are probably coupled on the X chromosome.

## SECONDARY HYPERIMMUNOGLOBULINEMIAS

### Hyperimmunoglobulinemia Secondary to Infections

Virtually all types of infection are followed by a rise in certain immunoglobulins; this can be determined by means of specific antibody titers. However, the rise does not always affect the overall immunoglobulin pattern. This subject has been discussed in detail in numerous reviews (Wuhrmann and Wunderly, 1957).

The acute phase of bacterial infection, characterized by local signs of acute inflammation, necrosis, fever, and leukocytosis—also called the primary inflammatory reaction—is accompanied by an increase in alpha glucoproteins (haptoglobin, orosomucoid), increase in fibrinogen, appearance of C-reactive protein and a decrease in albumin (Belfrage, 1963), but no change in immunoglobin on electrophoresis. This phase usually takes seven to ten days.

The secondary inflammatory reaction characterized by enlargement of lymph nodes, spleen, tissue and blood plasmacytosis, is paralleled by increase in gamma and beta globulins (true immunoglobulins) as well as specific antibodies. Duration of the secondary response depends on chronicity of infection.

This biphasic pattern of protein reaction in the face of a strong reaction to injury is seen in most acute bacterial infections, pneumonia, tonsillitis, streptococcal infections, and meningitis (Belfrage, 1963).

Infections with evident lymphoid proliferations such as infectious hepatitis, rubella, toxoplasmosis, typhoid, salmonellosis and subacute bacterial endocarditis exhibit a less pronounced first phase.

An increase of the immunoglobulins is usually noted early in the course and is marked and persistent. In viral hepatitis there is frequently an early elevation of IgM (Charmot and André, 1964). Elevation of both IgM and IgA normally disappears when liver function tests return to normal. However, in a study of an effect of infectious hepatitis on the immunoglobulin in mentally retarded children, persistent IgM and IgG elevation was noted up to seven months after liver-chemistry recovery; this abnormality was coupled with prolonged immuno-depression as evidenced by a lack of virus neutralizing antibody response (LoGrippo *et al.*, 1966).

In the exanthematous viral diseases of childhood there is little primary or secondary response.

Diffuse hyperimmunoglobulinemia is often found in protracted infections and infestations of various causes such as bronchiectasis, tuberculosis, histoplasmosis, coccidiomycosis, brucellosis, syphilis, kala-azar, leprosy, lymphogranuloma venereum, typhus, malaria, and certain chronic skin diseases. In some of these, such as trypanosomiasis caused by *T. gambiense* and in kala-azar (Silver *et al.*, 1961), the IgM's predominate. The increased globulin in kala-azar often has the properties of a cryoglobulin.

## Hyperimmunoglobulinemias Associated with Autoimmune Diseases

In the diseases grouped together as autoimmune disorders there is usually but not always an increase in immunoglobulins as well as presence of antibodies directed against the host's tissues. The significance of these autoantibodies is not fully understood. The concept of attributing etiology of these disorders to the presence of the autoantibodies is not accepted by many workers who feel that the autoantibodies may be secondary to certain destructive processes of the illness itself. However, these autoantibodies, although not the sole mechanism, may contribute to the pathogenesis of the disease.

### *Rheumatoid Arthritis*

In chronic rheumatoid arthritis there is frequently an increase in all immunoglobulins. However, the degree and frequency of elevation vary with each immunoglobulin class. Three- and four-fold increases have been found in IgA and IgG groups, but only two-fold increases in IgM (Tomasi, 1965). Claman and Merrill (1966), who studied serum immunoglobulins in seventy-two patients with rheumatoid arthritis, found that IgA levels were elevated in 51 per cent of sera up to 650 and even 800 mg per cent (normal 60–320 mg%). IgG levels exceeded the normal range of 660 to 1400 mg % in 25 per cent of patients and were as high as 1,900 mg %. IgM levels were elevated above the normal range of 100 to 320 mg % in only 17 per cent of patients and values of 700 and even 1,600 were infrequently encountered. Measurements were difficult and sometimes made inaccurate by the tendency of some rheumatoid factors (IgM) to form complexes with 7S globulins (so-called 22S complexes) and by *in vivo* interraction between 7S globulin molecules themselves forming complexes with sedimentation coefficients between 7S and 19S (Kunkel *et al.,* 1961). Finally the tendency of IgA to polymerize in some cases gave false low values for serum IgA.

However, similar findings were reported in rheumatoid sera by Hong and West (1964) : normal elevation of IgA in 55 per cent of cases and of IgM in 27 per cent.

There is correlation between IgA and IgG elevation and sedimentation rate values (Claman and Merrill, 1966; Sharp *et al.,* 1964). However, there is no correlation between duration of the disease and the serum globulins.

The significance of the changes in the serum globulins is difficult to determine. The IgM class contains most of the rheumatoid factor but is the class of immunoglobulins least often elevated in rheumatoid arthritis. IgA has been found to contain rheumatoid factor activity in a few patients. IgA and IgM are not found in normal synovial fluid but are frequently found in the synovial fluid of patients with rheumatoid arthritis.

The relationship between immunoglobulins and rheumatoid disease is further complicated by occurrence of a rheumatoid-like arthritis in patients with various types of hypoimmunoglobulinemia (see chapter on Hypoimmunoglobulinopathies).

The sera of most patients with rheumatoid arthritis contain what is commonly called the *rheumatoid factor* (RF). Rheumatoid factors are a heterogenous group of high molecular weight immunoglobulins which react with 7S immunoglobulin and are therefore referred to as "anti-gamma-globulin factors." Rheumatoid factors are primarily present in the 19S or IgM group, but RF in whole serum exists as a complex of a 19S and a 7S globulin with a sedimentation constant of approximately 22. In some rheumatoid sera, 7S globulins may be demonstrated to possess anti-gamma-globulin reactivity and are referred to as 7S rheumatoid factors. Complexes with intermediate sedimenting properties (7S to 19S) are formed as a result of interaction of 7S RF with other 7S gamma globulin. In a few patients the rheumatoid factor activity may reside to a certain degree in the IgA class.

The immunoglobulin with which RF reacts has been called the reactant (Christian, 1965). Various particles which are "coated" with the reactant serve as indicator system for RF. Agglutination systems may consist of sensitized bacteria, sensitized sheep cells (amboceptor coated), human Rh-positive cells coated with anti-Rh antibodies, and particles of polystyrene latex coated with human gamma globulin (latex fixation test). The specificity of various rheumatoid factors (taken from various individuals) for different genetic types of human immunoglobulin (reactant) is the basis for differentiating the human Gm and Inv groups of immunoglobulins (see Chap. 2).

The portion of the reactant immunoglobulin which reacts with the rheumatoid factor is Fc fragment obtained after papain digestion; the fragments which contain antibody-combining sites are nonreactive. While it is usually impossible to demonstrate a reaction between the reactant immunoglobulin alone and the rheumatoid factor, the reaction is facilitated by previous interaction between the reactant antibody and its respective antigen. It has been suggested that RF displays primary specificity for immunoglobulin which has been denatured in the course of combining with antigen. This is consistent with a hypothesis that there are several potentially "reactant" configurations of the immunoglobulin molecule which become exposed on the surface of the molecule only in the course of immune complex formation; thus their availabilities to react with rheumatoid factors are then revealed. Optimal reactivity of reactant globulins would result from either immune complex formation or other processes of denaturation (Christian, 1965). In summary, rheumatoid factors are antibodies with specificity directed against multiple antigenic determinants of 7S immunoglobulin.

While 70 per cent or more of sera of patients with clinical diagnosis of rheumatoid arthritis contain rheumatoid factor, less than 5 per cent of normal human sera will have this property. In rheumatoid arthritis there is high correlation between presence of RF and presence of subcutaneous nodules, symmetrical deforming arthritis of hands and wrists, and the severe systemic disease. Patients with the syndromes classified as variants of rheumatoid arthritis, such as juvenile rheumatoid arthritis, Marie-Strumpell spondylitis, psoriatic arthritis, arthritis associated with ulcerative colitis, regional enteritis and agammaglobulinemia usually do not have rheumatoid factors in their sera.

RF is present in a significant percentage of patients with other connective tissue syndromes and in a variety of illnesses (pulmonary tuberculosis, sarcoidosis, leprosy, syphilis, liver disease, leishmaniasis and bacterial endocarditis). In a number of the above conditions which are associated with diffuse hyperimmunoglobulinemia and presence of rheumatoid factor, small amounts of cryoglobulins may appear in the blood. These cryoglobulins represent complexes of the rheumatoid factor with the immunoglobulins (Meltzer and Franklin, 1966; Meltzer *et al.*, 1966) (see next subdivision—Rheumatoid Factor-Complex Hyperglobulinemias).

A significant number of patients with clinical rheumatoid arthritis exhibit antinuclear antibodies as shown by biologically false positive Wassermann reactions, positive LE cells preparations (0–27%) and positive immunofluorescence studies (14–65%). The antinuclear factors, both in the rheumatoid sera and in the LE sera, were found to be of IgG, IgA and IgM immunoglobulin classes (Barnett *et al.*, 1964).

### *"Rheumatoid Factor-Complex" Hyperglobulinemias ("Complex" or "Mixed" Cryoglobulinemia and "Complex" or "Spurious" Macroglobulinemia)*

This group of conditions includes mostly autoimmune disorders characterized by presence of rheumatoid factor and IgG-IgM complexes leading to cryoglobulinemia in some patients and to "spurious" macroglobulinemia in others.

Cryoglobulins, proteins which reversibly precipitate from blood on cooling, are most commonly encountered in multiple myeloma and macroglobulinemia but occur also in a variety of disease states including connective tissue disorders. Cryoglobulins can be composed of either IgG alone, of IgM alone, of IgG polymers, of IgG-IgM complexes (Meltzer and Franklin, 1966; Meltzer *et al.*, 1966) or of IgA-IgG complexes (Wager, Mustakallio and Räsäneu, 1968). The IgM cryoglobulins are all paraimmunoglobulins, have either a κ or a λ light chain but never both, and are found in Waldenström's macroglobulinemia, lymphatic leukemia, and in lymphosarcoma. These conditions are considered in the chapter on Paraimmunoglobulinopathies. The IgG cryoglobulins are primarily found in patients with multiple myeloma and in those with essential cryoglobulinemia. In these conditions the IgG cryoglobulins are also paraimmunoglobulins, having either the κ or λ light chain but not both. Rarely, heterogeneous IgG cryoglobulins are found in other conditions such as liver disease and purpura (Meltzer *et al.*, 1966).

In almost half of their twenty-nine patients with cryoglobulinemia, Meltzer and associates (1966) found the cryoglobulins to be composed of either IgG-IgM complexes or of IgG polymers. These cryoglobulins exhibited rheumatoid factor activity and contained both κ and λ light chains. On paper electrophoresis they migrated as a broad gamma globulin peak and there was moderate to marked hypergammaglobulinemia. The IgG-IgM complexes were found in nine patients with an unusual, yet readily recognizable, symptom complex consisting of purpura, weakness and arthralgias, and, in three patients, sudden onset of acute renal failure secondary to diffuse glomerulonephritis. Other associated findings in one or more of these patients were lymphadenopathy, hepatosplenomegaly, thyroiditis with a high antithyroglobulin titer, Sjögren's syndrome, vasculitis, presence of antinuclear antibodies and low or absent complement. One patient with IgG polymer cryoglobulinemia had severe rheumatoid arthritis and died of cerebral hemorrhages probably secondary to marked hyperviscosity of the serum.

The autoimmune nature of this disorder is suggested by the pathological findings of vasculitis, arteritis, diffuse glomerulonephritis, endocarditis, thyroiditis, and arthritis. The occurrence of Sjögren's syndrome and the presence of antinuclear antibodies and low or absent complement further supports this suggestion. However, similar cryoglobulins have also been described in patients with nonautoimmune disorders, such as proliferative disorders of reticulum cells and lymphocytes, cirrhosis, malignancies, sarcoidosis and aminoaciduria (Peetoom and van Loghem-Langereis, 1965; Buckley and Nagaza, 1965).

Complex cryoglobulins may be easily overlooked since they are not associated with a characteristic electrophoretic pattern, and precipitate only slowly at 0°C. This poor precipitability in the native state is probably due to the protective effect of other proteins especially the albumin, since in the isolated state these cryoglobulins precipitate almost instantaneously at temperatures between 20° and 30°C. The cryoprotein formation only means aggregation and precipitation in the cold of preexisting immune complexes. The rheumatoid factors (IgM) act as incomplete cryoglobulins, and precipitate in the cold in the presence of the IgG or the Fc fragment. These circulating autoimmune complexes may cause hemolysis by immune adherence reaction with red cells and leukopenia by a similar reaction with the white cells (Peetoom and van Loghem-Langereis, 1965). The deposition of the antibody-antigen complex in the tissues may initiate vasculitis, arteritis and kidney damage. When the IgM-IgG complex is dissociated *in vitro,* it is found that the IgG fails to complex with normal IgM, while the patient's IgM does complex with normal IgG. This points to the IgM as the abnormal specific autoantibody.

In the same group of autoimmune and some other disease processes, the IgG and IgM complexes may be non-cold-precipitable but may lead to "spurious" macroglobulinemia (Kunkel *et al.,* 1961; Ritzmann and Levin, 1963). This IgG-IgM complexing may similarly occur as a result of a fit of a rheumatoid factor for an antigenic site in the isologous IgG. The complexes dissociate with 6M urea but not with penicillamine, while in true macroglobulinemia the dissociation occurs with penicillamine.

### Systemic Lupus Erythematosus

In systemic lupus erythematosus there is primarily an increase in IgG with a lesser increase in the other immunoglobulins (Heremans, 1960; Tomasi, 1965). The immunoglobulin elevation is usually an expression of the duration of the disease rather than of its immediate severity (Hargraves and Opfell, 1956).

More than any other disease, systemic lupus erythematosus is characterized by circulating serum factors capable of reacting with various autologous tissue constituents. Some of these factors have been identified as the LE cell factor responsible for formation of the LE cells, the immunoglobulin which causes a positive Coombs test, an immunoglobulin which reacts with thromboplastin and thrombin and leads to prolonged clotting time, the

Wassermann reagin responsible for the biologically false positive reactions, and a factor capable of reacting with the desoxyribonucleohistone of the cell nucleus. Other antinuclear and anticytoplasmic antibodies have been identified through complement fixation, immunofluorescence, hemagglutination, flocculation, and passive cutaneous anaphylaxis (Holman, 1965). The antinuclear factors have been found in IgG, IgA and IgM classes of immunoglobulins (Barnett *et al.*, 1964).

Bence Jones proteinemia has also been described in systemic lupus erythematosus (Epstein and Tan, 1964). Its presence is explained as disproportionate light chain overproduction during disorderly immunoglobulin synthesis stimulated by an autoimmune process.

Since systemic lupus erythematosus is a disease characteristically associated with circulating autoantibodies, whenever a patient is found to have such autoantibodies, lupus erythematosus is suspected.

### Other "Autoimmune" Disorders

Patients with rheumatic fever frequently exhibit elevation of gamma globulin on serum electrophoresis which may reflect the rise in antibodies to streptococcal infection or the body response to chronic illness. No breakdown into various classes of immunoglobulins is available. Most patients with Sjögren's syndrome exhibit up to three-fold elevations of IgG and two-fold elevations of IgA and IgM. In seven out of seventy patients studied by Talal and Barth (1966), there was marked macroglobulinemia associated with cryoglobulinemia, lymphadenopathy, splenomegaly and purpura. The macroglobulin rise was of a homogeneous character but disappeared along with other manifestations of the disease on steroid therapy. Five of these patients also had reticulum cell sarcoma.

There is a generalized immunoglobulin increase in other autoimmune disorders: Hashimoto's thyroiditis (Green *et al.*, 1958; Roitt *et al.*, 1958), periarteritis nodosa, scleroderma, dermatomyositis, erythema nodosum, autoimmune hemolytic anemia, cold agglutinin disease (primarily IgM), and lupoid hepatitis (primarily IgG). The cold agglutinin frequently has specificity as an antibody to factor I in the red cell as well as type K specificity.

Matthews (1965) recently reported a case of Evans-Duane syndrome (idiopathic, autoimmune, acquired hemolytic anemia with thrombocytopenia) in a sixty-nine-year-old woman, associated with diffuse hypergammaglobulinemia, marked Bence Jones proteinuria, diffuse plasmocytosis as well as amyloidosis of primarily parenchymatous distribution.

### Hyperimmunoglobulinemias Associated with Malignancies

While diffuse hyperimmunoglobulinemia is occasionally associated with reticulum cell sarcoma, Hodgkin's disease and giant cell lymphoma, most of the patients with these diseases as well as those with various leukemias and carcinomatosis exhibit normal immunoglobulin pattern by electrophoresis and frequently generalized or selective hypoimmunoglobulinemia.

## Hyperimmunoglobulinemia Associated with Diseases of Unknown Etiology

### *Infectious Mononucleosis*

Infectious mononucleosis is a disease of protean manifestations and unknown etiology. Its diagnosis is greatly facilitated by presence of heterophile antibody in the sera of the patients. Heterophile antibody is any spontaneously occurring antibody reactive with tissues of another species. The heterophile antibody of infectious mononucleosis reacts with sheep red cells. Various heterophile antibodies reacting with sheep red cells occur in other conditions such as serum sickness and even in normal individuals (Forssman antibodies). The heterophile antibody of infectious mononucleosis, also called the Paul-Bunnell antibody, is distinguished from them in that it is absorbed with beef red cells but not by guinea pig kidney. This heterophile antibody is a macroglobulin as demonstrated by ultracentrifugation, by immunoelectrophoresis and incubation with an anti-IgM-macroglobulin serum. It is destroyed by mercaptoethanol (Carter, 1966a).

In addition to the Paul-Bunnell antibody, a number of other 19S antibodies may appear during the acute phase of infectious mononucleosis, including anti-i, rheumatoid factors, the Wassermann antibody, antinuclear factors, an antibody which may simulate antithyroglobulin, and possibly leukoagglutinins (Carter, 1966b). These are transient abnormalities usually present in low titer which appear at the time of maximal lymphoreticular proliferation. Each appears to occur separately in any one patient and, with rare exceptions, there is no correlation with other laboratory or clinical features of the disease. The exception is a rare hemolytic anemia with a lytic anti-i antibody.

In thirty-six patients with infectious mononucleosis no alteration was found in IgA, a 50 per cent increase in IgG and 100 per cent increase in IgM (Wollheim and Williams, 1966). The alterations regressed completely in three months, the IgG changes more slowly than those of IgM. A linear relationship was noted between the heterophile-antibody titers and IgM levels but none with the IgA and IgG.

The increase in immunoglobulins was not related to the severity of disease, evidence of hepatic involvement or fever. Cold agglutinins with anti-i-specificity were found in twenty-seven sera in titers of 1:5 to 1:640; they were all 19S and their presence paralleled to a certain degree a high heterophile-antibody titer. Absorption of high-titered serums with sheep cells resulted in no significant loss of IgM, indicating that heretophile antibody accounted for less than 5 per cent of the total IgM. Typing of the IgM from the patients with infectious mononucleosis, using five specific anti-IgM sera, resulted in a complex pattern different for each antiserum. Perhaps this was due to antigenic heterogeneity among IgM globulins.

It is likely that in the course of infectious mononucleosis a process alters the host's tissues and exposes antigenic sites normally hidden in human beings but present in other species (Wollheim and Williams, 1966).

### Sarcoidosis

Sarcoidosis, the noncaseating granulomatosis of lung, skin, and reticuloendothelial organs is a disease of unknown etiology. A few rare cases of associated hypoimmunoglobulinemia notwithstanding, the classical protein pattern in this disease is generalized elevation of all immunoglobulins. The highest elevation usually occurs in the IgG class; values four and six times the normal level are commonly seen. In addition, it is frequently possible to demonstrate in such a patient impaired delayed hypersensitivity and, if the lymphocytes are cultured, they exhibit impaired responsiveness to phytohemagglutinin. Positive latex fixation and other tests for rheumatoid factor-like proteins are common in this disorder.

Putkonen, Jokinen, and Mustakallio (1965) reported an unusually strong and rapid skin response to several Kveim antigens in a woman with sarcoidosis, associated with marked hyperimmunoglobulinemia, primarily of the IgG class, and marked plasmacytosis of the lymph nodes as well as a biologically false positive flocculation test for syphilis. Occasionally sarcoidosis presents with symptoms of macro- and cryoglobulinemia (Turkington and Buckley, 1966).

### Waldenström's "Benign" Hyperglobulinemic Purpura

In 1943 Waldenström reported three cases of a syndrome characterized by coexistence of a petechial rash and a diffuse increase of serum globulin. Numerous other cases have been added to the record since then, and it has become clear that this syndrome may be associated with a number of clinical conditions, many of them causes of diffuse hyperimmunoglobulinemia per se: chronic recurrent oral infections, severe rheumatoid arthritis (Lamotte *et al.*, 1965), Sjögren's syndrome (Fekete, Florescu, and Weiss, 1966; Birch *et al.*, 1964), sarcoidosis (Strauss, 1959), systemic lupus erythematosus (Larsson and Leonhardt, 1959; Waldenström, 1961), tuberculosis (Strauss, 1959) and a number of malignancies such as gastric tumor, hepatoma, reticulum cell sarcoma, thymoma (Birch *et al.*, 1964), two cases of multiple myeloma, and Mikulicz's syndrome (Waldenström, 1961). Out of twenty instances of this syndrome, Waldenström felt that only six were "essential" without associated conditions.

The rash of "hyperglobulinemic purpura" appears typically on the legs and is a chronic recurrent, seemingly nonprogressive disorder. The attacks are usually provoked by exercise, pressure, by carrying of heavy packages, by tight-fitting clothes, or by prolonged standing or sitting (Seiden and Kramer, 1958).

The attacks are often heralded by local itching, burning and pain. The rash attains its widest distribution and greatest intensity within a few hours of the onset. Some edema is usually present. Each lesion consists of a petechia with "pericapillaritis" on microscopy, similar to that seen in Henoch-Schönlein purpura (Birch *et al.,* 1964). After a few days the lesions become brown. The pigmentation may disappear or remain as permanent discoloration. With successive crops, which usually become more frequent as years go by, areas of permanent pigmentation may coalesce, resulting in a uniform brown color of legs which, after many years, slowly spreads up to the thigh and lower abdomen. Capillary fragility may be increased, as seen with the Rumpel-Leede test. The typical serum electrophoretic pattern is a broad-base increase in gamma globulin (not including IgM) with a rounded peak, not like the narrow-base homogeneous peak seen in multiple myeloma and Waldenström's macroglobulinemia. Other frequent clinical features include hepatosplenomegaly, anemia and occurrence of rheumatoid factor-like proteins and antinuclear factors in the blood (Schwartz and Fredd, 1964).

Benign hyperglobulinemic purpura must be distinguished from cryoglobulinemic purpura and from paraimmunoglobulinemia associated with purpura (also called "premyeloma") (Kyle and Bayrd, 1966). A few reports of late progression of the "benign" hyperglobulinemic purpura with generalized hyperimmunoglobulinemia to plasmocytoma (Sheon, Lewis, and Battle, 1966) and to multiple myeloma (Rogers and Welch, 1957) serve to obliterate the fine distinction between the paraimmunoglobulinemia and the hyperimmunoglobulinemia. When a paraimmunoglobulinopathy develops in a patient with a background of hyperglobulinemic purpura, chance coincidence could be at work or the same stimulus which was responsible for the reticuloendothelial stimulation might be held responsible for triggering the paraimmune response. Birch and coworkers (1964) reported hyperglobulinemic purpura associated with a benign thymic tumor, Sjögren's syndrome, Raynaud's phenomenon, hepatosplenomegaly, leukopenia and thrombocytopenia in a woman of fifty-six. Of these symptoms the purpura, hyperglobulinemia, leukopenia and thrombocytopenia were cured with thymectomy. Sjögren's syndrome and hepatosplenomegaly persisted. This interesting case adds to the linkage between hyperglobulinemic purpura and autoimmune disorders.

Although it is usually assumed that the "benign" hyperglobulinemic purpura is an autoimmune disorder (Waldenström, 1961), this is by no means proven and the pathogenesis of the condition remains obscure. Pathological examinations reveal "pericapillaritis," a pleomorphic vasculitis and spotty arteriolar necrosis. There is no good evidence to implicate antiintima antibodies, increased blood viscosity or inadequate protein coating of the capillary wall. Coagulation studies are usually normal, although the platelets may become coated with abnormal gamma globulin and give an abnormal thromboplastin generation test (Weiss *et al.,* 1963). Weiss tested the hypothesis of autosensitivity to patient's altered extravasated gamma globulin by injecting patients subcutaneously with their own serum, but no abnormal response was seen.

Henstell and Kligerman (1958) reported interference with the clotting mechanism by the elevated globulin. Complexes formed by the globulin with the prothrombin and with factor V and factor VII resulted in local decreases in the concentration of these clotting factors.

In treatment of hyperglobulinemic purpura, steroids and splenectomy have been ineffective (Strauss, 1959). Recently two patients with this disorder responded to intermittent therapy with thioguanine 40 to 100 mg a day for two to three weeks alternating with one or two weeks of no therapy (Weiss *et al.,* 1963). Purpura disappears, although there is not much change in the paper electrophoresis pattern of serum proteins. Thioguanine is thought to act by suppressing the abnormal vasculitic response, by decreasing the lymphocytic and monocytic reaction to inflammation; this drug probably exercises its effect around the blood vessels, where it may block the cellular response to whatever initiates the purpura. Chlorambucil has also been used in management of this syndrome (Sheon, Lewis, and Battle, 1966). However, the use of the potentially toxic drugs in this chronic and benign condition must be undertaken with great caution.

### Charmot's Syndrome

In twenty African patients with splenomegaly Charmot (Aron *et al.,* 1962) demonstrated presence of marked diffuse elevation of macroglobulins. No purpura, hemorrhagic tendency or adenopathy was observed. Anemia, fatigue, lymphocytosis and monocytosis were frequently present with occasional eosinophilia. Bone marrow examination revealed lymphoplasmacytosis of mature type. On biopsy of liver and spleen, a nonspecific reticuloendothelial hyperplasia was observed. This syndrome probably represents an inflammatory type of macroglobulinemia and predominantly splenic involvement. Exposure to many parasitic and bacterial antigens may be postulated in these African patients. However, etiology is not known. The term *tropical splenomegaly* with macroglobulinemia could be used. However, similar patients have been described in Europe, without tropical exposure.

### Liver Diseases

Changes in immunoglobulins in liver diseases vary with the type of liver lesion, with severity and duration of the ailment, and occasionally with the individual patient.

In Laennec's cirrhosis there is usually a markedly elevated IgA level, a moderately elevated IgG level and normal IgM globulins (Fahey, 1965). In hepatoma IgM levels drop (Heremans, 1960). In biliary cirrhosis IgM is elevated while IgA and IgG are normal. In viral hepatitis all immunoglobulins are usually elevated (Heremans, 1960); occasionally there is an elevation of just IgM (Charmot and Andre, 1964). In plasma cell hepatitis IgG may be elevated to five times normal while IgA and IgM may be only slightly increased.

The mechanism of these various forms of hyperimmunoglobulinemia with liver ailments is poorly understood. The rate of synthesis of the immunoglobulins in these conditions is increased (Andersen, 1964). It is not clear whether a decreased albumin is a stimulus to immunoglobulin production. Increased reticuloendothelial activity may be an irritative phenomenon in portal and biliary types of cirrhosis, while a response to infection is the cause of the hyperimmunoglobulinemia of viral hepatitis.

Autoimmunity undoubtedly plays a role in plasma cell hepatitis. This group of patients was first described by Kunkel and coworkers (1951) and consisted of young women with chronic liver disease, plasma cell infiltration of the liver and extreme hypergammaglobulinemia. Mackay, Taft, and Cowling (1959) noted that most of these patients had positive reactions to lupus erythematosus cell tests and coined the term *lupoid hepatitis*. As these antinuclear antibodies are secondary to the liver disease and as the incidence of liver disease in systemic lupus is rare, it is uncertain whether the association of LE cell phenomenon and the plasma cell hepatitis is of any etiological significance. It is of interest that plasma cell hepatitis usually responds well to steroids and to 6-mercaptopurine (Page, Condie, and Good, 1964).

To what extent the elevated immunoglobulin is involved in the etiology of hemolytic anemia which not infrequently accompanies liver disease is not well understood. Despite hyperimmunoglobulinemia, patients with severe liver disease suffer from immunological impairment; protracted and sometimes fatal infections are part of the clinical picture; Staphylococcus and Salmonella infections are common.

# Chapter 7

# PARAIMMUNOGLOBULINOPATHIES:
# INTRODUCTION AND GENERAL ASPECTS

*Definition.* The paraimmunoglobulinopathies are a group of diseases, usually neoplastic, which involve the immunocytes, cells that normally manufacture immunoglobulins. The neoplasm produces unusual homogeneous immunoglobulins which may appear in the blood, urine, and/or tissues. It is not entirely certain whether these strange immunoglobulins are qualitatively as well as quantitatively different from normal immunoglobulins. By

TABLE XXII

PARAIMMUNOGLOBULINOPATHIES

A. Multiple myeloma and its clinical variants
   1. Variants related to body distribution
      a. Solitary plasmacytoma
      b. Multiple plasmacytomas
      c. Extramedullary plasmacytomas
      d. Disseminated myelomatosis
      e. Plasma cell leukemia
   2. Variants related to physicochemical characteristics of the paraimmunoglobulins
      a. Cryoglobulinemia
      b. Pyroglobulinemia
B. Waldenström's macroglobulinemia, in which the paraimmunoglobulins are of the IgM variety
C. H-chain disease, which probably is a rare variant of myeloma in which the paraimmunoglobulins formed consist solely of heavy chains or portions of heavy chains
D. Paraimmunoglobulinopathies associated with other diseases
   1. Chronic lymphocytic leukemia, lymphosarcoma, reticulum cell sarcoma, and Hodgkin's disease.
   2. Other malignancies
   3. Nonneoplastic conditions more often characterized by diffuse hyperimmunoglobulinemia
      a. Severe chronic and subacute infections
      b. Liver disease
      c. Sarcoidosis
      d. Cold agglutinin disease
      e. Cold allergy
      f. Lupus erythematosus
      g. Rheumatoid arthritis
      h. Papular mucinosis
      i. Gaucher's disease
E. Paraimmunoglobulinopathies of unknown etiology
   1. Idiopathic paraimmunoglobulinemia
      a. Asymptomatic
      b. Symptomatic
   2. Idiopathic cryoglobulinemia
   3. Idiopathic pyroglobulinemia
F. Paraamyloidosis

this definition, purely reactive plasmacytosis, which is associated with a diffuse increase of all normal immunoglobulins (hyperimmunoglobulinopathy), is excluded from this discussion, although some clinical cases skirt the border between the reactive and the neoplastic groups.

*Classification.* We recognize the forms of paraimmunoglobulinopathies shown in Table XXII.

## ETIOLOGY

Most cases of paraimmunoglobulinopathy act as if they resulted from malignancies of the cells which produce the immunoglobulins. In the case of multiple myeloma, the malignancy usually involves the plasma cell or, in rare instances, closely related cells such as the reticulum cell or lymphocyte. In Waldenström's macroglobulinemia, the involved cell is usually the lymphocyte. Because these diseases are probably malignant, all the known causes of malignancy must be considered. Malignant cells are altered cells. There is growing evidence that the primary alteration occurs somewhere in the DNA→RNA→protein information system of the cell, probably with some change in the DNA. There is still considerable confusion in defining specific alterations of this system, since many of the possible types of alterations have not been named and even those that have, such as somatic mutation and induction, have not been defined specifically enough. It is generally agreed, however, that such changes may be brought about by many agents, including irradiation, viruses, and certain chemicals. Since DNA is found primarily in the chromosomes and is responsible for the genetically acquired information in the cell, the role of heredity must also be considered.

### Irradiation

The incidence of multiple myeloma, like that of myelogenous leukemia, was reported to be significantly increased among radiologists (Lewis, 1963). However, despite considerable work in mice on the production of leukemia by irradiation, only one reported tumor had the characteristics of myeloma (Potter and Fahey, 1960).

### Viruses

The evidence for possible viral etiology is sparse but important. Particles morphologically similar to virus particles were demonstrated in plasma cell tumors of mice under the electron microscope (Parsons *et al.*, 1961a), and apparent multiplication of virus in tissue culture of one of the tumors was demonstrated (Parsons *et al.*, 1961b). No virus-like particles were seen in normal plasma cells from the same strain of mice. There were no reports of successful cell-free transfers. Dalton, Potter, and Merwin (1961) described virus-like particles in a variety of primary and transplanted plasma cell tumors of mice. However, these workers did not consider the particles to be oncogenic viruses responsible for the plasma cell neoplasms. They failed to find similar particles in normal plasma cells or in myeloma cells from patients. On the other hand, Sorenson (1961) did demonstrate virus-like particles in cytoplasmic inclusion bodies within myeloma cells of man. Rask-Nielsen (1963) reported on a virus-induced reticulum cell neoplasm in mice which was associated with a slow gamma peak in the electrophoretic pattern of the serum proteins.

### Chemicals

The evidence that chemicals play an etiologic role is scanty. The spontaneous occurrence of plasma cell tumors has been noted in several strains of mice. The incidence of such tumors was increased following intrathymic injection of 9, 10-dimethyl-1, 2-benzanthracene into three strains of mice (Rask-Nielsen and Gormsen, 1956). However, no paraimmunoglobulinemia was found. Potter and Robertson (1960) produced plasma cell neoplasms and paraimmunoglobulinemia in BALB/cAn mice by the intraperitoneal injection of mineral oil or of an emulsion of incomplete Freund's adjuvant and heat-killed staphlococci (Potter and Boyce, 1962). Although the skin of some of the animals was painted with methylcholanthrene, this did not seem to be essential to the development of the neoplasm.

### Role of Heredity

**Family Studies.** Leoncini and Korngold (1964) reviewed the familial occurrence of multiple myeloma and Waldenström's macroglobulinemia. They found six kinships with multiple myeloma and two with macroglobulinemia and added a report of their own on two sisters with myeloma, each with proteins of type L. An additional report of myeloma in a brother and sister has appeared (Thomas, 1964). Seligmann and associates (Seligmann, Danon, and Fine, 1963; Seligmann, Danon, and Mihaesco, 1965) studied the sera of 208 relatives of sixty-two patients with Waldenström's macroglobulinemia and found a familial incidence of symptomatic and asymptomatic macroglobulinemia in six of the families. More recently, these studies have been enlarged and reported in a more readily available journal (Seligmann *et al.*, 1967). Waldenström's macroglobulinemia with cryoglobulinemia in one brother and cryoglobulinemia associated with Sjögren's syndrome in another brother have also been described (Biro, 1962). Familial cryoglobulinemia (Sitomer *et al.*, 1963), familial IgA-paraimmunoglobulinemia (Wysocki and Mackiewicz, 1965), and familial occurrence of chronic lymphocytic leukemia and multiple myeloma (Wirtschafter and Rapaport, 1960) have also been reported.

**Chromosome Studies.** Chromosomal abnormalities in the plasma cells similar to those seen in other forms of neoplasia have been found in a few patients with multiple myeloma (Lewis *et al.*, 1963). In some patients many of the plasma cells contained too few chromosomes, while in others the number of chromosomes exceeded the normal diploid number of forty-six but tended to be less than tetraploid. Das and Aikat (1967) have also reported deletions, translocations, giant chromosomes, and chromatid breaks and gaps. In several patients with Waldenström's macroglobulinemia, an extra large or giant chromosome has been reported (German, Biro, and Bearn, 1961; Ferguson and MacKay, 1963). In other patients no chromosomal abnormality was detected (Ferguson and MacKay, 1963). The chromosomes of the skin cells were normal (Ferguson and MacKay, 1963).

The chromosomal abnormalities observed may be the cause of the myelomatous transformation or may be the result of a nonspecific change in the cells affected by malignancy. These findings support the concept that the paraimmunoglobulinemias result from, or are at least associated with, abnormalities of the chromosomes of the somatic cells, which are probably the cells involved in the malignant process.

Further evidence favoring some role for heredity is to be found from the studies of mouse myeloma, where some inbred strains are highly susceptible to spontaneous myeloma tumors while other strains develop growths only after injection of a chemical agent. Chromosome abnormalities have been found in the spontaneous tumors (Fjelde, Lavan, and Rask-Nielsen, 1962).

### Role of Infection and Immunity

Patients with multiple myeloma frequently have infections, and it has been postulated that susceptibility to infection is increased because of the reduction of the normal immunoglobulins of the blood. Except for the possible viral etiology, there has been no evidence that other infections play an etiologic role.

The recognition that patients who have what appears to be a severe, protracted, benign proliferation of plasma cells related to the immune response but who later develop a picture indistinguishable from multiple myeloma raises the intriguing possibility that benign proliferation of the plasma cell may, under certain circumstances, become malignant (Osserman and Takatuski, 1965). The rapid multiplication of cells may increase the probability of somatic mutation and result in malignancy. Similar excessive benign stimulation of plasma cells may account for the myelomas which develop in mice injected with various agents (Potter and Robertson, 1960).

### Summary

While more evidence is needed, it is likely that many factors contribute to the etiology of the paraimmunoglobulinopathies. As with most malignancies, genetic susceptibility and environmental influences including irradiation, chemicals and infection are all probably important. The possibility that in some instances extreme benign stimulation of the cells producing the immunoglobulins may lead to the development of the malignant paraimmunoglobulinopathies must also be considered.

## INCIDENCE

Estimates of the incidence or mortality rate of the paraimmunoglobulinopathies are probably inaccurate because of the difficulty of diagnosis. Recent figures are more accurate because of the more general use of specific diagnostic procedures such as bone marrow aspirations and serum and urinary protein electrophoresis. Even allowing for the better diagnostic procedures, many physicians believe that the incidence of multiple myeloma is increasing and that it is no longer a rare disease. Waldenström's macroglobulinemia is even less well defined and has been recognized only within the last few years.

According to the United States Vital Statistics Reports, 1.5 to 1.7 deaths per 100,000 population were attributed to multiple myeloma and plasmacytoma each year for the years 1957 to 1961, with very little change during this period. This represents an increase over figures for 1949 to 1952, when 0.8 to 1.0 deaths per 100,000 population per year were reported (World Health Organization, 1955). These figures correlate well with the minimal estimates of incidence made by MacMahon and Clark (1956) in Brooklyn, New York, where it was estimated that from 1949 to 1952 there were 1.4 cases per 100,000 population per year. The incidence of multiple myeloma has been reviewed by Martin (1961). In Malmö, Sweden, the incidence was estimated to be 3 per 100,000 live population per year and in England, 2.6 per 100,000. These estimates probably reflect the actual incidence of the disease more closely than the death rates even though, essentially, all cases are eventually fatal.

The age incidence of the disease has not changed since 1931. In almost all series incidence reaches a peak at fifty to sixty years and falls sharply after age seventy. Only rarely is the disease found below the age of thirty. Review of several cases of plasma cell tumors reported in children and diagnosed as multiple myeloma did not reveal typical myeloma proteins or Bence Jones proteins. The sex incidence has changed markedly since 1921 when up to 70 per cent of the reported cases affected males. Most recent series show only a slight preponderance of males, about 55 per cent of the total, although in one series of 185 cases 66 per cent were males (Midwest, 1964). Negroes have a slightly higher incidence than Caucasians, and tend to manifest the illness at a younger age. The incidence varies considerably from country to country. The death rates reported from Norway, Sweden and Denmark are somewhat higher than in the United States, while those reported from Ireland, France, Italy, Finland, and Australia are lower (World Health Organization, 1955).

The incidence of Waldenström's macroglobulinemia, based upon a series of cases in which both macroglobulinemia and multiple myeloma were included, is estimated to be one fifth to one tenth that of multiple myeloma. In sixty cases reviewed (Dutcher and Fahey, 1959), two thirds were in men and two thirds of the patients were between the ages of fifty and seventy years at the time of diagnosis.

### Disease in Animals

Plasma cell tumors sometimes associated with disseminated myelomatosis have been found in domesticated animals such as the horse (Cornelius, Goodbary, and Kennedy, 1959), calf, pig, and dog, and in some laboratory animals including the mouse, rat (Bocciarelli and Violente, 1960), and Syrian hamster (Cotran and Fortner, 1962). Experimental work with transplantable multiple myeloma in mice has been particularly productive. Spontaneous plasma cell tumors occur in some strains of mice such as $C_3H$ but not in others (Cotran and Fortner, 1962). Other strains of mice, such as BALB/c, develop plasma cell tumors after intraperitoneal insertion of milli-pore filters (Merwin and Algire, 1959) or after intraperitoneal injections with mineral oil or incomplete Freund's adjuvant plus heat-killed staphylo-cocci (Potter and Boyce, 1962). The plasma cell tumors seem to arise from the reactive lipogranulomatous tissue. Accompanying the malignancies are protein abnormalities remarkably similar to those seen in patients with the paraimmunoglobulinopathies; these abnormalities include serum myeloma proteins, Bence Jones proteins, and amyloid deposits (Lehner, Rosenoer and Topping, 1966). Furthermore, these proteins have the same basic chem-ical and immunologic structure and interrelationships as their counterparts in human beings (Fahey and Askonas, 1962; Askonas and Fahey, 1962). A transplantable mouse leukemia with macroglobulinemia has been described (Clausen *et al.*, 1960; McIntire, Asofsky, Potter and Kuff, 1965). Mice with a transplantable reticulum cell sarcoma may develop plasmacytes and para-immunoglobulinemia (Wanebo *et al.*, 1966). Aleutian disease of mink is characterized by proliferation of plasma cells and diffuse hyperimmuno-globulinemia. In some mink, late in the course of this disease, a transition to paraimmunoglobulinemia with appearance of Bence Jones proteinuria has been observed (Porter, Dixon and Larsen, 1965).

### PATHOGENESIS

The pathogenesis of the paraimmunoglobulinopathies relates both to the malignant proliferation of the cell type involved, whether in a diffuse form or as a solid tumor, and also to the effects of the proteins produced by the tumor cells. Malignant proliferation does not necessarily mean rapid prolif-eration. The generation time (time from the end of one mitosis to the end of the next mitosis) of myeloma cells labelled with tritiated thymidine has been estimated to be from two to six days (Killmann *et al.*, 1962). For comparison, the generation time is one day for normoblasts, two days for normal myeloid precursors, and two to three days for leukemic myeloblasts. Because of this relatively long generation time and other factors, the disease cannot be explained solely as uncontrolled exponential growth but must be looked upon as an imbalance between production and destruction, resulting in an expanding mass of abnormal tissue.

In multiple myeloma, bone marrow infiltration and tumor masses are responsible for the bone pain and tenderness, which are the cardinal symptom and sign. Pathologic fractures and vertebral collapse are frequent results. Considering the large number of bones which may be involved in the process, the number of instances of pain in the region of the spine is disproportionately great (Innes and Newall, 1961), possibly because of the relatively poor adaptation of the spine to weight-bearing in the vertical position, we believe, or to its relative mobility (Innes and Newall, 1961). Anemia (which is common), thrombocytopenia, and leukopenia may result in part from the infiltration, as may enlargement of liver, spleen, and lymph nodes.

Extension of tumor from the area of the vertebra may cause compression of the spinal cord and result in paraplegia. For obscure reasons, vertebral collapse only rarely causes neurologic complications. It must be supposed that considerable vertebral collapse may occur without compromising the nerves or cord. Roentgenograms of these lesions usually show collapse involving in particular the anterior portion of the vertebral bodies, while posterior sections adjacent to the spinal cord remain relatively intact. When complete collapse occurs, paraplegia may result (Hagelstam, 1955).

Tumors and infiltrations of other organs may account for clinical findings in virtually any area of the body.

At one time considerable thought was given to the question of whether the extramedullary lesions of myeloma arose as an autochthonous growth or by direct transmission of myeloma cells. Present hypotheses of pathogenesis are best explained by direct transmission of tumor cells. However, it is possible that the sequence of events one sees from solitary plasmacytoma to disseminated multiple myeloma results from a train of etiologic events, such as somatic mutations, each occurring in a different cell of the same cell line.

Both the serum myeloma proteins and the Bence Jones proteins are formed in the abnormal plasma cells. The light and heavy chains are probably produced there under separate genetic control. There is evidence that normally light chains are synthesized in excess of heavy chains (Shapiro *et al.*, 1966). It has been suggested that the light chains release the heavy chains from the ribosomes (Askonas and Williamson, 1966 a and b). Some patients with multiple myeloma or macroglobulinemia are capable of producing and conjugating both light and heavy chains in approximately equal amounts and have only myeloma proteins and no Bence Jones proteins. In other patients the light chains are not all conjugated with heavy chains and are apparently transported in the blood and excreted very rapidly into the urine, where they appear as Bence Jones protein. In this situation the myeloma protein and the Bence Jones protein from the same patient have the same group specificity, i.e., either type K or type L, since the same light chain occurs in the serum myeloma protein and in the Bence Jones protein (Migita and Putnam, 1963; Edelman and Gally, 1962; Fahey and Solomon, 1963). Still other patients produce only light chains and have Bence Jones proteinuria without a serum myeloma protein but usually with hypoimmunoglobulinemia. Rarely, patients produce no demonstrable abnormal protein. Amyloid desposits, which are often seen in patients with myeloma, may be a manifestation of an abnormal protein which is deposited in the tissues in characteristic distribution.

As previously noted, there are two major immunologic types of light chains, only one of which is present in any myeloma or Bence Jones protein of a given patient. Four major classes of heavy chains, one specific for each family of immunoglobulins, have been distinguished: one characteristic of IgG, a second for IgA, a third for IgG, and a fourth for IgD (see Fig. 4 and Table III). Theoretically, we might expect to find some patients who are capable of producing disproportionately large amounts of heavy chains of any one of these four immunologic specificities. Franklin and coworkers (1964) and Osserman and Takatsuki (1964) have reported patients who excrete portions of heavy chains of IgG specificity without light chains. The five patients reported were clinically distinguishable from those with multiple myeloma. These patients had proteinuria with excretion of the fast Fc fragment or portions of the Fc fragment of heavy chains. These fragments do not give the Bence Jones heat test. Recently, Seligmann and Basch (1968) have described a patient who excretes heavy chains of IgA specificity. Patients who produce and excrete heavy chains of only IgM, or IgD specificity have not yet been discovered.

The proteins which may be produced in large amounts by the tumor cells may cause relatively little difficulty. In some cases the globulin level may increase to 12 gm per cent and the Bence Jones protein excretion may amount to as much as 50 gm per day. The high levels of the unusual homogeneous immunoglobulins may result from decreased destruction, increased production, or both. Actually, there is evidence that the abnormal protein in multiple myeloma is destroyed more rapidly than normal (Korman *et al.*, 1962), and it must then be supposed that there is greatly enhanced production to account for the high plasma levels reached. In Waldenström's macroglobulinemia the increased plasma level is also due to increased synthesis (Barth *et al.*, 1964).

If the serum protein produced by the tumor has the property of precipitating out or gelling in the cold (cryoglobulin), then many of the clinical findings may be related to this relatively rare phenomenon (cryoglobulinemia). The cryoglobulinemia may be demonstrated by precipitation at 4°C in serum collected at 37°C. The cryoglobulin characteristically goes back into solution when the serum is warmed to 37°C. When cryoglobulins are found in large amounts the patients usually have multiple myeloma or macroglobulinemia and the cryoglobulins may be either IgG or IgM (Meltzer and Franklin, 1966). However, cryoglobulinemia may also be found in many diseases involving the reticuloendothelial system, such as cold agglutinin disease, systemic lupus erythematosus, polyarteritis nodosa, rheumatoid arthritis, Sjögren's syndrome, rheumatic fever, cirrhosis, and chronic infections such as syphilis, kala-azar, bronchiectasis, and subacute bacterial endocarditis. Occasionally, no cause is found for the cryoglobulinemia and the disease is termed *essential* or *idiopathic*. In some of these patients unusual reticuloendothelial cells have been observed in the marrow during life even though they were not found at autopsy (Barr, Engle and Russ, 1957). This suggests that even in these "idiopathic" cases, the disease is closely related to multiple myeloma and to the proliferation of the cells producing the immunoglobulins.

Cryoglobulins may also result from aggregation of IgM and IgG, a reaction which has been interpreted as the IgM being an autoantibody to the IgG (Peetoom and van Loghem-Langereis, 1965). (See Idiopathic Cryoglobulinemia and Hyperimmunoglobulinemia.) When separated, neither the IgG nor IgM components alone have cryoglobulin properties, but mixing restored this property (Peetoom and and van Loghem-Langereis, 1965). In contrast to typical cryoglobulins these cryoglobulin IgG-IgM complexes may not redissolve upon heating to 37°C (Peetoom and van Loghem-Langereis, 1965).

Patients with cryoglobulinemia frequently have Raynaud's phenomenon, which in some cases may progress to frank gangrene of the fingers, toes, tip of the nose, and ears as a result of exposure to cold. The skin may show blotchy pigmentation and hemorrhage is common. In rare instances even slight reduction in temperature below 37°C may precipitate an attack. Other patients have no symptoms related to the cryoglobulinemia.

The symptoms and signs of cryoglobulinemia are probably produced by the *in vivo* precipitation or gelling of the cryoglobulin, resulting in sluggishness of the circulation and, in some instances, frank thrombosis. Secondary tissue reaction as manifested by chills and fever may develop (Volpe *et al.*, 1956) as may foreign body reaction. Histamine release, vascular spasm, and increased vascular permeability have also been implicated in the pathogenesis. Recently a cryoprecipitating factor which causes cold precipitation of normal plasma proteins has been found in the plasma of two patients with cryoglobulinemia (Manor, 1962).

The cryoglobulins differ in physicochemical properties from one patient to another. In some cases, the higher the concentration of the cryoglobulin in the blood, the higher the temperature approaching 37°C at which precipitation occurs (Volpe *et al.,* 1956) and clinical manifestations develop. In other instances the clinical syndrome appears even at relatively low cryoglobulin concentration (Barr, Engle, and Russ, 1957).

Cryoglobulins must be distinguished from cold agglutinins and cryofibrinogens (Ritzmann and Levin, 1961). It is interesting, however, that in some situations cryoglobulins occur in association with cold agglutinins or cryofibrinogens and, indeed, may be the cold agglutinin.

Sometimes when the serum is heated to 56°C for thirty minutes the serum protein precipitates and results in irreversible serum gelation (Lipman, 1964). Called pyroglobulinemia, this phenomenon is distinct from Bence Jones proteinemia (Engle and Woods, 1960). It does not seem to produce any clinical signs or symptoms. Pyroglobulinemia occurs most frequently in patients with multiple myeloma and other paraimmunoglobulinopathies, but may rarely occur associated with other conditions or even without any known association (Patterson *et al.,* 1968).

Paraproteinemia may increase the viscosity of the blood appreciably, resulting in thrombosis. This is especially true when the protein is a macroglobulin. While macroglobulins are usually found in Waldenström's macroglobulinemia, rarely a macroglobulin may be found in patients who have the clinical picture of multiple myeloma. Likewise, in some instances IgG myeloma proteins may aggregate *in vivo,* increasing the viscosity (Smith, Kochwa and Wasserman, 1965). Increased viscosity may produce impaired vision, epistaxis, and mucous membrane hemorrhages. Thrombosis of the central retinal artery or of any of the dural sinuses may result in neurologic symptoms. It is not unusual for a macroglobulin to be also a cryoglobulin, so that it is difficult to separate the properties of the two. Cryoglobulins increase the viscosity of the blood when subjected to cold.

Bleeding manifestations unrelated to thrombocytopenia often result from hyperglobulinemia, whether the protein is IgG, IgA, or IgM. However, bleeding manifestations are the most prominent when the macroglobulins are increased. Probably several different mechanisms are involved. Sometimes the proteins are thought to bind with certain of the coagulation factors, such as prothrombin, factor V, or factor VII (Henstell and Kligerman, 1958). It has also been postulated that in some cases calcium is so bound (Craddock, Adams, and Figueroa, 1953; Glueck, Wayne, and Goldsmith, 1962). Sometimes the globulins inhibit or otherwise interfere with the normal polymerization of fibrinogen to fibrin so that a faulty clot may be formed (Craddock, Adams, and Figueroa, 1953; Frick, 1955). In some instances this may be seen in the test tube when a fresh sample of blood is drawn and a fibrin gel is formed which fails to retract and express the serum. In other instances it has been thought that the proteins interfere with the action of platelets (Rebuck *et al.*, 1961). Sirridge, Bowman, and Garber (1958) reported increased fibrinolytic activity in multiple myeloma.

Amyloid deposits, sometimes called paraamyloid, usually of mesenchymatous distribution, occur in patients with multiple myeloma or macroglobulinemia. These deposits may cause gastrointestinal symptoms, myocardial and cardiac failure symptoms, as well as skin lesions, capillary bleeding, and neurologic manifestations (see Paraamyloidosis).

Almost all patients with paraimmunoglobulinopathy have reduction of the normal immunoglobulins. This is true whether or not a serum myeloma protein is present. As a result, disturbances in the immune reactions would be expected. The decreased normal immunoglobulins may play a significant, though not the only, role in the increased susceptibility to fungal and bacterial infections such as pneumonia. Fever may be related to such infections. Early in the course of the disease there is frequently no hypoimmuno-globulinemia, but sooner or later it eventually develops. The depression of the normal immunoglobulins may be due to either a suppression of production or increased destruction. It does not seem to be related to a physical crowding out of the normal plasma cells by the tumor cells, since it may occur before infiltration is so severe. Normal IgG proteins labelled with $^{131}$I have a biologic half-life of seventeen to thirty-two days with a mean of twenty-three days in normal individuals (Solomon, Waldmann, and Fahey, 1963). About 40 to 60 per cent of the body content of normal IgG is in extravascular compartments. Among patients with paraimmunoglob-ulinopathies, there is evidence that those with macroglobulin peaks, IgA myeloma peaks, Bence Jones proteinuria, or no serum myeloma protein all have normal or prolonged half-life of normal IgG globulin (Solomon, Waldmann, and Fahey, 1963; Lippincott *et al.*, 1960). This suggests that the decrease in normal plasma immunoglobulins found in these patients is related to faulty production. On the other hand, some patients with gamma$_2$ myeloma peaks have shortened survival of normal gamma$_2$ globulins (Solomon, Waldmann, and Fahey, 1963; Lippincott *et al.*, 1960). The decrease in normal immunoglobulins in these patients is probably related to decreased production as well as to increased destruction. The decreased production probably results from a humoral suppression related to a feedback mechanism involved in protein synthesis (Finkelstein and Uhr, 1964).

Recently, Gilbert *et al.* (1968), have described a patient who had plasma cell myeloma associated with thymoma, pure red cell aplasia, malabsorption syndrome, and presence of antimuscle antibodies. This case seems to bridge the gap between multiple myeloma and many other syndromes in which immunologic deficiency is found.

A number of workers have demonstrated in patients with multiple myeloma a diminished antibody response to a number of bacterial and other antigens (Zinneman and Hall, 1954; Lawson *et al.*, 1955; Larson and Tomlinson, 1952) as well as diminished type-specific agglutinins for human A and B erythrocytes (Lawson *et al.*, 1955; Linton, Dunnigan and Thomson, 1963). In general, the antibody production was least effective in those patients who had the largest amount of abnormal serum globulins. These would be the individuals who would probably have the most severe depression of the normal immunoglobulins (Zinneman and Hall, 1954). Antibody response was most nearly normal in those patients with normal or nearly normal electrophoretic patterns (Zinneman and Hall, 1954). The complement titer was normal in all patients studied (Lawson *et al.*, 1955). There was no correlation between patients with multiple myeloma who had hypoimmunoglobulinemia and those who developed recurrent pneumonia (Lawson *et al.*, 1955). From what we know of other types of patients who have hypoimmunoglobulinemia, we would expect deficient antibody response not only to bacterial organisms but also to fungi. On the other hand, these individuals should have a normal response to common viral infections and to smallpox vaccination. They should have normal ability to develop delayed type hypersensitivity of all types. Actually, their ability to respond normally to the Mantoux test has been demonstrated (Linton, Dunnigan and Thomson, 1963). Occasionally, however, there is decreased ability to reject homographs, although this response is variable. As a result of the inability to produce antibody, there is usually no response to diphtheria toxoid or vaccines. Silver (1963) has reviewed the role of infections, fever, and host resistance in neoplastic diseases.

Bence Jones proteins are ordinarily cleared from the blood very rapidly and appear in large amounts in the urine. Rarely, Bence Jones proteins may back up in appreciable amounts in the blood where they can be demonstrated by immunoelectrophoresis and the characteristic heat test. This retention of Bence Jones protein is probably related to a particular type of kidney damage. The excretion of large amounts of Bence Jones protein is undoubtedly one of the most important factors in the pathogenesis of the myeloma kidney. The Bence Jones protein is a constituent of the casts which mechanically block the tubules. However, the severity of renal impairment is not correlated with the amount or duration of Bence Jones proteinuria. Blackman and coworkers (1944) feel that Bence Jones protein has a direct harmful chemical effect on the renal tissue. Vassar and Culling (1962) described thickening of the glomerular basement membrane in a high proportion of patients with myeloma and suggested that it may result from Bence Jones proteinuria.

In the great majority of patients who excrete Bence Jones protein, only relatively small amounts of other serum proteins such as albumin are excreted. The kidney does an excellent job of separating the Bence Jones protein. In rare patients, probably related to a particular kind of kidney damage or in other instances to amyloidosis, the kidneys excrete into the urine all of the serum proteins, including even the serum myeloma protein if present. Factors which play a role in the pathogenesis of the kidney lesions include (1) infiltration with tumor cells; (2) amyloid deposits, either mesenchymatious or parenchymatous in type of distribution; (3) associated infection; (4) calcium deposits, either interstitially, in the tubular lumens, or in the calyces; (5) uric acid deposits; (6) solubility of the Bence Jones proteins under conditions (e.g., pH, ionic strength) prevailing in different parts of the kidney such as the glomerulus and parts of the kidney tubule; and (7) in rare cases, the destruction of proximal renal tubular epithelial cells by crystals, causing the functional failure of these cells and the clinical picture of the adult Fanconi syndrome (Engle and Wallis, 1957). Proteins, including Bence Jones proteins, may be secreted by the renal tubular epithelial cells (Shuster, Jones and Flynn, 1963) and, under certain circumstances, precipitate out in the cells. Likewise, they might precipitate out while being resorbed from the glomerular filtrate.

Hyperuricemia, frequently seen in paraimmunoglobulinopathies, probably results from enhanced purine and nucleic acid metabolism in this disease, as well as from chemotherapy. Increased RNA production antecedent to the synthesis of abnormal proteins by the proliferating plasma cells, as well as increased turnover of these malignant cells, is likely to result in elevation of the uric acid.

Myeloma is a malignant disease and as such some of the manifestations are best ascribed to "toxicity" for want of a better defined mechanism. Weight loss and fever without infection are often explained on this basis. Anemia may be caused by marrow infiltration or hemorrhage but may also develop without any significant degree of these phenomena. It has been shown that the anemia results from inadequate red cell production and increased red cell destruction, usually due to extracellular or plasma factors (Cline, and Berlin, 1962; Hyman, Gellhorn, and Harvey, 1956). These have also been ascribed to "toxicity" of the tumor. Other factors contributing to the anemia include renal insufficiency, radiotherapy, chemotherapy, infection, and iron deficiency. Anemia may become so severe that cardiac failure ensues with or without the added complication of myocardial amyloidosis. An unexplained peripheral neuritis may also result from "toxicity" (Victor, Banker and Adams, 1958; Kenny and Maloney, 1957).

In addition to the anemia and the occasional appearance of plasma cell leukemia, the blood may show evidences of myeloid metaplasia with many early myeloid and erythroid cells in the smear (Brody, Beizer and Schwartz, 1964). This is presumably due to the displacement of normal marrow by the tumor and, in some cases, fibrous tissue as well (Videbaek, 1956). In this situation, extramedullary hematopoiesis may be found in the liver, spleen, and other organs. In rare instances the red cell elements of the bone marrow may be megaloblastic, probably owing to a relative deficiency of vitamin $B_{12}$ (Forshaw, 1963) .

## INTERRELATIONSHIPS OF THE
## PARAIMMUNOGLOBULINOPATHIES

As clinical entities, paraimmunoglobulinopathies are closely related to each other and to other immunoglobulinopathies. Considerable overlap in the clinical manifestations of the various diseases has led to confusing nomenclature, especially as related to transitional forms. The interrelationships within this group have been both fascinating and perplexing to clinician and investigator alike. While there are several helpful ways of considering and clarifying these relationships, the following system has been useful to us.

The paraimmunoglobulinopathies are associated with, and probably result from, a malignant transformation or related dyscrasia of the antibody-producing system of the body. This system is composed of several morphologic cell types (the immunocytes) , including reticulum cells, plasma cells, and lymphocytes (see Fig. 31) (Maldonado *et al.*, 1966) . Reticulum cells develop into either lymphocytes or plasma cells. Lymphocytes are probably capable of changing into plasma cells. The proteins produced by these cell lines are unusually heterogeneous and there is some evidence that the most differentiated cell types are capable of producing only certain of these protein molecules and not others. It seems likely that the protein production is intimately related to the development or differentiation of these cell lines which, in turn, is under genetic control as modified by the turning on and off of certain genes during development (Nossal, 1962) . The cells involved in immunoglobulin synthesis may undergo a number of changes, anatomic, functional, physiologic and pathologic.

Malignancy of immunocytes results in the paraimmunoglobulinopathies which are being considered here. In some situations it is difficult to decide whether one is dealing with hyperplasia or with malignancy. In considering the malignant proliferation of these cell types, it is usually possible to define a disease on the basis of cell type involved and the rest of the clinical picture. Figure 31 illustrates the typical diseases at the corners of the triangle and the atypical overlapping syndromes in the circle. When reticulum cells undergo malignant proliferation, the usual clinical picture is that of reticulum cell sarcoma or Hodgkin's disease. In reticulum cell sarcoma usually there is no obvious abnormality of the immunoglobulins. Occasionally, there is hypoimmunoglobulinemia. In Hodgkin's disease the immunoglobulins are usually normal or increased. Usually delayed hypersensitivity reactions are profoundly depressed. Occasionally there is hypoimmunoglobulinemia. Rarely, in either situation, there may be a serum myeloma protein or Bence Jones protein and the clinical picture of multiple myeloma

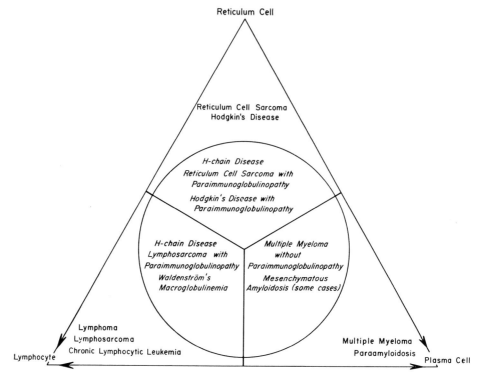

Triangle - cell types and the resulting classical diseases
*Circle - transitional diseases*

FIGURE 31. Malignant proliferation of reticulum cell, lymphocyte, and plasma cell and the resulting clinical syndromes.

(reticulum cell sarcoma and Hodgkin's disease with paraimmuno-globulinopathy). In rare cases heavy chains or fractions of heavy chains are found in the blood and urine (heavy chain disease). In malignant prolifera-tion of lymphocytes the picture is usually that of lymphosarcoma or lym-phatic leukemia. Often there is an associated hypoimmunoglobulinemia. In some instances there is also a Bence Jones proteinuria and even a serum IgG or IgA myeloma peak, and the clinical picture is indistinguishable from multiple myeloma (lymphosarcoma or lymphatic leukemia with paraimmu-noglobulinopathy). Rarely, heavy chains or fragments of heavy chains are found in the blood and urine. In most of these cases, however, the paraim-munoglobulin is a macroglobulin, and the disease picture is that of Wal-denström's macroglobulinemia. Finally, when the plasma cell is the malig-nant cell the clinical picture is usually that of multiple myeloma. There is almost always a depression of the normal immunoglobulins. Usually there is a serum myeloma protein and/or Bence Jones protein. Sometimes the clini-cal picture of primary amyloidosis is associated with the myeloma. There is no difficulty in defining the characteristic diseases but sometimes there is great difficulty in defining the atypical syndromes represented in the circle. There is no general agreement concerning what to call these cases, since many physicians put great stress on the cell type in making a diagnosis while others stress the clinical picture.

In certain conditions associated with hyperplasia of the immunoglobulin-producing cells with a generalized hyperimmunoglobulinemia, the electrophoretic pattern may show a superimposed homogeneous peak which is indistinguishable from the peak seen in the paraimmunoglobulinopathies of malignant origin. This may make it very difficult to distinguish benign physiologic hyperplasia from malignant proliferation. The borderline between benign and malignant is often poorly delineated. The homogeneous peak probably represents a manifestation of somatic mutation with proliferation of one cell clone. When this should be called premalignant or malignant or benign has not been clearly defined. Two examples illustrate this point.

A patient coming tc the attention of the physician because of a high titer cold agglutinin in the blood has all the features of autoimmune hemolytic anemia of cold agglutinin type, including the macroglobulin spike in the electrophoretic pattern of the serum proteins. However, bone marrow aspiration reveals infiltration with lymphoid cells which the pathologist has difficulty defining as benign or malignant. There may also be other evidence of lymphoid proliferation in the lymph nodes or spleen. In this situation there are two possibilities: (1) either the patient has autoimmune hemolytic anemia with cold agglutinins and, since the cold agglutinins must be manufactured somewhere, the lymphoid hyperplasia is merely the manifestation of their production; or (2) the patient has Waldenström's macroglobulinemia, a malignancy of the lymphoid cells, and the abnormal protein produced happens to have the properties of a cold agglutinin. With our present definitions not even the most careful study of the degree of homogeneity of the proteins produced or of the specificity of the cold agglutinin for red cell factors will permit differentiation.

Another patient presents with what appears to be early classic rheumatoid arthritis. However, electrophoresis of the serum proteins reveals a spike in the pattern superimposed on a relatively normal or slightly depressed gamma globulin peak. The bone marrow aspirate contains about 20 per cent plasma cells, some abnormal. No abnormalities of the bones are demonstrable by x-rays. Again there appear to be two possibilities: (1) the patient has rheumatoid arthritis and the relatively homogeneous protein spike upon electrophoresis is related to this disease; or (2) the patient has early multiple myeloma and the rheumatoid arthritis disease picture is secondary to it. In rare cases it is virtually impossible to be certain which of the two to choose.

In general, if the abnormal protein can be shown to be of just one immunologic type, a malignancy is favored. Nonetheless, it is quite probable that specific antibodies against a single immunologic determinant are also of just one immunologic type and might under certain circumstances be produced in large amounts by nonmalignant stimuli. Osterland *et al.* (1966) have reported the production of such relatively homogeneous group specific streptococcal antibodies in rabbits hyperimmunized with streptococcal vaccines.

# Chapter 8

# PARAIMMUNOGLOBULINOPATHIES:
# MULTIPLE MYELOMA

*Definition.* Multiple myeloma is a neoplastic condition of plasma cells which results in local tumors, particularly in bones, as well as in dissemi-nated infiltration of the bone marrow and other tissues. It is associated with the presence of abnormal proteins which circulate in the blood, may be excreted in the urine, or be deposited in the tissues.

## PATHOLOGY

Multiple myeloma is essentially a malignancy of the plasma cell and closely related cells. In rare situations the clinical picture of multiple mye-loma is associated with proliferation of the reticulum cell or even the lymphocyte and in still other situations mixtures of these cell types may be seen (Maldonado *et al.,* 1966). Normal plasma cells produce antibodies, and malignant plasma cells, such as those seen in multiple myeloma, pro-duce the serum myeloma proteins and Bence Jones urinary proteins. There is now considerable evidence that the myeloma proteins and Bence Jones proteins are closely related, if not identical, to antibodies.

### Morphology of the Myeloma Cell

The cell that is characteristic of multiple myeloma has been called the myeloma cell. It is seen by pathologists in sections of tumor stained with hematoxylin and eosin or eosin-methylene blue. In these preparations the tumor is characterized by sheets or infiltrations of cells having a basophilic cytoplasm, eccentric nucleus, and often one or more nucleoli. The nuclei may or may not have the typical spoke-wheel pattern of chromatin charac-teristic of the Marschalko type plasma cell. The paranuclear clear zone is poorly defined. The degree of maturity of the cells varies from patient to patient.

Hematologists make bone marrow smears, spicule smears, or bone mar-row touch preparations stained with a Romanovsky stain such as Wright's stain (see Fig. 32). The morphologic features of the myeloma cells are best seen in these preparations. Typically, the cells have abundant, strongly basophilic cytoplasm which is not absolutely homogeneous but which has a granulated appearance as a result of the endoplasmic reticulum so clearly seen upon electron microscopy (see Fig. 14). The paranuclear clear zone may be absent. Cytoplasmic inclusions (Zucker-Franklin, 1964; Bessis, 1961) which may rarely be present, are the acidophilic disks called Russell bodies (see Fig. 15), finer acidophilic granules, clear round vacuoles which are sometimes basophilic and called Mott bodies, acidophilic rods, and acidophilic plate crystals. Sometimes the cytoplasm may be filled with Mott bodies and these cells have been called Mott cells, morula cells, and "grape cells." Rarely, iron-containing inclusions have been found (Lerner and Parker, 1968). Most of these inclusions are not absolutely diagnostic of myeloma and may be seen in the cytoplasm of plasma cells in certain nonmalignant situations. In many cases of myeloma, cytoplasmic fragments without nuclei are seen in the blood smears and bone marrow smears. The nuclei of myeloma cells are usually eccentric but may rarely be centrally placed. The nuclear chromatin is relatively fine and homogeneous, in contrast to normal plasma cells, which have a coarser chromatin pattern. Depending upon the degree of immaturity of the cells, there may be nucleoli. Often one large nucleolus is present, but there may be two to four. Occasionally, vacuoles or Mott bodies may be found in the nucleus. These may lie in portions of the cytoplasm which have invaginated into the nucleus. Giant forms of myeloma cells are frequently seen.

FIGURE 32. Morphology of plasma cells and closely related cells in bone marrow smears stained with Wright's stain. Magnification X1,000 (approximately). Typical cells were selected. (A) Normal plasma cells from patient with rheumatic fever. (B) and (C) Plasma cells from patient with multiple myeloma. (D) Plasma cells from patient with multiple myeloma. Note Mott bodies in one of the cells. (E) Small plasma cell with ragged cytoplasmic border from patient with multiple myeloma. (F) Giant plasma cell with pink staining cytoplasmic border from patient with multiple myeloma. Because of staining qualities these cells are sometimes called flame cells or thesaurocytes. (G) Plasma cell from patient with idiopathic cryoglobulinemia. (H) Plasma cell (? reticulum cell) from patient with idiopathic cryoglobulinemia (same patient as G). (I) Plasma cell with rod-shaped inclusions in cytoplasm from patient with multiple myeloma and the secondary adult Fanconi syndrome. (J) Predominance of lymphocytes and paucity of plasma cells from a patient with multiple myeloma who had large amounts of a myeloma protein in the serum and Bence Jones protein in the urine. (K) Plasma cells with Russell bodies in cytoplasm and with reticulated cytoplasm from patient with multiple myeloma and paraamyloidosis. (Patient of Dr. L. W. Diggs, University of Tennessee.) (L) Plasma cells rather than the usual lymphocytes from a patient with Waldenström's macroglobulinemia.

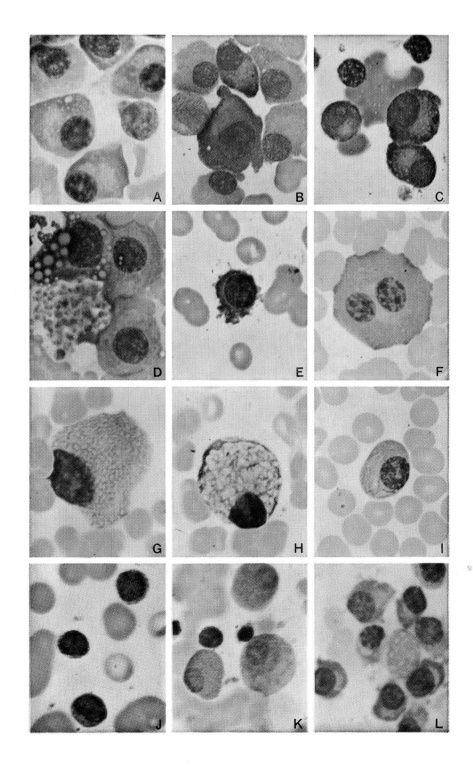

Single cells that answer to the description of myeloma cells may be found rarely in normal bone marrow aspirates. Moderate and large numbers of similar cells, even giant forms, may be found in the marrow of patients who have a marked hyperimmunoglobulinemia from any cause, such as liver disease, severe drug reaction, malignant tumor, chronic infection, Boeck's sarcoidosis, and lupus erythematosus. These cells may be indistinguishable from cells seen in some patients with multiple myeloma, though they do not have the degree of immaturity or developmental nuclear-cytoplasmic dissociation seen in some patients with myeloma. Large numbers of very immature myeloma cells with developmental nuclear-cytoplasmic dissociation are virtually diagnostic of multiple myeloma.

A number of morphologic variants may be seen. The primary cell type may be indistinguishable from small lymphocytes or may have the appearance of a myeloma cell but with the cytoplasm almost entirely ripped off. At the other extreme the cells may be unusually large, resembling reticulum cells with basophilic cytoplasm. Cells intermediate between lymphocytes and plasmacytes are frequently found.

Normal bone marrow aspirates usually contain 3 per cent or less of plasma cells. There are many conditions in which the number of plasma cells in the marrow is increased, so number of cells alone is not diagnostic. In addition, plasma cells in reactive plasmacytosis may resemble myeloma cells. However, it is unusual to have over 20 per cent plasma cells in a cellular marrow in anything other than myeloma. When increased numbers of plasma cells, particularly over 20 per cent, are associated with typical myeloma morphology, the diagnosis of multiple myeloma is likely. It is usually neither necessary nor wise to make the diagnosis on bone marrow examination alone.

Attempts to correlate morphology of myeloma or plasma cells with clinical picture or prognosis have not been uniformly productive. Most workers have found no correlation between cell morphology and protein type (Kubota, Schwartz, and Putnam, 1956). There is some evidence that the more immature and anaplastic cells are found in patients with the poorest prognosis. Likewise, Paraskevas, Heremans, and Waldenström (1961) have described cell types which are found only in myelomas of IgA type. However, most patients with IgA type myeloma do not have the distinctive cells. The characteristic cells have a large amount of cytoplasm, the edges of which stain pink with Wright's stain, and have been called flame cells or thesaurocytes. Cells from patients with IgA type myeloma are thought to have increased amounts of periodic acid-Schiff positive materials in their cytoplasm very much like the cytoplasm of cells from patients with macroglobulinemia. This relates to the fact that IgA and IgM molecules have markedly increased carbohydrate components as compared to the IgG.

The morphology of the myeloma cells differs from one patient to another and is virtually patient specific. The morphology is relatively stable from one stage of the disease to another.

### Distribution of Tumor Cells

The tumor cells may be localized in a single tumor mass or solitary myeloma found usually in the medullary cavity of bone in an area of red marrow formation such as the skull, mandible, ribs, vertebrae, pelvis, sternum, clavicle, scapula, humerus, and femur. In some cases multiple tumor masses are found. Extramedullary solitary tumors have been found in any portion of the upper part of the respiratory tract, where they most frequently occur about the larynx, palate, nose, and accessory nasal sinuses (Figi, Broders, and Havens, 1945). Other extramedullary sites of solitary and multiple plasmacytomas include the pleura, thyroid gland, lacrimal gland, ovary, stomach, intestines, kidney, spermatic cord, skin (Hellwig, 1943), and lymph nodes (Suissa, LaRosa, and Linn, 1966). Essentially, all of these tumors eventually develop into disseminated multiple myeloma. Plasma cell tumors of the conjunctiva represent a special situation. These are apparently granulomas and do not metastasize (Hellwig, 1943). These tumors occur in young individuals as well as older people. Conjunctival plasmomas are composed of dense sheets of plasma cells, often arranged perpendicular to the surface; there is no capsule. The plasma cells may contain Russell bodies and, in some instances, amyloid deposits are associated with the plasma cells (Hellwig, 1943).

Patients with disseminated multiple myeloma may have tumor cells in any organ. The red bone marrow is usually infiltrated throughout the body. In many regions the marrow may be solid tumor with typical punched-out lesions seen in x-rays. The lesions frequently result in vertebral collapse and pathologic fractures. In some instances the infiltration of the marrow is so diffuse that x-ray examination may show no abnormalities or only just a diffuse osteoporosis. The combination of multiple solid tumors and diffuse infiltration is commonly seen. Next in decreasing frequency to bone lesions is infiltration of liver, spleen, lymph nodes, kidney, lung, heart, and pancreas (Hayes, Bennett, and Heck, 1952). Infiltration of these organs may be slight or may result in complete replacement of the normal structures of the organ (spleen, lymph node) or partial replacement (liver, kidney, lung, heart, pancreas). Histologically, there is a higher proportion of primitive reticulum cells in the lymph nodes than in the bone lesions in the same case. Of interest are cases of proved multiple myeloma with lymph nodes revealing a picture of reticulum cell sarcoma and Hodgkin's disease. Are these instances of coexistence of two separate diseases of the reticuloendothelial system or one disease with diverse manifestations, depending on the organ involved?

Until recently it was thought that peripheral neuritis was rarely a result of involvement by myelomatous tissue. Barron (Barron, Rowland, and Zimmerman, 1960) performed careful pathologic examinations on three patients with myeloma and symmetric sensorimotor polyneuropathy. He found numerous focal endoneurial, penineurial, and interfascicular deposits of myeloma cells in the peripheral nerves of the extremities. At the site of metastatic infiltration, there was focal degeneration of myelin sheaths and less severe degeneration of axons. There was associated propagation of demyelination beyond the site of the focal involvement, probably representing Wallerian degeneration. No amyloid deposits were found in the peripheral nerve studies even though one patient also had generalized amyloidosis. Other investigators (Clarke, 1956) feel that neuropathy in patients with multiple myeloma may also arise from direct infiltration of nerve roots and peripheral nerves by amyloid. The muscles may also be infiltrated by tumor cells. Extramedullary tumors may be found.

In patients with disseminated disease, tumor cells in small numbers may be found in the blood. In some instances there may be a large number of tumor cells in the blood, giving the picture of plasma cell leukemia. Rarely, this is the primary manifestation of the disease.

### Amyloid

When amyloid deposits occur in association with multiple myeloma or other paraimmunoglobulinopathies, the term *paraamyloidosis* is used. It has been estimated that 10 to 20 per cent of patients with myeloma also have amyloidosis (Bayrd and Bennett, 1950; Magnus-Levy, 1952). The distribution of the deposits is that of mesenchymatous amyloidosis. The walls of blood vessels are involved in 100 per cent of cases of paraamyloidosis. In half the cases there are deposits in the heart muscle and in the lung. The gastrointestinal tract, including the tongue, esophagus, stomach, small intestine, and colon, is frequently involved. Amyloid deposits also occur in the skin, kidney, and skeletal muscle. Although there have been no good pathologic studies demonstrating it, it has been postulated that amyloid deposits along the nerves may account for the neuropathy sometimes present (Dumas, Rentschler, and Earle, 1957). Median neuritis due to amyloid deposition in the carpal tunnel has been described (Grokoest and Demartini, 1954). Rarely, there is also involvement of the liver, spleen, lymph nodes, adrenals, thyroid, and pancreas. In contrast to the amyloid found in patients with chronic infections and rheumatoid arthritis, in myeloma the amyloid usually does not stain well with Congo red or crystal violet.

### Kidney Lesions

The pathologic lesions of the kidney vary. There is usually some infiltration of the kidney with tumor cells. The characteristic lesion is the presence of many large casts in the renal tubules, some of the casts being associated with foreign body giant cells. The casts may be extremely large, concentrically laminated, and may have sharply outlined refractile edges (Zinneman, Glenchur, and Gleason, 1960). In rare instances they may stain metachromatically with methyl violet, just like amyloid (Clinicopathological Conference, 1962). Fluorescent dyes with a selective affinity for amyloid stain the casts in the majority of instances of kidney involvement (Vassar and Culling, 1962). The number of such casts does not correlate with the acute renal failure which may develop in some patients (Healy, 1963). The renal tubular epithelium may show degenerative changes and some of the tubules contain red cells. In rare instances there may be crystalline deposits in the tubules. In a few instances there have been rod-shaped crystalline deposits in the epithelial cells of the proximal convoluted tubules, associated with marked destruction of these cells. This rare lesion occurs in patients who show clinical evidence of proximal renal tubular failure, the so-called adult Fanconi syndrome, associated with the multiple myeloma (Engle and Wallis, 1957). Resorption of protein is thought to occur in the cells of the proximal convoluted tubules, and in these cells Oliver and MacDowell (1958) have demonstrated droplets which may become unusually prominent in patients with multiple myeloma. Rarely, crystalline deposits associated with foreign body giant cells have been seen in the glomeruli (Sickel, 1959). There may be some sclerosis of glomeruli, but it is not clear how directly this is related to the myeloma. Some patients have calcium deposits in the kidney, either in the parenchyma or in the calyces. Both casts and the surrounding tubular epithelium may be calcified. This usually occurs in those patients who have hypercalcemia. Other patients have uric acid deposits in the kidney similar to those seen in gout. Pyelonephritis is not uncommon. When amyloid deposits appear, the deposition is characteristically in the blood vessel walls and around the tubules. However, in some instances the deposits may be in the glomeruli and virtually indistinguishable from the lesions seen in parenchymatous amyloidosis.

## CLINICAL MANIFESTATIONS

### Bone Pain

This is usually the presenting symptom in multiple myeloma, appearing in 75 to 90 per cent of patients. In patients with diffuse myelomatosis without discrete punched-out lesions, bone pain is not a frequent complaint (Innes and Newall, 1961).

Kenny and Maloney (1957) distinguish among three general categories of pain in multiple myeloma. They are (1) the boring pain of the expanding lesion in the marrow cavity, (2) aching pain due to nerve compression, and (3) acute stabbing pain associated with a pathologic fracture. Whitelaw

(1963) surveyed seventy-two patients with multiple myeloma at the British Columbia Cancer Institute (Toronto) with respect to the causation of pain. He felt that pain, especially of acute onset, was almost always due to a fracture, although not necessarily apparent on x-ray. The great majority of osteolytic lesions were painless.

The onset of pain may be gradual over the course of weeks or months; more commonly it is abrupt, with sudden severe back or chest pain associated with a compression fracture of a thoracic or lumbar vertebra or with a rib fracture. Case histories often cite specific activities associated with the onset of bone pain. An elevator came to a sudden stop and an individual with unsuspected myeloma suffered a vertebral fracture and excruciating pain. A house painter made a misstep on a ladder with a similar result. A taxi driver who twisted awkwardly in his seat broke a rib and developed severe pain. A housewife who opened a window and fractured her right humerus suffered from excruciating pain.

Bone pain is most commonly located in the back, ribs, or pelvis, less commonly in the legs, shoulders and arms. In the adult there is a definite tendency for the disease to develop first in the axial skeleton, which houses the blood-forming marrow, but eventually the myelomatous proliferation involves the extremities as well. The intensity varies from mild ache and soreness to unbearable excruciating pain which may require frequent administration of narcotics. Pain is usually increased with motion and weight bearing. The pains may be so severe that the patient becomes completely immobilized. Coughing, sneezing, or turning in bed may provoke excruciating pain. Pain may fluctuate concomitant with healing of pathologic fractures and occurrence of new ones. There is, however, an overall tendency to progression in intensity and extension of pain in the untreated, and in many of the treated, patients. Bone tenderness may or may not accompany bone pain; it is usually not seen with back involvement, while the sternum and ribs are likely to be very tender. While palpable plasmacytomas of skull, clavicle, and mandible may be painful on motion of the part, they are seldom, if ever, tender to outside pressure.

Bone pain constitutes so much a part of the picture of myeloma that if it is missing the diagnosis is difficult. In general, patients with diffuse myelomatosis fall into this category; in these cases the main manifestation is anemia, purpura, amyloidosis, renal involvement, or increased susceptibility to infections. "Premyeloma" patients who have a myeloma-type protein in the serum or urine are also in this category. Absence of bone pain is also characteristic of the macroglobulinemia of Waldenström variant.

### Fracture

Pathologic fractures occur in 50 to 60 per cent of patients with multiple myeloma (Snapper, Turner, and Moscovitz, 1953; Yentis, 1961). They may come about after a minimal trauma or strain, either as the initial presenting manifestation or later in the course of the disease. There are three different types of fracture occurring in myeloma.

Compression fractures of thoracic or lumbar vertebrae due to diffuse infiltration or tumor formation may lead to spinal cord compression, paraplegia, neurogenic bladder, and terminal urinary tract infection.

Other true fractures occur in femur, pelvis, humerus, clavicles, sternum, and ribs. These lead to a flail chest, interfere with breathing, and are conducive to respiratory infections.

"Milkman's fractures" are usually bilaterally symmetric "pseudofractures" of ribs, pelvis, clavicles, or femora associated with osteomalacia and are observed in patients suffering from the adult Fanconi syndrome complicating myeloma (see Renal Manifestations).

Fractures heal at a normal rate, according to Snapper (Snapper, Turner, and Moscovitz, 1953); however, immobilization, common in this disease, slows down the healing process through osteoporosis. In addition, plasma cells infiltrate the callus and slow down effective healing.

With progression of the process, marked skeletal deformities develop. Multiple compression fractures cause shortening of the patient's stature, described as the "concertina effect," occasionally as much as 15 cm. Fractures of thoracic structures lead to kyphoscoliosis and flail chest. Sternal fractures in myeloma are a bad prognostic sign, as fatal ventilatory failure often follows. With pelvic and femoral fractures the gait is affected and becomes like that of a "waddling duck."

### Tumor Formation

*General Characteristics.* The incidence of plasma cell tumor formation in patients with multiple myeloma varies from 90 per cent (Geschikter and Copeland, 1928) to 20 per cent (Snapper, Turner, and Moscovitz, 1953) to 5 per cent (Innes and Newall, 1961). The discrepancy is probably due to early diagnosis of less advanced cases in the more recent series.

The tumors frequently form over the involved bone. Palpable nodules over the skull may sometimes be correlated with areas of rarefaction on x-rays. Palpable "beads" over the ribs and sternum may be areas of past fractures where the plasmacytoma has broken through the periosteum and grown out into the soft tissue. Masses over ilium, sacrum, clavicle, humerus, mandible, and maxilla have been observed.

In addition, visceral plasmacytomas may occur without contiguity to bony involvement. They have been noted to arise from upper respiratory passages, lung, lymph nodes, gastrointestinal tract, ureters, kidneys, nerve roots, and spinal cord.

Plasmacytomas vary in size from that of a pea to that of a grapefruit. When they develop within and expand the bone, they form a hard swelling.

When they perforate the cortex and spread into the subcutaneous tissue, they are usually soft and may be fluctuant. Some of these may appear warm, red, and tender and mimic an abscess. After a biopsy a bruit may sometimes be observed (Snapper, Turner, and Moscovitz, 1953). A thin shell of over-lying bone may give the plasmacytoma a crepitant consistency.

*Solitary Plasmacytoma.* This is a term reserved for cases of a single plasma cell tumor, proved by biopsy or excision, with a normal bone marrow and x-rays showing no other lesions in the rest of the skeleton. The final diagnostic criterion for this designation is that on adequate follow-up no evidence of generalization is found (Bichel and Kirketerp, 1938). The requirement of absence of protein abnormality was in the original criteria for diagnosis of solitary plasmacytoma. However, Lane (1952) reported a case of single plasmacytoma of the mandible in which an abnormal gamma globulin peak disappeared after excision of the tumor. Solitary plasma cell tumors have been reported in the pelvis, spine, clavicle, and other bones. On x-ray examination they appear as a destructive bone lesion, often are of a "soap bubble" variety (Case Records, 1960), and must be differentiated from a giant cell tumor of bone (which rarely occurs in flat bones), hemangioma, and carcinomatous metastasis from breast or kidney. In most patients who start out with what seems to be solitary plasmacytoma, multiple foci eventually appear elsewhere in the skeleton, and a generalized stage indistinguishable from multiple myeloma develops. Occasionally, solitary plasmacytomas are extramedullary, as in a lymph node (Suissa, LaRosa, and Linn, 1966) or breast (Richards, Katzmann, and Coleman, 1958).

A true solitary plasmacytoma is rare. Christopherson and Miller (1950) compiled twenty-two cases and reported three of their own with solitary tumor without generalized disease followed three years or more; five cases were followed longer than ten years; twelve cases were proved solitary at autopsy. Innes and Newall (1961) reviewed forty-six patients with solitary plasmacytoma at Edinburg Royal Infirmary. Of these, one patient was followed ten years and four patients longer than five years; five patients died of unrelated causes. Björnberg (1962) followed his patient for $1\frac{1}{2}$ years after surgical excision and radiotherapy of a small, solitary extramedullary plasmacytoma of the orbit. There was no sign of recurrence or generalization. Wright (1961) reported a patient with solitary plasmacytoma of the femur in good health and without evidence of recurrence twenty-two years after amputation. Another patient with solitary plasmacytoma of the humerus was followed for thirty-five years without recurrence. After careful follow-up of reported patients, Wright felt that only three similar cases had been reported previously; two by Christopherson and Miller (1950) (20 years after hemimandibulectomy and 19 years after curettage and radiotherapy of tibia) and one by Chesterman (1948) (16 years after amputation for plasmacytoma of tibia). These five cases carefully followed sixteen and thirty-five years substantiate the hitherto doubted concept of a true solitary plasmacytoma of bone.

**Multiple Plasmacytomas.** Multiple plasmacytomas are the form of myeloma intermediate between solitary plasmacytoma on the one hand and generalized myelomatosis on the other. This form is characterized by the presence of several isolated plasmacytomas. The term multiple myeloma technically applied to this form of the disease. It is, however, usually applied to the more generalized stage with diffuse involvement between the foci.

**Extramedullary Plasmacytomas.** The exact incidence of extramedullary plasmacytomas is difficult to determine because of the overlap between the benign inflammatory plasmacytosis of a nonosseous organ and the true tumor-like plasmacytoma. In various series the incidence has varied between 2 and 20 per cent of the total myeloma cases. Innes and Newall (1961) studied records of 188 cases of myeloma and found six cases in which extramedullary tumor formation was the first manifestation of the disease. Hellwig (1943) reviewed 128 cases of extramedullary plasmacytomas. In sixty-three cases extramedullary plasmacytomas originated in the upper respiratory passages (nasal septum, turbinates, nasopharynx, larynx, pillars, uvula, soft palate, floor of the mouth, and sublingual region). Initially, most of these were single noninvasive tumors (polypoid, pedunculated, sessile, elevated, or diffuse) ; some were multiple noninvasive tumors; some showed local destructive properties; nine had lymph node metastases, nine tumors of air passages metastasized to bones. The symptoms varied from those of entirely mechanical nature (nasal obstruction, difficulty in breathing, cough, hoarseness, sensation of a foreign body in the throat) to pain due to invasion of nerve, hemorrhage, foul discharge from necrotic areas in the locally invasive group, to a rapidly progressive downhill course and death within two years of the diagnosis. The survival in the initially noninvasive group was five to eighteen years. The patients were treated with surgery, x-rays, or both.

While extramedullary myelomas, when they occur, are frequently found in the upper part of the respiratory tract, these are still rare lesions. In a study covering fourteen years, Figi, Broders, and Havens (1945) of the Mayo Clinic found that of 360 milignant neoplasms in the pharynx, only two were plasma cell tumors; of 300 malignant growths in the nasopharynx, two were myelomas; of 625 malignancies involving the nose and accessory sinuses, six were plasma cell myeloma; and of 1,620 neoplasms of the larynx, only one was plasma cell myeloma.

Other less frequent locations of extramedullary plasmacytomas are lymph nodes, (Suissa, LaRosa, and Linn, 1966) , lacrimal gland, orbit (Björnberg, 1962) , the gastrointestinal tract (stomach [Couret, 1946], intestine [Esposito and Stout, 1945], pancreas) , pleura, thyroid, urogenital tract (kidney, spermatic cord, vulva, ovary) , and skin (especially scalp) .

Cutler (1934) and more recently Rosenberg, Attie, and Mandelbaum (1963) reported a case of multiple myeloma in which the first sign of the disorder was a plasmacytoma of the breast. Rosenberg's patient was a forty-one-year-old woman with multiple bilateral breast lesions simulating fibrocystic disease. After an investigation, the generalized character of the illness became apparent. Histologic study of the breast tumor revealed plasmacytoma. The sternal marrow was diagnostic of multiple myeloma. The protein abnormalities and later bone lytic involvement were also discovered.

A special instance of extramedullary plasmacytoma is the "benign plasmacytosis pudendi," or benign primary erythroplasia of Queyrat. The lesions are bright red plaques of the vulva or penis which on biopsy reveal plasmacytic infiltration of the upper cutis. Most cases show no progression and probably represent chronic inflammation. Hyman and Leider (1961) feel that some instances may represent a forme fruste of multiple myeloma in extramedullary location. They may, on the other hand, be premonitory of ultimate development of a more complete picture of multiple myeloma (Lightstone and Cohen, 1960).

In fifty of the 128 cases of extramedullary plasmacytomas reported by Hellwig (1943), the tumors originated in the conjuctiva of one or both of the eyelids or in the bulbar conjunctiva. They appeared as diffuse swellings or a cylindric mass, bright or bluish red, smooth, and firm. Conjunctival plasmoma is entirely benign; it was first reported in association with trachoma and considered an inflammatory lesion (Chojnacki, 1935). It may be one of the causes of hyaline and amyloid degeneration of the conjunctiva. After surgical excision a few of the tumors recurred several times, but there was no further invasion or dissemination.

From the prognostic viewpoint, localization and gross appearance are more reliable criteria than the histologic structure. Tumors of conjunctiva and of vulva are benign while those of identical cytologic character in the respiratory passages are highly destructive.

In summary, apart from the few benign tumors of extramedullary plasmacytosis (conjunctiva and pudendal region), most extramedullary plasmacytomas have the tendency to invade and metastasize. Once invasion occurs the clinical picture follows that of generalized myelomatosis. Good reviews of all recorded extramedullary plasmacytomas are presented by Dolin and DeWar (1956) and by Edwards and Zawadzki (1967).

### Diffuse Infiltration

Widespread infiltration of the skeletal system with plasma cells is much more commonly seen than solitary or multiple plasmacytomas. Most patients with this form have, in addition, multiple discrete tumors scattered throughout the bone, and the term *multiple myeloma* is classically applied to this most common form of the disease. Some patients present with diffuse skeletal dissemination which roentgenologically appears as normal or as demineralization without discrete lesions. Both forms of generalized disease, with or without discrete lesions, have been termed *disseminated myelomatosis*. Extramedullary structures (skin, lungs, liver, spleen, kidneys, mucous membrances [Lightstone and Cohen, 1960], and eye [Allen and Straatsma, 1961]) may also become diffusely infiltrated with plasmacytes.

### Lung Involvement

This occurs in about 50 per cent of patients with myeloma. Recurrent pneumonias may be an early presenting complaint, may characterize the entire course of the disease, or may be the terminal event. They are correlated with a great increase in abnormal globulins. The increased incidence of pneumococcal pneumonia in these patients suggests that there is difficulty in antibody formation against this organism. Indeed, it has been shown that patients with multiple myeloma fail to develop antibodies against pneumococcal capsular polysaccharides (Lawson *et al.*, 1955). The phagocytosis prompting action of the myeloma serums is also diminished. In addition, patients with multiple myeloma reveal patchy but severe immunologic deficiency and poor antibody response when challenged with various antigens (Linton and Dunnigan, 1963) (see Pathogenesis). It is assumed that the predominant synthesis of the abnormal myeloma globulins at the expense of true antibodies predisposes the immunologically impoverished individual to recurrent infections. Another possibility is that the high protein interferes with phagocytosis. Increased blood viscosity due to elevated globulins and to the *in vivo* rouleau formation probably decreases the pulmonary circulation and renders the lung particularly susceptible to infection.

Because of rib and sternal fractures, ventilation and clearance of secretions are frequently painful and diminished in these patients. Kyphosis resulting from compression of thoracic vertebrae may lead to emphysema. It is easy to see how a bout of unresolved pneumonia leads to bronchiectasis and thus further predisposes the patient to subsequent recurrent episodes of pneumonia. Pulmonary infarcts are not infrequent in patients bedridden from any cause. Bedrest may also lead to hypostatic pneumonia.

Finally, the underlying neoplastic process itself, plasmacytic tumor or infiltration, sometimes involves the intrathoracic structures. Following a pathologic rib fracture a subpleural tumor may grow into the chest cavity (see Fig. 36 *Right*) ; mediastinum and hilar nodes may become involved; in some cases, pleural tumors were observed without contiguous bony involvement (Innes and Newall, 1961). Plasmacytic infiltration of lung parenchyma has also been observed.

### Neurologic Symptoms and Signs

About 17 per cent (Kenny and Maloney, 1957) to 40 per cent of patients with multiple myeloma have symptoms and signs referable to the central nervous system. The clinical manifestations include hemiplegia, convulsions, psychotic episodes, cranial nerve palsies, Horner's syndrome, herpes zoster, paraplegia, degenerative cord disease, peripheral neuropathy, glove and stocking type paresthesias, ulnar nerve palsy, median neuritis, and interosseous atrophy.

The neurologic manifestations may arise from direct involvement of the nervous structure by the myelomatous tissue and from compression of the nervous structure by the involved bone. Involvement or compression of the eye may produce proptosis. More commonly, compression of the spinal cord by an involved vertebra leads to paraplegia. Peripheral nerve involvement has also been documented (Barron, Rowland, and Zimmerman, 1960).

Neurologic symptoms may also result from indirect involvement. One type of indirect involvement is through thrombosis such as that of the central retinal artery and of any of the dural sinuses. The other type is the not well understood "toxic polyneuritis" or "myeloma neuropathy," well described by Victor and associates (1958). This symmetric polyneuropathy shows a predilection to lower extremities and distal segments; it manifests itself as marked atrophy of involved muscles, with impairment of all sensory modalities. Pathology consists of striking degeneration of the myelin sheaths and axis cylinders of the peripheral nerves and to a lesser degree of the anterior and posterior spinal roots. Frequently, the cerebrospinal fluid protein is markedly elevated. In some cases of persistent peripheral neuritis, repeated biopsies failed to reveal any pathologic lesion except nerve atrophy (Kenny and Maloney, 1957). Of great significance is the fact that the clinical manifestations of the neuropathy may precede those of multiple myeloma. Likewise, the neurologic manifestations may dominate the clinical picture. Even so, the myelomatous involvement may be minimal and go unnoticed until autopsy. Some students of this problem think that the "myeloma polyneuropathy" is causally related to the toxic effect of abnormal globulins on the nerve tissue, but there is no good evidence to support this belief. "Myeloma polyneuropathy" is actually similar clinically and pathologically to the mixed sensory-motor type of neuropathy observed in association with other neoplastic diseases, especially bronchogenic carcinoma. Victor and associates (1958) make a distinction between the myelomatous and carcinomatous neuropathy just described and the sensory carcinomatous neuropathy in which degeneration of dorsal root ganglion cells is the most prominent change. All these neurologic signs and symptoms may long precede the manifestations of the associated neoplasm; therefore, in patients with obscure neuropathies a careful search should be made for carcinoma and multiple myeloma.

Progressive multifocal leukoencephalopathy has been reported in two cases of multiple myeloma (Bethlem, van Gool, and den Hartog Jager, 1964; DelDuca and Morningstar, 1967). Most of the fifty cases of progressive multifocal leukoencephalopathy have been associated with an underlying chronic disease, usually lymphoma, leukemia, carcinoma, or granuloma. In this syndrome multiple foci of demyelination occur in cerebrum, cerebellum, brain stem, and basal ganglia. Clinically, progressive focal neurological signs and dementia lead to death in two to six months. The cerebrospinal fluid is usually normal and the electroencephalogram is diffusely and nonspecifically abnormal.

Cerebral toxoplasmosis in a patient with multiple myeloma has been reported (Theologides, Osterberg and Kennedy, 1966). This unusual infestation is probably related to lowered resistance to infection.

### Renal Manifestations

Renal and urinary signs and symptoms of multiple myeloma are many and diverse and occur in 60 to 90 per cent of patients with this disease (Sanchez and Domz, 1960).

Myelomatous infiltration of kidneys may be asymptomatic; it may result, however, in distortion of the calyceal structures, giving on intravenous pyelography the appearance of a cystic kidney. Renal shadows are not infrequently enlarged in myeloma (Recant and Hartroft, 1961).

Two discrete clinical syndromes are associated with excretion of Bence Jones protein. One is correlated with the finding of a classic myeloma kidney with eosinophilic casts and giant cells blocking the tubules, resulting in degeneration of tubular cells; the term *internal hydronephrosis* has been applied to this condition (Macalister and Addison, 1961). Clinically, it is characterized by progressive and severe renal failure with proteinuria, cylindruria, hematuria, pyuria, decrease in all renal functions (especially PSP excretion), and profound uremia with a striking absence of hypertension. Multiple myeloma is not an uncommon cause of chronic renal failure in patients over forty and should also be considered in differential diagnosis of albuminuria and elevated blood urea nitrogen in the setting of a normal blood pressure. Renal insufficiency is responsible for 43 per cent of deaths in multiple myeloma (Allen, 1951).

The other clinical syndrome associated with Bence Jones proteinuria is correlated with more subtle changes produced by a crystalline material (suspected but not proved to be Bence Jones protein) deposited in the cells of the proximal convoluted tubule. These changes result in interference with the resorptive functions of the proximal tubule through a mechanical displacement, a competitive saturation of the resorptive enzymes, or a direct toxic effect on the enzymes involved (Wallis and Engle, 1957). The resulting clinical symptom complex bears the name of the adult Fanconi syndrome (Engle and Wallis, 1957; Sirota and Hamerman, 1954; Dragstedt and Hjorth, 1956; Muntendam, 1958; Short and Smith, 1959; Dedmon, West, and Schwartz, 1963; Costanza and Smoller, 1963; DaCosta *et al.*, 1960) and is seen in a number of other conditions associated with a proximal tubular defect. It is characterized by hypophosphatemia, osteomalacia with multiple fractures and pseudofractures, elevated alkaline phosphatase, massive generalized amino-aciduria, renal glycosuria, albuminuria, mild systemic acidosis, occasional hypokalemia, and hypouricemia. The blood urea nitrogen is almost always normal. Sometimes only the renal tubular acidosis is found (Sanchez and Domz, 1960).

Acute or chronic pyelonephritis is a common complication of multiple myeloma with or without Bence Jones proteinuria. The susceptibility to infections must play a predisposing role in the kidney as well as in the lung. Renal abscess may form.

Nephrocalcinosis is common in patients with myeloma, is probably related to hypercalcemia, may be evident radiologically, and may contribute to renal failure. Hyperuricemia is present in about 40 per cent of patients with myeloma (Osserman, 1959). Uric acid nephropathy and stones occur with variable frequency.

A picture indistinguishable from acute glomerulonephritis or nephrotic syndrome may be seen as well as acute tubular necrosis and water-losing nephritis (Sanchez and Domz, 1960). Nephrosclerosis, an independent finding in some of the elderly patients with multiple myeloma, further complicates the renal picture.

Associated amyloidosis with or without renal vein thrombosis may lead to a classic nephrotic syndrome with massive albuminuria, hypoalbuminemia, edema, and hypercholesterolemia.

Hematuria, microscopic to massive, may, in addition, be caused by the bleeding diathesis in myeloma (see Laboratory Findings).

Acute anuria has been reported by Healy (1963) in three patients with multiple myeloma; he also reviewed eight previously recorded case histories with this syndrome. The cause of acute anuria in this situation is not clear. Obstruction to flow by Bence Jones protein casts has been held responsible in most cases. However, the histology in Healy's patients revealed so few Bence Jones protein casts as to suggest that they may be coincidental and not the basic cause of the anuria. Two patients with acute oliguric renal failure had no Bence Jones proteinuria. It is likely that the acute anuria is precipitated by a fall in hitherto compromised glomerular filtration in myeloma. Dehydration due to gastrointestinal loss, febrile illness, or preparation for pyelography was present in eight of eleven cases. Anuria followed intravenous pyelography in five of eleven cases (Healy, 1963; Killmann, Gjorup and Thaysen, 1957). This procedure has been incriminated because of its tendency to lower glomerular filtration rate by dehydration and abdominal compression. Renal vasoconstriction may also occur as a reaction to the dye and further lower the filtration rate. Acute renal failure in multiple myeloma need not always be fatal as demonstrated by Bryan and Healy (1968) ; in their case considerable improvement in renal pathology was accomplished with a combination of dialysis, supportive therapy as well as melphalan.

In summary, renal symptomatology varies greatly in patients with multiple myeloma. It ranges from asymptomatic cases through those with hematuria, pyuria, cylindruria, renal colic, adult Fanconi syndrome, and nephrotic syndrome, to chronic renal failure and acute anuria.

### Hepatosplenomegaly and Lymphadenopathy

In about 40 per cent of patients with myeloma, hepatomegaly has been noted (Snapper, Turner and Moskovitz, 1953). Although plasmacytic infiltration of the liver is rare, amyloid deposits are not infrequent. Hepatomegaly with hepatic failure may occur as a result of urethan toxicity. In about a quarter of cases hepatosplenomegaly has been described (Snapper, Turner and Moskovitz, 1953). Ascites is rare. Though the incidence of lymphadenopathy is not well documented, it is not uncommon.

### Gastrointestinal Symptoms

Anorexia, nausea, vomiting, and diarrhea are frequent symptoms in myeloma prior to any treatment. Gastrointestinal symptoms are more marked in azotemic patients but may be present in the absence of renal disease. In spite of the frequency of gastrointestinal complaints, myelomatous lesions are seldom found in the gastrointestinal tract at autopsy (Kenny and Maloney, 1957). More frequently amyloid deposits occur in this system. Amyloid deposits are responsible for the macroglossia occasionally seen in this disease.

Rarely, an extramedullary plasmacytoma may be found arising in the pancreas or in the stomach (Richards, Katzmann, and Coleman, 1958). Wuketich and Maehr (1963) reported a case of myelomatosis massively involving the stomach and to a lesser degree the pancreas, spleen, one adrenal, and the thyroid.

Loss of weight occurs preterminally in all cases of multiple myeloma. Since many patients survive a number of years with this disease, weight loss may not be present at the time the diagnosis is made and may not occur until much later in the course of the illness. It varies from no more than a couple of pounds to forty and sixty pounds. In Kenny and Maloney's (1957) series, weight loss of a few pounds to fifty pounds occurred in sixty-three per cent of the patients.

### Cardiac Manifestations

Congestive heart failure seen in multiple myeloma may be due to the incidentally associated arteriosclerotic heart disease aggravated by concomitant anemia or may be due to amyloidosis of the heart (See Paraamyloidosis). The usual striking absence of hypertension despite urinary findings and renal impairment has been commented on previously.

### Manifestations of Associated Cryoglobulinemia

When cryoglobulins are present, patients suffer from impairment of blood flow through arterioles, resulting in epistaxis, bleeding gums, purpura, hypersensitivity to cold, cyanosis, and Raynaud's syndrome. Cryoglobulinemia is sometimes responsible for thromboses, peripheral as well as those of dural sinuses and of the retinal vessels (see Fig. 33). Visual disturbances due to increased viscosity of the blood, to massive dilatation of the tortuous veins, or to thromboses are frequent. Rouleaux formation and red cell autoagglutination which are common in peripheral smears of myeloma patients are accentuated in the presence of cryoglobulinemia and may interfere with blood typing at room temperature. For further discussions see under Pathogenesis of the Paraimmunoglobulinopathies in Chapter 7.

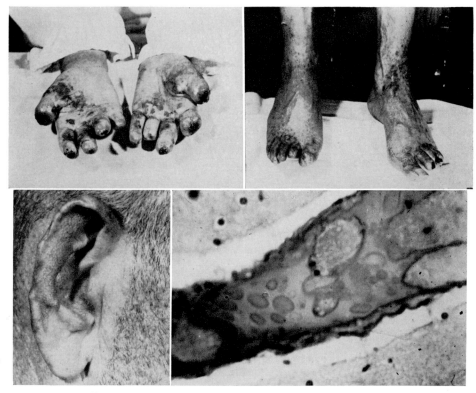

FIGURE 33. Manifestations of cryoglobulinemia. (*Upper left*) Gangrene of hands. (*Upper right*) Gangrene of feet. (*Lower left*) Detail of ear. (*Lower right*) Longitudinal section of a blood vessel of the brain, showing dense precipitate within the lumen. H & E stain, X400. (Reprinted with permission from BARR, D. P.; ENGLE, R. L., JR., and RUSS, ELLA M.: *Ann Inter Med, 47*:1225, 1957.)

### Hyperviscosity Symptoms

Aggregation of IgG globulin and IgG polymer formation elevates serum viscosity and may lead to symptoms which resemble those of macroglobulinemia (Smith, Kochwa and Wasserman, 1965). These symptoms are bleeding, especially from the mucous membranes of nose and mouth, and disturbed vision, dilatation and segmentation of retinal veins, round hemorrhages, and papilledema. Also, decreased pulse pressure, vertigo, electroencephalographic changes, syncope, convulsions, distention of dependent veins and capillaries and dependent plethora and edema may be present.

### Skin, Vascular Tissues, Extremities

The findings include amyloid infiltration of skin and joints (see Clinical Manifestations of Paraamyloidosis), clubbing, disappearance of lunulae (crescents on fingernails) (Snapper, Turner and Moskovitz, 1953), appearance of Beau's lines (transverse bands on the fingernails) (Aberg and Craig, 1966), and xanthelasma. Raynaud's phenomenon may occur owing to the presence of cryoglobulinemia. Abnormal proteins in the plasma may be partly responsible for thromboses, peripheral as well as of the dural sinuses and the central retinal artery. Bleeding diathesis is due to thrombocytopenia, interference with the clotting process by the abnormal proteins, or to capillary damage caused by abnormal proteins such as cryoglobulin. Hemorrhagic tendencies in myeloma occur in about 10 per cent of patients (Kenny and Maloney, 1957) but are usually not severe. Purpura and epistaxis are the most common of these manifestations. However, massive subcutaneous hemorrhages, gastrointestinal hemorrhage, and hematuria may occur.

A skin condition which is probably (but not certainly) related to plasma cell myeloma is papular mucinosis or "lichen myxedematosus." In this unusual form of tissue proteinosis the deposits may give rise to generalized lichenoid form of the disease with many small discrete flesh colored nodules 2 to 3 mm in diameter distributed over the entire body but with a predilection for the hands, forearms, upper part of the trunk, face and neck. The papules eventually coalesce and with time massive furrows form over the face and brow, giving the patient a saddened look, with reduction of facial expressiveness and impairment of movements of the jaw. Heavy, disabling and disfiguring folds form over the trunk and extremities interfering with walking. Other forms of papular mucinosis are characterized by larger papules and anular lesions, flesh colored to red, lichenoid plaques which resemble lichen planus, urticareal plaques and nodular eruptions.

The histological changes consist of marked edema of upper cutis with splitting and fragmentation of collagen fibers into a loose fibrillar network and a fine granular material around the fibrils. Similar changes occur about the hair follicles. Large stellate cells resembling fibroblasts are interspersed among the fibrils. In older lesions fibroblasts become more numerous—cellular infiltrate chiefly lymphocytes, variable number of mast cells, histiocytes and polymorphonuclear leukocytes may or may not be noted about the blood vessels and skin appendages. The fibrillar material stains metachromatically with toluidine blue but not with methyl violet and does not take the Congo red stain. As hyaluronidase pretreatment changes the material so that it is no longer metachromatic with toluidine blue, it was thought that the deposits represent mucin, hence the appellation "papular mucinosis." "Lichen myxedematosus" is derived from purely gross resemblance to localized pretibial myxedema. However, thyroid function tests are normal in the lichen myxedematosus. Perry, Montgomery and Stickney (1960) were the first to report a case of this disease associated with multiple myeloma with an abnormal peak migrating in the beta region on electrophoresis. Osserman and Takatsuki (1965) studied another patient with this association and postulated that the fundamental disorder was a paraimmunoglobulinopathy and that the skin deposits consisted of an exceptionally basic IgG bound to the acidic mucopolysaccharides of the connective tissue ground substance.

### Systemic Manifestations

These include weight loss, generalized weakness, and fever. Fever is usually associated with infections, clinically obvious or occult. Occasionally, low grade vacillating fever may persist. When vigorous diagnostic efforts fail to discover infection, the fever is attributed to the malignancy itself.

### Radiologic Manifestations

In diffuse myelomatosis x-ray studies are often negative. Radiologically, resorption of bone can be recognized only after 20 to 40 per cent of the calcium has disappeared (Snapper, Turner and Moscovitz, 1953). The invaded skeleton may appear normal, as quite large areas of bone destruction may occur without x-ray evidence of bone involvement (Yentis, 1961).

In about 25 to 40 per cent of cases of myeloma x-ray films show diffuse demineralization of the skeleton (see Fig. 34 *Left*) or coarse trabeculation (Lewin and Stein, 1958). These findings probably represent diffuse infiltration of bone marrow spaces by myeloma cells, leading to thinning and destruction of trabeculae (Starcich, 1957). These microradiologic lesions usually coalesce later to result in frank osteolysis. In addition, disuse osteoporosis, resulting from the immobilization seen so frequently in this disease, contributes to the radiologic picture of demineralization. The disease usually progresses faster in individuals with diffuse demineralization with or without lytic lesions than in those with discrete lytic lesions alone. Patchy demineralization may be the only radiologic finding in myeloma.

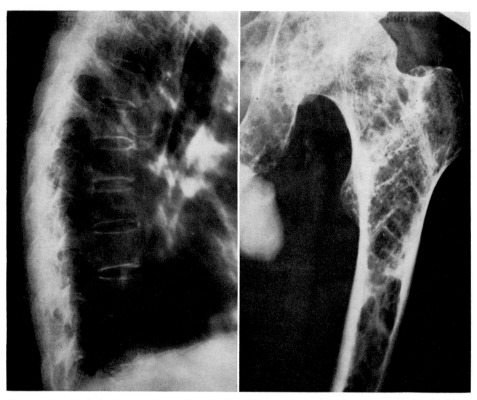

FIGURE 34. Radiologic manifestations. *(Left)* Thoracic spine, lateral, showing diffuse demineralization. *(Right)* Head of femur. (Prepared in consultation with Dr. Mordecai Halpern.)

The characteristic punched-out areas of increased translucency of the involved portion of bone, and especially of the skull, have been recognized as the x-ray lesion par excellence of multiple myeloma and occur in about 50 per cent of cases. However, punched-out areas as the exclusive type of bone lesion are rather exceptional and occur in only 13 per cent of cases (Lewin and Stein, 1958). These lesions usually have a clear-cut margin, sometimes a "soap bubble" or septate appearance (see Fig. 34 *Right*). Their distribution is wide and includes the skull (see Fig. 35 *Upper*), where they are best seen, pelvis (see Fig. 35 *Lower*), spine, ribs, clavicles, sternum, and proximal long bones of the extremities (see Fig. 36 *Left*). A predominant involvement of the distal ends of the extremities and the phalanges has been described in a patient with an alpha myeloma and hemolytic anemia (Osserman, 1959).

The radiologic features, which correlate with the pathology, are multiple. They arise primarily in the medulla either as nodules or as diffuse infiltration. In the skull, early lesions are confined to the diploe, and tangential views are necessary to visualize them; later, lesions coalesce and invade both inner and outer tables (Galgano, 1955). They destroy bone trabeculae.

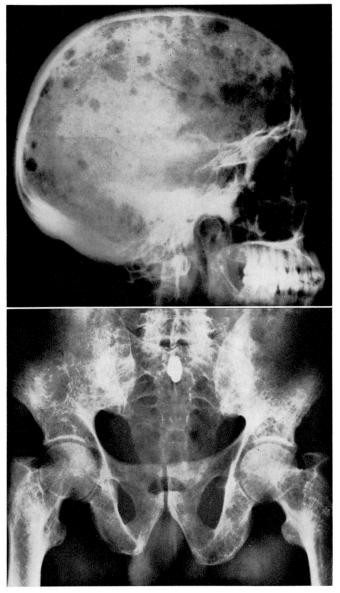

FIGURE 35. (*Upper*) Skull. (*Lower*) Pelvis. (Prepared in consultation with Dr. Mordecai Halpern.)

They erode the cortex from within and may lead to a sharply scalloped appearance. They tend to expand bone. They often reach the periosteum and form soft tissue masses, such as subpleural masses arising from the ribs (see Fig. 36 *Right*) and subcutaneous masses arising from the clavicles. The osteolytic foci tend to coalesce, forming large areas of destruction inviting pathologic fractures which occur in 62 per cent of patients (see Fig. 36 *Left*) (Yentis, 1961). Compression fractures of thoracic and lumbar vertebrae are

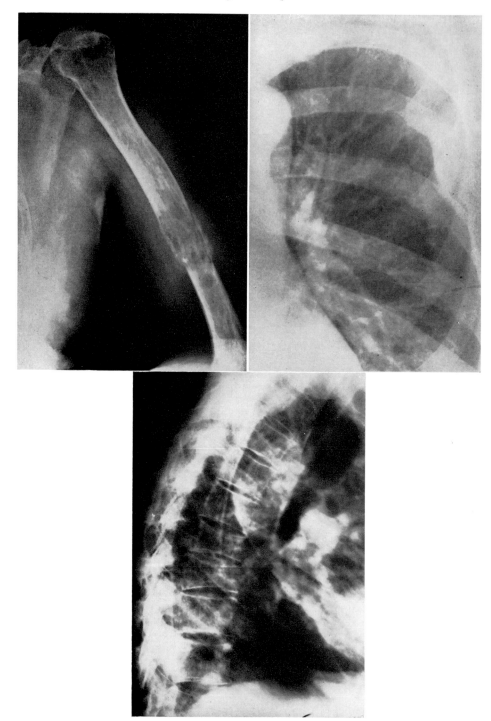

FIGURE 36. Radiologic manifestations. (*Left*) Humerus showing punched-out lesion, fracture, and callus formation. (*Right*) Subpleural mass. (*Lower*) Thoracic spine showing compression fracture. (Prepared in consultation with Dr. Mordecai Halpern.)

common (see Fig. 36 *Lower*). Milkman's pseudofractures due to osteomalacia of the adult Fanconi syndrome associated with multiple myeloma have been mentioned. They are symmetric, usually multiple bands of radiolucency occurring in ribs, pelvis, clavicles, and upper and lower extremities. No displacement is noted. These bands are localized areas of osteomalacia in the vicinity of encircling arteries. Lesions in the mandible are common in multiple myeloma; this is helpful in the differential diagnosis. Soft tissue extension, also frequently seen in myeloma, helps to distinguish these lytic lesions from those of metastatic carcinoma.

In the past, many authors emphasized as the most important feature the complete lack of hypercalcification and new bone formation in myeloma (Schinz *et al.*, 1952a; Carson, Ackerman, and Maltby, 1955). X-ray evidence of sclerosis or new bone formation would suggest to them that the process is other than myeloma. However, in recent years Krainin, D'Angio, and Smelin (1949), Lewin and Stein (1958), Odelberg-Johnson (1959), and Langley, Sabean and Sorger (1966) described untreated cases of myeloma with sclerotic lesions on x-ray in the absence of fractures. In addition, they found lytic lesions having sclerotic margins. New bone deposition in the callus after a fracture has been described (see Fig. 36 *Left*). Localized areas of sclerosis in myeloma may occur in the presence of paraamyloid (Schinz *et al.*, 1952b). Radiologic evidence of recalcification has also been reported after x-ray therapy (Russo and Brown, 1956) and after urethan therapy (Rundles and Reeves, 1950).

In summary, multiple myeloma has no characteristic x-ray features that will result in a definite diagnosis although the diagnosis is frequently suspected on the basis of x-ray findings. The punched-out lesions formerly held to be characteristic are present in less than half the cases. Specimens of bone marrow or bone biopsy and in some cases autopsy specimens are essential to make a definite diagnosis.

### Association with Other Diseases

Of great interest are several reports of cases of multiple myeloma associated with coexistent or preexistent rheumatoid arthritis (Galli and Chiti, 1955; Davis, Weber, and Bartfeld, 1957; Perl, 1958). The exact relationship of the two entities in each case is not well understood from the available data. However, the following several possibilities present themselves.

1. An initial erroneous diagnosis of rheumatoid arthritis is made on the basis of osteoarthritis and associated anemia, splenomegaly, subcutaneous masses, and elevated sedimentation rate, while in reality these associated findings are manifestations of unsuspected myeloma (Perl, 1958) occasionally complicated by paraamyloidosis (Goldberg, Brodsky, and McCarty, 1964).

2. Reactive plasmacytosis and the diffuse type of hyperglobulinemia

with an increase of the macroglobulin, "rheumatoid factor," are simply manifestations of rheumatoid arthritis. Parenchymatous amyloidosis is not infrequently seen in this disease and all these manifestations of rheumatoid arthritis may sometimes be mistakenly diagnosed as multiple myeloma.

3. Rheumatoid arthritis associated with an excessively stimulated reticuloendothelial system with plasmacytosis and hyperglobulinemia may have modified the "biologic background" so as to predispose to development of myeloma (Galli and Chiti, 1955).

4. The abnormal serum proteins in myeloma may be the cause of articular damage as suggested by Chini (1950).

5. Joint manifestations found in myeloma might be the result of paraamyloid infiltration of articular and periarticular structures.

6. The two processes may be unrelated.

Coexistence of Paget's disease of bone and multiple myeloma is rare. Of 1 million patients admitted to Veterans Administration hospitals between 1949 and 1953, 1,136 (1:880) were diagnosed as having Paget's disease, and 900 (1:1,111) were found to have multiple myeloma. In only two cases both diseases occurred in the same patient, an incidence of 1 in 500,000 (Rosenkrantz and Gluckman, 1957). Since then, Serre and Simon (1959) and Grader and Moynihan (1961) have reported one more case each. The authors have been observing a patient with asymptomatic paraimmunoglobulinemia and Paget's disease for ten years. This makes a total of five cases. This incidence is probably lower than chance occurrence. Though both multiple myeloma and Paget's disease involve bone destruction, there are a number of interesting differences in their effect on bone. In multiple myeloma there is little osteoblastic activity and the alkaline phosphatase is rarely elevated. In Paget's disease both osteoclasia and bone formation occur with a high alkaline phosphatase and there is a remodelling of the bone rather than progressive bone destruction.

Although hyperuricemia occurs in about 40 per cent of patients with multiple myeloma (Osserman, 1959), an associated acute gouty arthritis is extremely rare. Only seven cases have been reported in the literature (Talbott, 1959). These cases may have manifested a totally unrelated gouty diathesis.

Development of myeloma in three patients with chronic osteomyelitis of twenty-seven to forty-three years' duration has been recorded (Baitz and Kyle, 1964). In two of these, plasma cell tumors developed in the osteomyelitic sinus tract. This interesting association may lead to speculation that the chronic irritation of the tissue by infection could have been an oncogenic factor.

Blanchard and Olin (1961) reported a case of diffuse histoplasmosis associated with multiple myeloma. The relationship may have been simply that the malignant transformation of the reticuloendothelial system altered the host's ability to deal with the fungal infection.

In about 20 per cent of fifty-seven cases of multiple myeloma autopsied at the Mallory Institute of Pathology from 1930 to 1956, a second neoplasm was found (Weitzel, 1958). This compared to 8 percent of 365 cases of lymphoma and leukemia and 4 per cent of 3,398 cases of another primary carcinoma. The need for thorough clinical examination of patients with known primary cancer and a coexistent osteolytic lesion must be emphasized. Because of the bone lesion the patient may not be offered a chance of surgical or other curative treatment of the primary cancer on the assumption that the osteolytic lesion represents a metastasis. The life expectancy of a patient with multiple myeloma may be appreciably longer than that of a patient with metastatic carcinoma. If the osteolytic lesion is due to myeloma, curative therapy for any incidentally associated carcinoma should be considered. For this reason, patients with plasma cell myeloma must be thoroughly examined for a possible coexistent carcinoma. Association of osteogenic sarcoma and multiple myeloma has been reported by Grader and Moynihan (1961). Association of various malignancies with paraimmunoglobulinemia is discussed under Paraimmunoglobulinopathies Associated with Other Diseases—Other Malignancies in Chapter 9.

The relationship of multiple myeloma to diseases of lipid metabolism has been of great interest. Strikingly low cholesterol (Lewis and Page, 1954) and low total lipid (Kanzow, 1958) values in patients with multiple myeloma and macroglobulinemia have been commented on repeatedly. Hypercholesterolemia occurs when the nephrotic syndrome develops in these conditions (Osserman and Takatsuki, 1963a; Waldenström, 1952). In addition, the degree of atherosclerosis found in patients with multiple myeloma is remarkably decreased as compared with the expected degree in this age group (Spain *et al.*, 1956). However, records of ten cases of multiple myeloma associated with familial hyperlipidemia, hypercholesterolemia, and xanthomatosis (Osserman and Takatsuki, 1963a; Heremans, 1960; Lennard-Jones, 1960; Marten, 1963; Frame, Pachter, and Nixon, 1961; Levin *et al.*, 1964; Cohen *et al.*, 1966) and one case of Gaucher's disease associated with paraimmunoglobulinemia are found in the literature.

Association of multiple myeloma with myeloproliferative disorders such as polycythemia vera and myelofibrosis with myeloid metaplasia has been observed on several occasions (Brody, Beizer and Schwartz, 1964; Heinle *et al.*, 1966).

### Asymptomatic Patients

In the early stages of multiple myeloma, some patients present with only a typical paraimmunoglobulin spike in the serum electrophoretic pattern. These individuals may be entirely asymptomatic. A number of these may have an unexplained elevation of the sedimentation rate, although some show a surprisingly normal sedimentation rate despite an abnormal globulin peak. Some of these patients suffer from an increased susceptibility to infection; others have a mild bleeding disorder with occasional purpuric eruptions. Bone marrow examinations, skeletal x-rays, and urinalyses are repeatedly normal. Other patients may have an unexplained proteinuria.

Electrophoretic studies of large series of presumably normal individuals followed over many years may throw light on the duration and further significance of the premyeloma stage. Routine urinary protein electrophoresis in patients with unexplained proteinuria might identify some of these cases in an early stage. The larger topic of asymptomatic paraimmunoglobulinemia is considered later, in Chapter 9.

## LABORATORY FINDINGS

### *Peripheral Blood*

On initial examination of patients with myeloma, in about 30 per cent there is no anemia; 45 per cent have a moderate degree and 25 per cent a severe degree of anemia (Innes and Newall, 1961). In about 5 per cent the presenting symptoms are those of anemia alone. Anemia is commoner in the group with diffuse myelomatosis (Innes and Newall, 1961) than in multiple plasmacytoma. With progression of disease, anemia appears in virtually all cases (Osserman, 1959). The severity of anemia is variable. In some cases moderate anemia persists without progression and is well tolerated; in others it attains a severe degree and requires frequent blood transfusions.

Generally, anemia is normocytic and normochromic but may be macrocytic. Anemia of multiple myeloma may be due to a combination of factors. The major factor is an incompletely compensated hemolytic process, manifested by inadequate erythropoiesis in the face of a moderately shortened red cell life span (see Pathogenesis). This basic defect is frequently complicated by extravascular blood loss, iron deficiency, and by a more marked hemolytic component.

The white blood count is usually unremarkable. However, in about a quarter of the cases moderate to severe leukopenia may be present. As in anemia, the exact etiology is unknown but leuko-agglutinins have been implicated as well as the impaired ability of the partially replaced bone marrow to respond adequately to the accelerated leukocyte destruction. Leukopenia may contribute to the increased susceptibility to infections. Lymphocytosis up to 60 per cent has been observed. Leukemoid reaction may occur with a shift to the left in the myeloid series and a significant increase in myelocytes and promyelocytes. In a small number of cases unexplained eosinophilia up to 46 per cent has been noted in the absence of manifest allergy or parasitic infestation (Snapper, Turner, and Moskovitz, 1953).

Plasma cells can be seen in the peripheral blood in the majority of cases if buffy coats are examined (Ginsberg, 1962). Sometimes cytoplasmic fragments of plasma cells are seen in blood smears. *Plasma cell leukemia,* which represents the rarest and most malignant clinical variant of myeloma, should be considered not as a separate entity but as a part of the spectrum of primary plasma cell dyscrasia or as a phase in the generalized disease process. Up to 1957 only fifty cases had been reported (Bichel *et al.,* 1952), but several have been reported since then (Thorling, 1962; Gjerlow, 1959; A case, 1962). Plasma cell leukemia is characterized by white cell counts up to 38,000, of which 20 to 90 per cent are plasma cells. The disease terminates fatally; its average duration is from six to eight months, while the duration of the aleukemic forms averages eighteen to twenty-four months. Clinically, these patients suffer from anemia, thrombocytopenia, bleeding diathesis, generalized lymphadenopathy, hepatosplenomegaly, and varying degrees of bone pain. Renal involvement occurs in 50 per cent of the cases. In most cases of plasma cell leukemia only slight changes are seen in the distribution of the serum proteins (Thorling, 1962), although according to Bichel (Bichel *et al.,* 1952) Bence Jones proteinuria, increased sedimentation rate, and abnormal serum proteins occur in plasma cell leukemia with the same frequency as in other myeloma variants. Plasma cell leukemia with the rare IgD peak has been recorded (Ben-Bassat *et al.,* 1968). Bence Jones protein-emia has also been reported (Mullinax, Mullinax, and Himrod, 1967). Most commonly, hypogammaglobulinemia is seen in this form and the total protein concentration may be normal or even reduced. Punched-out lesions are usually not seen in the bones.

Platelet counts are usually normal in most cases of myeloma. In about a quarter of the cases, thrombocytopenia may be observed; this may contribute to the bleeding diathesis. The etiology of thrombocytopenia in myeloma is obscure, but it may be similar to that of the anemia and leukopenia; namely, enhanced platelet destruction (possibly by platelet agglutinins) and an incompletely compensating thrombocytopoiesis by a partially replaced bone marrow.

Rouleaux formation on the slide and "red sand" or agglutination in the red cell pipette are the oldest observed phenomena in the clinical pathology of myeloma. Rouleaux formation can be observed in half the patients. Agglutination in the red cell pipette is less frequent. Both phenomena are related to the presence of an abnormal globulin in blood.

Grossly elevated sedimentation rates are found in 51 per cent of patients, moderately increased rates in 34 per cent, and normal sedimentation rates in 15 per cent of 122 cases (Innes and Newall, 1961). Normal sedimentation rates occurred most frequently in solitary plasmacytomas. There is a general but not wholly consistent correlation between an elevated sedimentation rate and the degree of hyperglobulinemia.

### Bone Marrow

The uneven distribution of lesions in the bone marrow of patients with multiple myeloma requires that this organ be examined repeatedly before this disease is ruled out. In Innes and Newall's (1961) study of 130 patients in whom bone marrow punctures were done, initial findings were characteristic of multiple myeloma in only 108. Twenty-two patients initially had a normal bone marrow; half of these had a solitary plasmacytoma, three had only extramedullary lesions. However, eight were later found to have multiple plasmacytomas. This diagnostic difficulty is characteristic and in some patients three or four bone marrow examinations are done before the diagnosis is established. In some cases, the difficulty in obtaining a representative bone marrow sample is related to inability to aspirate because of dense packing of plasma cells and to dilution by peripheral blood because of associated hemorrhage. Repeated bone marrow aspirations or even a bone biopsy may be necessary to reach an unequivocal diagnosis. In Silver's (1965) series, a posterior iliac crest biopsy using the Vim-Silverman needle was at least as helpful as open sternal biopsy. In most cases it is unnecessary to perform splenic punctures for diagnosis of myeloma, although plasmacytes are often present in that organ as well (Watson *et al.,* 1955) .

The characteristic findings on the bone marrow aspiration are described in detail under Pathology. The bone marrow contains a large number of abnormal-appearing plasma cells (see Fig. 32) . If the marrow aspiration contains sheets of myeloma cells, the diagnosis is likely. With a smaller number of scattered myeloma cells, the diagnosis may be less certain, especially if the cells are of the more mature type. While some patients with reactive, benign plasmacytosis may have as many as 10 to 15 per cent plasma cells in the marrow, an increase of more than 3 per cent should be considered suspicious, especially when coupled with abnormal morphology (nucleocytoplasmic dissociation, nucleoli, absence of paranuclear clear zone, presence of Russell bodies, Mott cells, giant multinucleated cells, and cytoplasmic fragments) .

Yet another finding on bone marrow aspiration is rouleaux formation which parallels that of peripheral blood. Megakaryocytes may be increased in early stages of myeloma, especially in the face of active bleeding. Late in myeloma, megakaryocytes may be decreased or absent, in keeping with general failure or invasion of the bone marrow. With bleeding or hemolysis, erythroid hyperplasia may be present; in the late stages of the disease hypoplasia occurs.

Of special interest in some cases of myeloma is the tendency toward macrocytosis and megaloblastosis. Forshaw (1963) reported a patient with multiple myeloma and megaloblastosis of the bone marrow whose anemia responded partially to vitamin $B_{12}$ injections. This patient had free acid in the stomach, a borderline Schilling test, and a somewhat lowered serum vitamin $B_{12}$ level. In our series a few patients with multiple myeloma had previously been misdiagnosed as having pernicious anemia. The relationship of myeloma and megaloblastosis is not well understood. One may speculate that the enhanced purine metabolism of the plasma cells may direct all the enzymes and building blocks involved in synthesis of nucleic acids, including vitamin $B_{12}$ and folic acid, toward the plasma cells, creating a relative deficiency in the erythroid cells.

### Serum Proteins

Total serum protein is increased in most patients with myeloma. Albumin is usually normal or decreased, and globulin is usually increased as determined by the Howe fractionation technique. However, in some patients total protein and albumin/globulin ratio may be completely normal because the technique does not discriminate adequately among the various globulins and albumin or because the abnormal protein may precipitate out with the fibrin as a cryoglobulin during the preparation of the sample for analysis.

The most generally used technique for analysis of the serum proteins is filter paper electrophoresis which gives results similar to those of the classic boundary electrophoresis of Tiselius and of electrophoresis in agar and in starch blocks. In paper electrophoresis, albumin and the various globulins separate out on the filter paper according to their mobility in an electric field. The proteins are stained on the paper and quantitated by photometry (see Fig. 37). The characteristic finding in multiple myeloma is the presence of a sharp spike or homogeneous peak in the electrophoretic pattern, found somewhere between the slow gamma globulin region and the region of the alpha globulins (Osserman and Lawlor, 1955) (see Figs. 37, 38, 39). This spike represents the paraimmunoglobulin or serum myeloma protein in the blood and is usually associated with a suppression of all the normal immunoglobulins. Such a spike is observed in 60 to 80 per cent of patients with myeloma, but it is not diagnostic of myeloma since it may be seen in many other paraimmunoglobulinopathies. Some patients with myeloma lack the serum myeloma protein but excrete Bence Jones protein in the urine. In this situation hypogammaglobulinemia is usually evident in the serum protein electrophoretic pattern. A few patients with myeloma have been reported who have a hypogammaglobulinemia without evidence of any abnormal serum, urinary, or tissue protein such as amyloid. In about

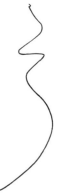

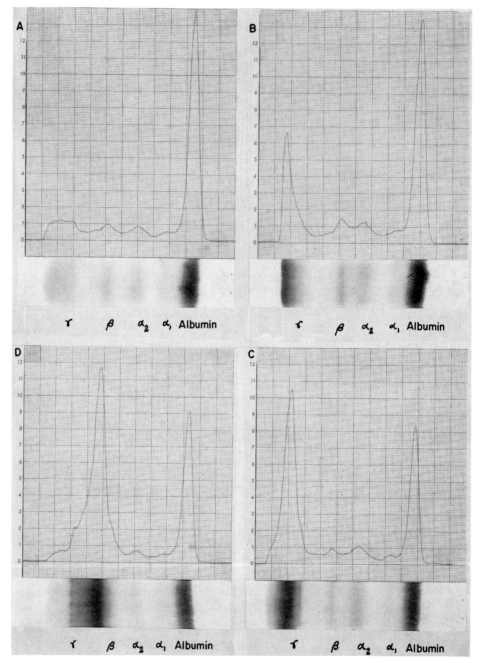

FIGURE 37. Filter paper electrophoresis of sera. (A) Normal pattern. (B) IgG myeloma protein of slow gamma mobility. (C) Waldenström's macroglobulinemia with a macroglobulin of midgamma mobility and of type K. (D) IgA myeloma protein of type K; mobility is fast gamma or beta. (Prepared by Dr. Roy Bonsnes)

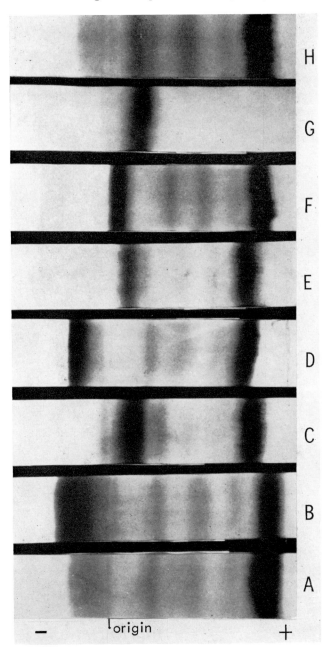

FIGURE 38. Filter paper electrophoresis of sera and urine. (A) Normal serum. (B) Diffuse hypergammaglobulinemia. (C) Multiple myeloma serum with an IgA myeloma protein. (D) (E) and (F) Multiple myeloma sera with IgG myeloma proteins. (G) Urine with Bence Jones protein. (H) Serum from the same patient as G, showing Bence Jones proteinemia.

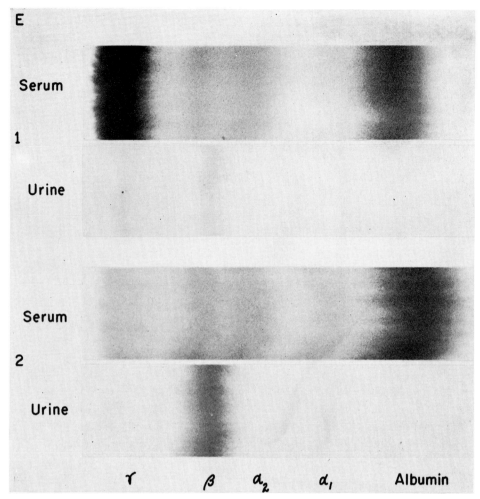

FIGURE 39. Filter paper electrophoresis of serum and urine in same patient. (1) Patient with multiple myeloma with gamma myeloma protein in the serum and a Bence Jones protein of beta mobility in the urine. Note that the serum myeloma protein is also seen in the urinary pattern. (2) Patient with multiple myeloma with slight hypogammaglobulinemia in the serum and Bence Jones protein of beta mobility in the urine.

one per cent of well-documented cases of multiple myeloma no paraimminoglobulinemia or paraimmunoglobulinuria is detected (Coltman, 1967). Rarely the serum protein electrophoretic pattern is entirely normal.

Electrophoresis in starch gels or in acrylamide may be used to resolve more serum protein components than can be identified with the techniques already mentioned (see Figs. 40 and 41). Heterogeneity of the serum myeloma protein spikes is best seen with starch gel and acrylamide electrophoresis. Otherwise, the patterns are comparable to those seen on paper electrophoresis. Starch gel electrophoresis of serum proteins of myeloma patients may reveal multiple abnormal spikes (Engle *et al.*, 1961). In some cases a double spike may result from malignancy of two clones of plasma cells. In other situations, the additional peaks may be due to polymerization of the primary protein, aggregation of the primary component with other serum proteins or, in rare instances, the presence of Bence Jones proteinemia (Solomon and Fahey, 1964; Williams, Brunning, and Wollheim, 1966). Rarely the starch gel pattern shows a spike which was not obvious in the filter paper pattern. In other instances an obvious spike on filter paper will be completely missed by the starch gel method.

A still more sophisticated method for analysis of the serum proteins is immunoelectrophoresis (Osserman and Lawlor, 1961) (see Fig. 42). In this technique the serum proteins are first separated by electrophoresis in agar. The separated proteins are then allowed to interact with antibody to human

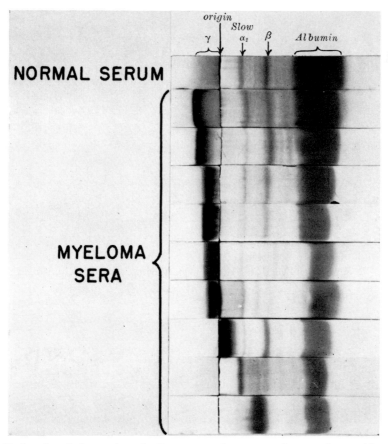

FIGURE 40. Starch gel electrophoresis. Serum protein patterns from patients with multiple myeloma, showing variability in migration of myeloma peak. This photograph is a composite of several individual patterns, making comparison of exact mobilities difficult. (Figs. 40 and 41 are reproduced with permission from ENGLE *et al.*: *J Lab Clin Med,* *58*:1–22, 1961, The C. V. Mosby Co., St. Louis, Mo.)

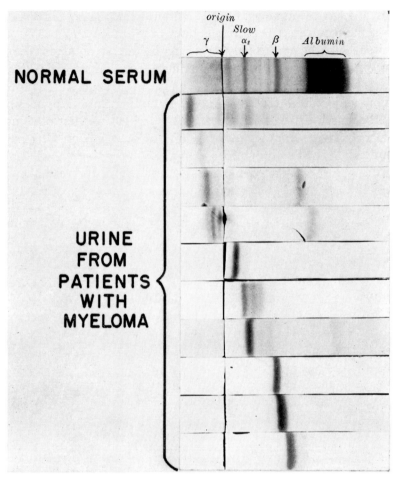

FIGURE 41. Starch gel electrophoresis. Urinary Bence Jones protein patterns from patients with multiple myeloma. Note multiple bands of some Bence Jones proteins. This photograph is a composite of several individual patterns, making comparison of exact mobilities difficult.

serum proteins placed in a trough along the side of the electrophoretic strip. Precipitin reactions occur as antigen and antibody diffuse through the agar in a direction perpendicular to that of the electrophoretic separation. It is by means of immunoelectrophoresis that the four families of immunoglobulins, IgG, IgA, IgM, and IgD have been identified. Each family gives a characteristic precipitin arc. The homogeneous serum myeloma protein is identified in the pattern by an aberration which occurs in a portion of the IgG or IgA arc. There is a thickening of a restricted region of the arc. The arcs for the immunoglobulins not representing the serum myeloma protein are indistinct or absent because of the generalized hypoimmunoglobulinemia.

Another useful technique for studying the serum proteins is double im-

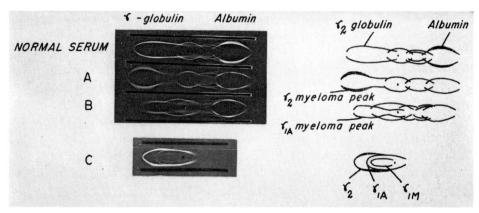

Figure 42. Immunoelectrophoresis of serum proteins. (A) Pattern from patient with $\gamma_2$ myeloma protein in serum. Note aberration in $\gamma_2$ curves. Antiserum used with rabbit antihuman serum. (B) Pattern from patient with $\gamma_{1A}$ myeloma protein in serum. Note increased intensity of $\gamma_{1A}$ arcs and decrease in $\gamma_2$ globulins. Antiserum used was rabbit antihuman serum. (C) The three families of immunoglobulins, $\gamma_2$, $\gamma_{1A}$, and $\gamma_{1M}$, are shown. Antiserum used was rabbit antihuman gammaglobulin. (Courtesy of Dr. Leonhard Korngold.)

munodiffusion in agar gels using the Ouchterlony plate method (Korngold, van Leeuwen, and Engle, 1962). With proper selection of antisera it is possible to obtain information similar to that obtained by immunoelectrophoresis and, in addition, to detect subtle differences among antigens. Korngold has developed this relatively simple technique as a useful procedure for the diagnosis of the various paraimmunoglobulinopathies (Korngold, van Leeuwen, and Engle, 1962).

By whatever technique it is studied, a serum myeloma peak is specific for an individual patient. Once it is observed, it does not ordinarily change in physicochemical characteristics during the course of the disease. Skoog (1965), however, has observed a patient who developed an entirely different protein peak during relapse after a successful course of therapy with suppression of the original peak. It is not unusual for the quantity of the abnormal protein to vary with treatment or progression of the disease. New peaks appearing late in the course of myeloma have been described (Engle and Wallis, 1957).

Patients with solitary plasmacytoma frequently have either a normal pattern or a very faint peak. As the disease becomes more generalized, repeated studies may show a gradual change to the highly abnormal pattern with an intense peak, and decrease in other immunoglobulins (Innes and Newall, 1961). A case has been recorded of a patient with a solitary plasmacytoma with an abnormal peak in the serum which disappeared after excision of the tumor (Lane, 1952).

Of all electrophoretic mobilities of the peak in myeloma, the alpha pattern is the rarest (Tidstrom, 1962). Before the advent of immunoelectrophoresis there was difficulty in distinguishing between an alpha₂ homogeneous peak and the diffuse nonspecific increase in the alpha₂ mucoproteins so commonly seen in many wasting diseases, including carcinoma and myeloma. Because of this difficulty many cases were misdiagnosed as alpha₂ myeloma.

The presence of cryoglobulins in the serum is of clinical importance in evaluating the patient with multiple myeloma. In order to detect cryoglobulins in the serum, a warm syringe is used for the venous puncture. The blood is removed, allowed to clot, and centrifuged, all at 37°C. The serum is separated at 37°C and then placed in the refrigerator at 4°C. A precipitate or gel which forms on cooling of the serum and goes back into solution on warming is cryoglobulin.

### Urinary Findings

About 60 per cent of patients with myeloma manifest proteinuria, and about 35 per cent (Kenny and Maloney, 1957) have Bence Jones protein in the urine. While most patients with multiple myeloma and proteinuria are found to have almost pure Bence Jones protein in the urine, in some cases appreciable amounts of albumin are also found, and in rare instances virtually all of the serum proteins, including even the serum myeloma protein, may be found. In this last situation, the patient usually has para-amyloidosis.

Bence Jones protein is a low-molecular-weight protein which precipitates on heating at 40° to 60°C at pH 5 and dissolves on boiling at 100°C at pH 3. Bence Jones proteins may migrate in the paper electrophoretic pattern anywhere between the slow gamma and the alpha globulin regions. When Bence Jones protein is present in the urine of a patient with paraimmunoglobulinemia, it usually migrates faster than the corresponding serum protein. Sometimes the urine must be concentrated before electrophoresis in order to detect the Bence Jones protein.

If urine containing Bence Jones protein is studied by electrophoresis in starch gels, two to five bands are seen in place of the single band seen on filter paper electrophoresis (Engle *et al.*, 1961) (see Fig. 41). At least part of the heterogeneity is related to the presence of monomers and dimers of the basic Bence Jones protein unit.

Bence Jones proteins may also be detected by immunoelectrophoresis (Osserman and Lawlor, 1961) and the Ouchterlony plate method (Korngold, van Leeuwen, and Engle, 1962). By using appropriate antisera in either technique, it is possible to determine the immunologic type of a given Bence Jones protein.

The chemical peculiarities of the Bence Jones protein may be responsible for the damage Bence Jones proteinuria produces in these patients. In the presence of Bence Jones proteinuria, the blood urea nitrogen is elevated in 50 per cent of patients. Renal impairment in myeloma signifies grave prognosis.

To demonstrate the presence of Bence Jones protein by the heat test, fresh urine is collected and centrifuged. A screening test with 5 per cent sulfosalicylic acid is first run on the supernatant. If no precipitate develops, no protein of any kind is present. Uristix is an unsatisfactory test for Bence Jones protein as the bluish discoloration is weak even in the presence of large amounts. If sulfosalicylic reaction is positive, the pH of another specimen of the urine is adjusted to 5 with 4 per cent acetic acid and the urine is heated slowly to 60°C. If precipitate forms between 40° and 60°C, the presence of Bence Jones protein is very likely. An equal amount of 5 per cent sulfosalicylic acid is added. This precipitates all the protein in the urine and brings the mixture to pH 3. The urine is boiled. If the precipitate dissolves during boiling and returns during cooling, the presence of Bence Jones protein is likely. Transferrin has similar thermal properties, though the temperature of initial precipitation is more than five degrees higher than that of Bence Jones proteins (Bernier and Putnam, 1964b). Transferrin is excreted in the urine only with larger quantities of albumin. Rarely, a urinary Bence Jones protein may have properties of a cryoprotein (Varriale, Ginsberg, and Sass, 1962). Recently, the definition of Bence Jones protein has been enlarged to include all homogeneous light chains, either κ or λ, whether or not they give a positive heat test. Apart from the Bence Jones protein, patients with multiple myeloma may excrete a number of other proteins in the urine. With progressive renal damage, albumin and, to a lesser extent, the entire spectrum of serum globulins may appear in urine.

When the adult Fanconi syndrome complicates the clinical picture of myeloma, the urine is frequently alkaline and may contain glucose and even acetone despite a normal blood sugar level. Hematuria, sometimes massive, may be the only manifestation of the coagulation defect in myeloma. Pyuria is not infrequent in view of complicating urinary and renal infections. Cylindruria may be present.

### Renal Function Tests

Phenolsulfonphthalein excretion is usually impaired early with renal involvement in myeloma. Urea clearance is decreased later in the disease. Elevation in blood urea nitrogen may be moderate, 25 to 40 mg%, for a period of time and severe terminally.

Intravenous pyelography and the antecedent preparatory dehydration may lead to acute and fatal anuria. While only thirty-one deaths were reported in 3.8 million urographies, acute fatal anuria following intravenous pyelography has been reported in five patients with multiple myeloma (Healy, 1963; Killmann, Gjörup, and Thaysen, 1957). In view of the increased risk, this procedure should be done with great care, if at all, in patients with multiple myeloma. Multiple myeloma should be ruled out before intravenous pyelography is carried out in cases of proteinuria of unknown etiology.

### Coagulation Studies

Blood clotting is frequently abnormal in multiple myeloma. The bleeding disorder is occasionally related to thrombocytopenia, to amyloid infiltration, or to capillary damage from impaired blood flow secondary to increased viscosity. The tourniquet test and sometimes the bleeding time are positive in these situations.

In addition, certain myeloma proteins and macroglobulins may interfere with blood coagulation. The following tests may be abnormal: recalcification time, clotting time, clot retraction, clot fragility, and prothrombin time. Because of poor or absent clot retraction in some cases, it may be virtually impossible to obtain serum for various laboratory procedures.

### Blood Chemistries

Serum calcium is frequently normal in multiple myeloma. It is elevated in about 5 to 10 per cent of cases. This increase has been ascribed to enhanced binding by the abnormal protein. Hypercalcemia is more often related to massive osteolysis; it is enhanced by defective glomerular filtration and in itself contributes to renal damage. Manifestations of hypercalcemia (disorientation, coma, cardiac arrhythmia, and renal failure) may dominate the clinical picture or be the presenting symptom complex.

Serum calcium is decreased in 10 to 30 per cent of cases. This decrease may be related to a low serum albumin, which is the major calcium-binding protein. More frequently, hypocalcemia is a manifestation of renal failure and is associated with hyperphosphatemia. Tetany rarely if ever occurs in this setting.

The conspicuous absence of alkaline phosphatase elevation in the presence of osteolytic lesions is a curious fact, helpful in diagnosis and in differentiation from metastatic cancer involving bones. The alkaline phosphatase may become elevated in the course of myeloma, in the presence of an acute fracture, and when an adult Fanconi syndrome complicates myeloma. The serum acid phosphatase may be abnormal in multiple myeloma, and the diagnosis of prostatic carcinoma metastatic to the bone must be ruled out (Goldberg, Takakura and Rosenthal, 1966).

As previously mentioned, the serum uric acid is frequently increased in myeloma as a result of enhanced purine, RNA, and protein synthesis. On the other hand, hypouricemia associated with hypokalemia, hypophosphatemia, renal glycosuria, and amino-aciduria are manifestations of the adult Fanconi syndrome, which may complicate multiple myeloma (Engle and

Wallis, 1957) . When renal failure and uremia complicate myeloma, hyper-phosphatemia, hyperkalemia, hyperuricemia, hyponatremia, and acidosis (low $CO_2$ and pH) may be present.

### Miscellaneous Tests

Loutsides (1962) described a urethan-gel reaction in which urethan added to myeloma sera causes gel formation. However, this reaction was found to be nonspecific (Huhnstock and Distler, 1963) .

The Sia euglobulin test involves precipitation upon addition of distilled water to an abnormal serum. It is frequently but not always positive with macroglobulinemia (see Waldenström's Macroglobulinemia) and occasionally positive in IgA and IgG myeloma.

The abnormal proteins may impart to the serum anticomplementary activity in the Wassermann test.

### Biopsies

Biopsy of bone marrow has been discussed. Biopsy of skin, gums, kidney, and rectum may be helpful in establishing the diagnosis of amyloid involvement. Biopsy of enlarged lymph nodes may reveal plasmacytic infiltration. In some cases of proved multiple myeloma, the biopsy may be compatible with Hodgkin's disease, reticulum cell sarcoma, or lymphocytic lymphosarcoma. Splenic biopsies for diagnosis of multiple myeloma have been described but are not widely used (Watson *et al.*, 1963) . When acute anuria occurs, renal biopsy may be of help in establishing the site and extent of obstructive involvement and in differentiating among prerenal, renal, and postrenal oliguria.

### PROGNOSIS

Multiple myeloma is a universally fatal disease with the average time of survival in most large series (Kenny and Maloney, 1957; Snapper, Turner, and Moskovitz, 1953; Geschikter and Copeland, 1928; Lichtenstein and Jaffe, 1947) being less than two years. Average survival following diagnosis is about ten months and following onset of symptoms, 18.5 months (Heini-vaara and Eisald, 1960) . Survival data reported by various investigators are not truly comparable because of different methods used in avoiding the usual inaccuracies inherent in survival estimates. Osgood (1960) obtained a survival curve from time of diagnosis in 192 patients and found that 90 per cent survived approximately one month, 50 per cent approximately seven months, and 10 per cent approximately sixty months. He found that survival from onset of symptoms in 600 cases, including 192 from his own series, was 90 per cent for five months, 50 per cent for sixteen months, and 10 per cent for sixty months.

The Study Committee of the Midwest Cooperative Chemotherapy Group reported similar data (Study Committee, 1964). From time of diagnosis 90 per cent survived one to two months, 50 per cent survived seven to eleven months, and 10 per cent survived thirty to eighty-four months. From onset of symptoms 90 per cent survived four to seven months, 50 per cent survived fifteen to twenty months, and 10 per cent survived forty to eighty months. Feinleib and MacMahon (1960) obtained a 96 per cent follow-up on 238 Brooklyn residents diagnosed as having multiple myeloma during the years 1943 to 1952. They reported a shorter survival after onset of symptoms: 90 per cent survived two months, 50 per cent survived 9½ months, and 10 per cent survived forty-five months. This difference may be related to the fact that this group was of generally lower socioeconomic status and thus may have minimized symptoms. In Innes and Newall's series (1961), 53 per cent survived three years; eight patients lived over five years, three patients over eight years, and none over ten years. In two patients there were spontaneous remissions.

All investigators note a slightly longer survival in young patients with myeloma than in the older group (Study Committee, 1964; Feinleib and MacMahon, 1960). Women may have a better prognosis from the time of diagnosis than men (Heinivaara and Eisald, 1960; Feinleib and MacMahon, 1960). Attempts to correlate duration of survival with cell type and the electrophoretic pattern have been unsuccessful. While Kenny's (Kenny and Maloney, 1957) patients with the most anaplastic cells survived seven months or less and those cases surviving over nine years had mature myeloma cells, the remainder showed such a discrepancy between cell type and survival that any prognostic statement from cell type alone seems unwarranted.

Survival is usually longer in those who present with a solitary lesion. Although the majority of patients with what seems to be solitary tumor survive only one or two years, extremely long survivals have been noted in this group. Survival of seventeen and thirteen years after onset of symptoms has been reported in two patients starting out with a solitary lesion (Kaye *et al.*, 1961). Cohen, Svien, and Dahlin (1964) studied fifty-five patients with myeloma of the vertebral column and recorded a survival of five to twenty-one years for eighteen patients of the forty-four who had either a normal bone marrow or no marrow examination.

As long as the tumor is localized and restricted to the soft tissues, clinical cure may be achieved by surgical or radiologic treatment alone or in combination. However, no known method prevents the eventual fatal outcome after the tumor has either invaded the bone structure or spread to the lymph nodes.

Anemia and renal dysfunction indicate a poor prognosis. Once severe anemia develops, patients deteriorate rapidly without remissions and are unaffected by treatment. Renal function is another useful prognostic determinant. Survival is longest in the group with no pathologic renal findings, shorter in patients with proteinuria, and shortest in the group with proteinuria and either pathologic sediment or elevated blood urea nitrogen or both (Kenny and Maloney, 1957; Osserman, 1959).

## COMPLICATIONS AND MODE OF DEATH

The most frequent causes of death (Study Committee, 1964) in myeloma patients are infections, noninfectious cardiopulmonary conditions, uremia, and malignancy itself. Other complications leading to death are pathologic fractures, spinal cord compression, cerebrovascular accidents, and complications of therapy.

Pneumonia accounts for most infectious complications. Urinary tract infections and septicemia are next in frequency. Pulmonary edema accounts for half the noninfectious cardiopulmonary complications. Myocardial involvement occurs through either ischemia secondary to anemia or atherosclerosis, or is related to paraamyloid deposits. Cerebrovascular accidents are not infrequent in patients with myeloma. Cerebral thromboses are facilitated by increased blood viscosity and cerebral hemorrhages, by thrombocytopenia and other hemorrhagic tendencies. Occasionally, a patient with multiple myeloma lapses into an unexplained coma without localizing signs. The cerebrospinal fluid reveals a high level of abnormal protein, and no hemorrhage or thrombosis is detected at autopsy. These cases are frequently referred to as "paraproteinemic coma," and an assumption is made that the high protein and the coma are causally related.

Pathologic fractures are a leading indirect cause of death in myeloma. Spinal cord compression due to tumor or compression fractures of vertebrae may lead to death via neurogenic bladder and urinary tract infection. Pathologic fractures also lead to immobilization and frequently to pneumonia.

Renal death in myeloma occurs either abruptly with acute anuria or gradually in the face of chronic uremia.

Complications of therapy include liver failure from urethan and bone marrow failure from any chemotherapeutic agent.

Pregnancy did not seem to affect the course of the disease in the only patient reported (Kosova and Schwartz, 1966); a normal pregnancy in a 35-year-old Negro who received urethan for her multiple myeloma resulted in the birth of a normal baby with a normal serum electrophoretic pattern.

## DIAGNOSIS AND DIFFERENTIAL DIAGNOSIS

The most common manifestations of myeloma are pain, weakness, fatigue, anemia, cardiopulmonary symptoms, and neurologic and renal complications. Findings which most frequently lead to a suspicion of myeloma are anemia, bone pain, bone lesions, and abnormal serum proteins. The most common combination of symptoms is bone pain plus anemia. Diagnosis is established with the finding of a characteristic bone marrow abnormality and protein abnormality.

Because of the diverse manifestations of multiple myeloma, the list of differential diagnoses is long and varied.

When bone pain is present, differential diagnosis includes osteoarthritis, rheumatoid arthritis, Marie-Strumpell arthritis, osteoporosis, osteomalacia, and metastatic bone cancer. In a number of patients with physical stigmata of rheumatoid arthritis, back pain is thought to represent another manifestation of their previous rheumatoid arthritis and the diagnosis of multiple myeloma is missed or delayed. A similar situation exists in elderly patients in whom a diagnosis of senile or postmenopausal osteoporosis is made. Osteoarthritis is frequently used as a wastebasket diagnosis of the back pain in the elderly. Metastatic disease is commonly suspected. X-rays may or may not be helpful in differentiation. Apart from bone marrow examination and protein studies, which establish the diagnosis, absence of alkaline phosphatase elevation in the face of widespread bone involvement may be of help in the diagnosis of multiple myeloma.

The list of differential diagnoses of roentgenologic findings in myeloma is very long. Epidermoid cysts of the skull may produce lytic lesions; these, however, have a scalloped, dense margin. Osteoporosis circumscripta may produce x-ray findings in the skull similar to those of multiple myeloma. Eosinophilic granuloma usually occurs in a younger age group. Hydatid disease of bone is rare in this country; it involves vertebrae and ilium. The malignant giant cell tumor usually presents a distinct soap bubble appearance. Metastatic carcinoma, especially that secondary to carcinoma of the thyroid, is the most difficult lesion to differentiate. In metastatic carcinoma the absence of extension of the lesion into the soft tissue is helpful in diagnosis. Diffuse skeletal hemangiomatosis with preponderance of lytic lesions must also be considered (Wallis, Asch, and Maisel, 1964). Other possibilities are sarcoidosis, osteoporosis, and even hyperparathyroidism.

A number of hematologic disorders must be considered when a patient presents with anemia, bleeding disorder, or both. These include leukemia, lymphoma, and thrombocytopenic purpura.

Given a patient with a homogeneous protein peak in the serum, it is essential to consider, in addition to multiple myeloma, Waldenström's macroglobulinemia and all the other paraimmunoglobulinopathies (see Table XXII).

## PREVENTION

Since the etiology of multiple myeloma remains obscure, no method of prevention is known. Future discoveries may indicate that prevention is possible by avoiding specific precipitating stimuli.

In the present state of knowledge, prevention means avoidance of complications in a patient in whom the diagnosis of myeloma is made. Given a patient with a serum "premyeloma" peak, the greatest benefit lies in preventing infections and treating them promptly if they occur. In a patient with Bence Jones proteinuria, prevention consists of hydration and maintenance of electrolyte balance. In a patient with diffuse skeletal involvement, prevention of complications implies prevention of disuse osteoporosis through judicious activity, avoidance of sudden strenuous movements and fractures, and avoidance of hypercalcemia through hydration.

Since the disease is invariably fatal, the concept of prevention must be altered. No amount of prophylactic effort can ward off the progress of the disease. However, many patients can be kept comfortable and socially and economically productive through a great part of the course of their illness by means of supportive measures designed to prevent complications, as well as by means of chemotherapeutic agents described in the next section.

## MANAGEMENT AND TREATMENT

Management of patients with multiple myeloma is a difficult and challenging problem. Myeloma is a universally fatal disease and any treatment is, therefore, palliative. Usually, the diagnosis is established following development of an acute complication of the disease (anuria, fracture, hypercalcemia, infection) and specific and nonspecific measures directed at the complication are indicated. Occasionally, chemotherapy directed at the basic disease can be started concomitantly with the supportive treatment and may favorably influence the complication. However, the efficacy of chemotherapy cannot be meaningfully evaluated until the complicating features such as electrolyte imbalance, uremia, and infection are corrected.

The criteria of improvement include decrease in pain, improvement in anemia, decrease in abnormal proteinemia and proteinuria, shrinking of soft tissue masses, decrease in plasmacytosis of the marrow, and recalcification of bone lesions.

### Supportive Measures and Treatment of Complications

With renal impairment in myeloma, attention must be directed at hydration to correct the electrolyte imbalance and hypercalcemia. Hypercalcemia usually responds to a regimen of hydration, low calcium diet, and corticosteroids; occasionally, chelating agents are used. The responsiveness of the hypercalcemia of myelomatosis to corticosteroids has been noted (Merigan and Hayes, 1961). When acute anuria occurs, the functional impairment prior to its onset may be only slight. This encourages the use of more vigorous therapy such as hemodialysis or peritoneal lavage (Healy, 1963). Renal biopsy, by demonstrating few obstructive casts, may be helpful in screening patients who, despite the diagnosis of myeloma, have a fairly good prognosis. These patients should be offered every chance of survival, including hemodialysis and peritoneal lavage, provided that other disabilities from multiple myeloma are not great.

Infections, which so frequently complicate the course of multiple myeloma, call for proper use of antibiotics and gamma globulin. The choice and the dose of the antibiotic depend on the type and sensitivity of the offending microorganism and the severity of infection. While the report of the cultures is being awaited, the patient may be placed on 1 to 1.5 gm a day of a broad-spectrum antibiotic orally (tetracycline, erythromycin); in more fulminant infections the patient is placed on 1 to 10 million units of penicillin intramuscularly or intravenously and 1 gm of streptomycin intramuscularly daily. When the cultures and sensitivities are reported, the therapy is adjusted accordingly. The use of human gamma globulin in treating infectious complications of multiple myeloma has gained acceptance despite its high cost because of the realization of the immunologic impoverishment of these patients. Although various "priming" and "maintenance" schedules have been used, we have administered a daily dose of 2 cc of human gamma globulin intramuscularly for a week or two, or longer, until the patient has overcome the infection.

With widespread bony involvement, fractures, and associated disuse osteoporosis, a judicious use and balance of bed rest, mobilization, and ambulation are of great importance. Various supports, corsets, and braces may be helpful to keep the patients ambulatory. In some bedridden patients, an intensive antiosteoporotic regimen helps achieve a transition to full activity. This treatment includes calcium lactate 3.6 gm a day in divided doses, strontium lactate 2.1 gm a day, vitamin D supplements 50,000 units every other day, high protein diet, estrogens such as Premarin® 1.25 mg a day (used cyclically in women), and androgens. Recently, nonandrogenic anabolic steroids have been added to the regimen with some success: either norethandrolone (Nilevar®) 20 to 30 mg a day orally, stanozole (Winstrol®) 2 to 6 mg a day orally or nandrolone phenylpropionate (Durabolin®) 25 to 50 mg intramuscularly each week or equivalent doses of other agents. When cord compression occurs, laminectomy and cord decompression usually result in complete restoration of function (Kenny and Maloney, 1957).

Corticosteroids have been helpful in treatment of associated anemia, thrombocytopenia, and hypercalcemia (Merigan and Hayes, 1961). These agents reverse the hypercalcemia by reducing the accelerated bone breakdown (Lazor and Rosenberg, 1964). Equivalents of 40 to 60 mg of prednisone per day in divided doses have been used in the initial stages of treatment; this has been followed by tapering the dose gradually. Maintenance amounts of 10 to 15 mg a day have been used over long periods of time. Adverse effects of larger doses of steroids, especially the increase in susceptibility to infection, have limited their usefulness. Dexamethasone-induced

fatal necrotizing polyarteritis of coronary and renal vessels has been recorded in the course of treatment of multiple myeloma with this agent
(Skoog and Adams, 1963).

Androgens have been found to exert a marrow-stimulating effect in myeloma complicated by anemia. Weekly doses of 200 to 600 mg of testosterone
enanthate intramuscularly or daily oral doses of 75 to 100 mg of methyltes-
tosterone have been followed by striking improvement in anemia in 60 per
cent of patients (Gardner and Cohen, 1966). The mode of action seems to
be nonspecific stimulation of erythropoiesis. The effect is less pronounced on
the granulocyte and platelet formation. Gardner and Cohen (1966) advo-
cate an initial six-week period of androgen treatment prior to extensive
skeleton irradiation; this course may be helpful in preventing the onset of
postirradiation anemia.

Blood transfusion is another supportive measure in the anemia patient
with multiple myeloma. When iron deficiency is present, anemia responds
to iron administration. The dosage used has been 0.6 gm of ferrous gluco-
nate or its equivalent three times a day after meals.

In the rare patients with hyperviscosity syndrome associated with multiple myeloma plasmapheresis is indicated (see under Waldenström's Macroglobulinemia).

Recently, attention has been given to use of sodium fluoride in treatment
of skeletal lesions of multiple myeloma (Gardner and Cohen, 1966; Reutter
and Siebenmann, 1965 Carbone *et al.,* 1968). Administration of sodium
fluoride induces radiologically detectable increase in bone density within
six to eighteen months, concomitant with relief of pain in half of the patients. At first there is coarsening of the trabecular pattern in vertebral
bodies best seen in lateral projections of the lumbar and thoracic spine,
Stage I fluorosis. Later the changes progress to Stage II fluorosis with apparent fusion of the thickened trabeculae and a striking increase in bone
density. Calcium balance becomes markedly positive; bone biopsy shows
thickened trabeculae with thicker cortices.

Sodium fluoride is given by mouth in 50 mg doses twice or three times a
day one half hour before meals (Gardner and Cohen, 1966). If no hypercalcemia is present calcium lactate is added to the regimen, one hour after
the meals three times a day in 1.0 gm to 3.6 gm doses.

The mode of action of fluoride is unknown and appears to be complex.
Fluoride is concentrated in bone where crystals of fluorapatite are formed
instead of the usual hydroxyapatite. The fluoride-containing crystal is less
reactive with body fluids and less susceptible to resorption. Sodium fluoride
is being used in osteoporosis of any cause, including the steroid-induced
osteoporosis and the senile osteoporosis (Rich and Ivanovich, 1965; Cohen
and Gardner, 1966).

Adverse effects include nausea and diarrhea, occurring in one third of patients; this is managed by reducing the dose to 50 mg a day for one week and then gradually increasing it by 50 mg increments weekly until 150 mg per day dose is reached again. Some patients tolerated 800 mg a day for three months. Fifty mg a day was tolerated by all patients. To date no important toxic action of this dose of fluoride has been reported. One case of optic neuritis was seen in a patient taking 20 mg sodium fluoride a day for six weeks; however, it was difficult to determine in that case if there was causal relationship between the optic neuritis and the medication (Rich and Ivanovich, 1965).

While the question arises whether the fluorotic bone is conceivably not as strong as normal bone, no pathological fractures were encountered in endemic fluorosis in India (Singh *et al.*, 1963) and in sporadic chronic flouride intoxication in Texas (Sauerbrunn, Ryan and Shaw, 1965). Experimental work also suggests that bone strength in fluorosis is normal.

In chronic fluoride intoxication fluorotic radiculomyelopathy is the presenting symptom. There is excellent reason, therefore, to use the smallest effective dose of fluoride, as higher doses may combine the desired effect on bone with increasing interference with the metabolism of the central nervous system. The dose recommended for senile osteoporosis is 50 mg a day (Rich and Ivanovich, 1965). Doses used in multiple myeloma varied between 100 and 150 mg a day.

### Specific Measures

Indications for specific therapy of patients with myeloma are bone pain, anemia, tumor mass, encroachment of tumor mass on a vital organ, or hyperviscosity syndrome.

X-ray therapy to a painful skeletal site is the most promptly effective mode of treatment for relief of pain (Bromley, 1961). X-ray therapy may also cause shrinkage of plasmacytomas. However, because of the wide dissemination of lesions in myeloma, x-ray therapy suffers from limitations.

Urethan was the first fairly effective agent in myeloma; it was used extensively in the 50's (Kenny and Maloney, 1957; Rundles and Reeves, 1950; Harrington and Maloney, 1950; Luttgens and Bayrd, 1951; Rundles, Dillon and Dillon, 1950). It can be quite effective in patients who can tolerate 1 to 3 gm. or more daily. Unfortunately, gastric irritation makes it unacceptable to 60 to 75 per cent of patients. Rectal suppositories of urethan in similar doses provide another mode of administration. However, rectal irritation is a limiting side effect. When well tolerated in a syrup of wild cherry or in an enteric-coated capsule, urethan relieves bone pain and seems to arrest the course of the disease of some patients for a time. Urethan therapy may be rarely associated with spectacular recalcification of skeletal lesions (Rundles and Reeves, 1950; Rundles, Dillon and Dillon, 1950) and improvement in anemia. However, there is no evidence that there is significant prolongation of survival in patients on urethan. Some recent work casts doubt on the efficacy of urethan. A controlled study indicated that urethan may be no better than a placebo and that patients on this agent had a shortened survival (Holland *et al.,* 1966). With prolonged urethan therapy, hepatic damage and subacute yellow atrophy may occur (Ohler, Houghton, and Maloney, 1950).

With the advent of new chemotherapeutic agents, trials of many of these substances in patients with multiple myeloma were recorded.

Stilbamidine and 2-hydroxystilbamidine were introduced by Snapper in 1945 (Snapper, Turner and Moskovitz, 1953) for treatment of multiple myeloma because of their effect in kala-azar, a condition likewise characterized by hyperglobulinemia. Toxic effects of these compounds have precluded their general use. Similarly, another diamidine compound, 4-4-diamidino-diphenylamine dihydrochloride, an antifungal agent closely related to stilbamidine, was tried in multiple myeloma with disappointing results (Denman and Ward, 1959; Skinner, Bergsagel, and Truax, 1963).

Radioactive phosphorus is not beneficial except in rare instances (Bayrd, 1955; Lawrence and Wasserman, 1950). Bayrd (1955) reported a single case of acute plasma cell leukemia in which a remission of over nine years followed the administration of radioactive phosphorus. Use of vinblastine in myeloma has been disappointing (Costa *et al.,* 1963).

Rivers and others of the Veterans Administration Cancer Chemotherapy Group (Rivers, Whittington, and Patino, 1963); Solomon, Alexander and Steinfeld (1963), Tourtellotte and Call (1964), and Skoog and Adams (1966) used cyclophosphamide in patients with multiple myeloma and reported significant improvement and prolonged survival time in some. Cyclophosphamide, a cyclical phosphodiamine (Cytoxan® is unique among alkylating agents in that it is inactive *in vitro. In vivo,* enzymatic cleavage of the phosphamide group releases the active portion of the compound. The drug can be given orally or parenterally. The initial dose used has been 200 mg a day until the white cell count falls to between 2,000 and 2,500 per cu mm. Cyclophosphamide is temporarily discontinued and resumed when white cell count rises again above 2,500 at maintenance dose of 50 to 100 mg per day. With weekly leukocyte counts, the dose is adjusted to keep the leukocyte count above 2,500.

About a third of the patients exhibit dramatic subjective and objective evidences of improvement: disappearance of bone pain, increase in appetite, return to normal activity, fall in paraimmunoglobulin level, disappearance of Bence Jones urinary proteins, rise in the hematocrit, change in the negative calcium balance to positive and improvement in negative nitrogen and phosphorus balance. However, improvement in the appearance of bone on roentgenograms is rare.

The side effects include leukopenia, nausea, alopecia and, rarely, hemorrhagic cystitis. Nausea is usually dose-related and is not a significant problem. Alopecia is reversible despite maintenance doses of the drug. The degree of leukopenia is used as a guide to therapy as it is a very sensitive indicator which helps the physician protect marrow erythroid elements and megakaryocytes.

Androgenic therapy, as well as steroid therapy in some cases, has been found a good additive to cyclophosphamide administration (Skoog and Adams, 1966).

L-phenylalanine mustard is the treatment of choice in multiple myeloma. The racemic mixture of D-phenylalanine and L-phenylalanine mustard (bischloroethylaminophenylalanine) was first reported to be effective in multiple myeloma by Russian workers in 1958 (Blokhin *et al.*, 1958). Favorable results from use of the L-isomer (melphalan, L-sarcolysin, Alkeran®) have been reported widely (Swan, 1961; Bergsagel, 1962; Bernard, Seligmann, and Danon, 1962; Osserman, 1963; Waldenström, 1964a).

In those patients who show a response, the alleviation of bone pain is usually immediate and often dramatic. In about half the patients there is objective evidence of disease suppression. A decrease in the serum and/or urinary paraimmunoglobulins is frequently associated with an increase in the serum albumin and an increase in the normal immunoglobulins. Reduction of plasma cell counts and qualitative changes in plasma cells from repeated bone marrow aspirations have been described (Waldenström, 1964a). Improvement in anemia is also seen. The functional status of patients is often remarkably improved. Remissions, when they occur, last six to thirty-six months or longer.

In a few cases there is x-ray evidence of skeletal improvement; in other patients some lesions regress and others progress simultaneously. Preliminary evidence suggests that the survival of these patients may be prolonged (Waldenström, 1964a), but because of the great variability in the natural history of myeloma, further studies will be necessary to confirm this point.

Various dosage schedules of L-phenylalanine mustard have been used (Osserman, 1963; Waldenström, 1964a). The recommended initial dose is 4 to 6 mg a day orally. It is adjusted, as required, on the basis of blood counts done at weekly intervals. The amount is usually decreased after two to three weeks to a dose of 1 to 3 mg a day, which is maintained as long as the white blood cell count is above 3,000 and the platelet count is greater than 100,000 per cu mm. The initial dose is reduced if leukopenia or thrombocytopenia is present.

The alternate schedule aims at a more vigorous suppression of the myelomatous bone marrow. Initial doses of 6 to 10 mg a day are given for seven to ten days and then stopped. White blood cell count and platelet count are usually maximally suppressed within three to five weeks. When the counts are recovering, maintenance therapy of 1 to 3 mg daily is instituted, aiming at a leukocyte count range of 3,000 to 3,500 per cu mm. Patients are followed and blood counts obtained at intervals of two to three weeks. The initial dose of L-phenylalanine mustard should be reduced if there is leukopenia or thrombocytopenia. Occasionally, the response is very gradual over several months and therapy should not be abandoned too soon. As is the case with many chemotherapeutic agents used as maintenance therapy, L-phenylalanine mustard should not be abruptly discontinued as severe relapse may result. The chief untoward reactions to L-phenylalanine mustard are bone marrow depression and occasionally nausea and vomiting.

Combined phenylalanine mustard and corticosteroid therapy has been the most effective treatment to date. The alternate phenylalanine mustard schedule is being used along with prednisone 1.25 mg/kg per day to a maximum dose of 100 mg per day. After two to three weeks the prednisone dose is reduced to about 40 mg per day. After five to six weeks the dose is further reduced to a maintenance of 20 mg a day or lower. Side effects of prolonged corticosteroid administration, especially osteoporosis, must be watched for during the combined therapy.

# Chapter 9

# OTHER PARAIMMUNOGLOBULINOPATHIES

## WALDENSTRÖM'S MACROGLOBULINEMIA

*Definition.* Waldenström's macroglobulinemia results from a proliferation of lymphoid cells, probably neoplastic, causing lymphocytosis, enlargement of lymph nodes and spleen, and infiltration of bone marrow and other tissues; it is associated with the presence of abnormal macroglobulins in the blood and, occasionally, Bence Jones proteins in the urine.

### Pathology

Just as multiple myeloma is usually associated with proliferation of plasma cells, Waldenström's macroglobulinemia is usually associated with proliferation, probably neoplastic, of lymphoid cells throughout the body. In rare instances, the predominating cell type may be a plasma cell or reticulum cell. Regardless of the cell type, the characteristic feature is the presence of increased amounts of large-molecular-weight macroglobulins in the blood and, occasionally, Bence Jones proteins in the urine.

### Morphology of Characteristic Cell

There has been considerable discussion about the exact nature of the cell seen in most cases of Waldenström's macroglobulinemia. One of the difficulties has been getting general agreement on the definition of the disease. In the first cases described by Waldenström, the lymphoid nature of the disease was recognized because the predominating cell was the lymphocyte. In the bone marrow there are often small pyknotic lymphocytes whose nuclei are almost denuded of cytoplasm (Zucker-Franklin, 1964). In the peripheral blood the lymphocytes may be indistinguishable from those seen in chronic lymphatic leukemia. In other cases, the characteristic cell seems to be midway between a lymphocyte and a plasma cell, and, rarely, cells indistinguishable from plasma cells predominate. Under the electron microscope, it has been shown that both the lymphoid cells and the lymphoid plasma cells are equipped with endoplasmic reticulum for protein synthesis (Zucker-Franklin, 1964), even though the usual small lymphocyte is not so equipped (Fig. 16). With the periodic acid-Schiff stain, positive staining granules and bodies may be seen in the cytoplasm and sometimes in the nucleus. These, however, are not diagnostic of macroglobulinemia.

### Tissue Lesions

The bone marrow, spleen, liver, and lymph nodes are infiltrated with the characteristic cells in varying degrees (Dutcher and Fahey, 1959). Sometimes the reticulum cells are also increased in number. In the spleen the infiltrates may be in the cords of Billroth. Sometimes the lymphoid follicles are large and increased in number. In the liver the infiltrations occur at the portal triads. Such infiltrations may occur in almost any organ. When the central nervous system is involved (Bing-Neel syndrome) (Bing and Neel, 1936), the meninges and nearly all the perforating meningeal vessels of the cerebral hemispheres, cerebellar hemispheres, midbrain, pons, and medulla oblongata are infiltrated with the characteristic cells filling the Virchow-Robin spaces and infiltrating the vessel walls. In some rare cases the bone lesions may develop into punched-out lesions. Paraamyloidosis occasionally accompanies the macroglobulinemia (see Multiple Myeloma and Paraamyloidosis).

### Clinical Manifestations

Patients may come to the attention of the physician for any one of several reasons. There may be localized or generalized enlargement of lymph nodes and/or enlargement of the spleen indistinguishable from similar findings in lymphosarcoma or lymphatic leukemia. Lymphadenopathy, hepatomegaly and splenomegaly alone or in combination occur in thirty to fifty per cent of the patients (Cohen, Bohannon, and Wallerstein, 1966). Hemorrhagic manifestations may predominate, and have been reported in 60 per cent of cases. Purpura, epistaxis, mucosal bleeding, and massive gastrointestinal hemorrhage are common. Thrombotic episodes are a serious consideration and may involve the eye (Ackerman, 1962) or other critical locations. Eye grounds typically present distended, tortuous venules and hemorrhages; "link-sausage" appearance of retinal veins and frank retinal vein thromboses are not uncommon. These changes have been attributed to the abnormal levels of circulating macroglobulins producing increased viscosity of the retinal blood flow with sludging and stagnation. Symptoms of systemic disease such as fatigue, weakness, lassitude, anorexia, and malaise are often present. Congestive heart failure and pulmonary hypertension, when present, are usually due to increased blood viscosity.

Neurological symptoms which accompany macroglobulinemia have been classified into five groups (Logothetis, Silverstein, and Coe, 1960). Strokes and acute unifocal brain syndromes are difficult to differentiate from each other. Encephalopathies or multifocal diffuse brain syndromes are sometimes associated with patches of demyelination. Neuropathies are not rare. Tinnitus, vertigo and deafness are common complications. Subarachnoid hemorrhage may be the culmination of generalized bleeding diathesis. The fifth group is mixed. The combination of neurologic abnormalities and hyperglobulinemia has been called the Bing-Neel syndrome (Bing and Neel, 1936).

Renal insufficiency is an infrequent complication (Argagni and Kipkie, 1964). Bone pain is usually not a complaint unless osteoporosis is severe. There is an increased susceptibility to infections, but not as high as in multiple myeloma. Rarely, manifestations of accompanying generalized amyloidosis may be present (Forget, Squires, and Sheldon, 1966; Cohen, Bohannon, and Wallerstein, 1966). About one sixth of patients will have no symptoms when the macroglobulinemia is first detected (Bayrd, Hagedorn and McGuckin, 1965).

Roentgenograms characteristically reveal generalized osteoporosis. Only rarely seen are the punched-out lesions of bone indistinguishable from those in myeloma (Welton *et al.,* 1968). If the macroglobulin is also a cryoglobulin, all of the manifestations of cryoglobulinemia may be present, with Raynaud's phenomenon and cutaneous ulcers in exposed areas.

## Laboratory Findings

Anemia occurs in over 80 per cent of the patients with macroglobulinemia. It is normocytic and may be caused by hemolysis, blood loss, or disturbed erythropoiesis secondary to the proliferation of abnormal cells in the marrow. Cline and coworkers (1963) found a shortened red cell life span in six of their ten patients. White blood cell counts are usually normal; occasionally leukopenia occurs as part of a pancytopenia. Relative lymphocytosis is found in 37 per cent (Cohen, Bohannon and Wallerstein, 1966). Leukocytosis with lymphocytosis may suggest lymphatic leukemia. Thrombocytopenia severe enough to explain bleeding is found in half the patients with clinical evidence of bleeding (Cline *et al.,* 1963). Rouleaux formation of red cells is common and clumping of red cells in the counting chamber often makes counting difficult. Sedimentation rate is usually elevated. Studies have revealed coagulation defects involving fibrinogen, prothrombin, factor V and factor VII with no consistent pattern (Henstell and Kligerman, 1958).

The bone marrow aspirate usually contains large numbers of the characteristic cells, usually lymphocytes, occasionally lymphoid plasma cells, or even plasma cells. Tissue mast cells are seen frequently. The lymph node biopsy specimen and splenic aspirate are often indistinguishable from those of lymphosarcoma.

The urine may be normal. In rare instances, Bence Jones proteins, even in large amounts, may be found.

Characteristic abnormalities of the plasma proteins are seen. The globulins are usually elevated and upon electrophoresis a characteristic spike is seen in the region of the immunoglobulins, usually between the beta and gamma peaks; this is a result of the IgM elevation. This spike is indistinguishable from the spike in myeloma. As in the case of multiple myeloma, there is usually a decrease in all the other immunoglobulins and albumin is usually diminished. Under ordinary circumstances the macroglobulins that are immunoglobulins do not migrate into starch gels unless the gels are prepared with an unusually large pore size; this property helps to distinguish them from the 7S immunoglobulins of the IgG and IgA families. The size of the macroglobulin may be determined in the ultracentrifuge, where one, two or more fast sedimenting components may be seen with sedimentation coefficients of 19 or 21S, or higher. However, the macroglobulins may be more easily distinguished by immunologic techniques when characteristic findings are seen both in immunoelectrophoresis (Osserman and Lawlor, 1961) and in the Ouchterlony immunodiffusion technique (Korngold, Van Leeuwen, and Engle, 1962). By either technique the characteristic intensity and position of the precipitation line when appropriate antisera are used demonstrate that one of the IgM family is markedly increased and that the increase is usually due to a single type, either type K or type L. Macroglobulins usually constitute up to 5 per cent of serum gamma globulins. Increase of macroglobulins between 5 and 15 per cent occurs in association with nephrosis, lupus erythematosus, rheumatoid arthritis and a variety of other conditions. Elevation in excess of 15 per cent is highly suggestive of Waldenström's macroglobulinemia (Ritzmann *et al.*, 1960). The macroglobulin may be a cryoglobulin.

A positive Sia water test, wherein a rapidly settling precipitate forms when a drop of serum is dropped into 10 cc of water, is not diagnostic and may be negative, even though the macroglobulins are elevated (Bernard *et al.*, 1961).

### Differential Diagnosis

Diagnosis depends upon the finding of the characteristic macroglobulin elevation.

Lymphosarcoma and lymphatic leukemia may be indistinguishable from Waldenström's macroglobulinemia except for the presence of the increased macroglobulin peak in the latter.

Macroglobulins may be elevated in many conditions, both benign and malignant. However, the eponym, *Waldenström's macroglobulinemia,* is reserved for those associated with lymphoid hyperplasia or usually lymphoid malignancy, not related to other known cause. The distinction from multiple myeloma may be difficult and in some intermediate cases impossible.

Cold agglutinin disease may be difficult to distinguish from Waldenström's macroglobulinemia and may in some instances be indistinguishable unless an arbitrary decision is made. The disease may be discovered because of the high titer cold agglutinins and hemolytic anemia. The lymphoid changes in the marrow and lymph nodes may be similar in both conditions. If the change is malignant or if the protein produced has type specificity, the diagnosis of Waldenström's macroglobulinemia is favored and it must be supposed that the macroglobulin happens to have the properties of a cold agglutinin. On the other hand, the cold agglutinin frequently has specificity as an antibody to factor I in the red cell as well as type K specificity and, if there is no evidence of frank malignancy, a diagnosis of cold agglutinin disease of autoimmune type is made. In rare instances it is impossible to decide between the two diagnoses.

## Prognosis

The prognosis of Waldenström's macroglobulinemia is better than that of multiple myeloma. Exact figures are difficult to obtain because the disease has not been recognized until relatively recently. According to one report, its course is one of progressive deterioration and, as a rule, is concluded in thirty-eight to forty months (Ritzmann *et al.,* 1960).

In another series (Cohen, Bohannon, and Wallerstein, 1966), the duration of survival from the estimated date of clinical onset of the disease varied from twenty-three to 152 months with a mean of fifty-five months. The duration of survival from the date of diagnosis ranged from seven to eighty-two months, with a mean of thirty-four months. Most untreated patients with progressive disease become severely anemic, ultimately debilitated and die in four to five years (Bayrd, Hagedorn, and McGuckin, 1965). On the other hand, in some patients the condition is essentially benign, static, and asymptomatic at least for many years. Survivals of eight and eighteen years have been documented (Bayrd, Hagedorn, and McGuckin, 1965). High incidence of a second malignancy has been noted in patients with Waldenström's macroglobulinemia.

## Complications and Mode of Death

Thromboses and hemorrhage are the major complications which may in themselves lead to death. Death may also result from the lymphoid malignancy, anemia and uncontrollable infection. In those rare instances of Bence Jones proteinuria, a myeloma kidney and renal failure may develop. Amyloidosis is a rare complication. Very frequently, death is due to unrelated causes such as coronary thrombosis or another malignancy.

## Treatment

Some patients do well for long periods of time without treatment. Supportive measures such as blood transfusions and antibiotics when needed are indicated. Since many of the patient's problems are related to the large amounts of circulating macroglobulins, resulting in increased viscosity of the blood, efforts may be needed to reduce them either by drugs or by plasmapheresis.

Plasmapheresis is the procedure of draining large amounts of blood and returning to the patient his own red cells, thereby removing the plasma (Skoog, Adams, and Coburn, 1962; Solomon and Fahey, 1963). Symptoms usually develop when relative viscosity goes above 7 (relative to water), but the threshold may vary as much as from 4 to 12, depending on the vascular bed and other factors. By plasmapheresis it is possible to remove as much as 1,000 cc of plasma a week and maintain the patient at a blood viscosity below his symptom threshold (Solomon and Fahey, 1963). Plasmapheresis is indicated when bleeding, renal impairment, congestive heart failure, pulmonary hypertension, neurologic symptoms, or Raynaud's phenomena occur. Plasmapheresis is also used in the interim when time is needed to institute chemotherapy. Thrombocytopenia, leukopenia, and Coombs-positive hemolytic anemia are not benefited by plasmapheresis. The chief disadvantage of plasmapheresis is the short duration of benefits. Macroglobulin levels return to pretreatment levels in ten days.

Drugs which split the macroglobulins into smaller components have been tried but their use is in the experimental stages. Penicillamine (dimethylcysteine) is a chelating agent and a sulfhydryl reducing agent; hence it can cleave the disulfide bonds of certain high-molecular-weight proteins (Deutsch and Morton, 1957). It has been demonstrated that with daily, oral divided doses of 1 to 2 gm of DL or D-penicillamine it is possible to break up the high-molecular-weight proteins, thereby reducing serum viscosity and relieving a number of clinical symptoms in patients with macroglobulinemia (Glenchur, Zinneman and Briggs, 1958; Ritzmann, Coleman and Levin, 1960; Levine, Hammack, and Frommeyer, 1960). However, the long-term administration of this substance, such as is used for Wilson's disease, is not without dangers. Skin rashes, especially a maculopapular rash and rarely a desquamation of skin on the face and trunk, have been described. Leukopenia and thrombocytopenia which may occur with the DL form of the drug have been shown to be due to the L component, which is an antimetabolite to pyridoxine (Scheinberg and Sternlieb, 1960). Corcos and others (Corcos *et al.*, 1964) reported two cases of neutrophilic agranulocytosis during administration of D-penicillamine. At times a generalized reaction with fever and adenopathy follows. Nephrotic syndrome associated with penicillamine therapy has been described in three patients (Adams *et al.*, 1964).

As with most malignancies, one of the most effective forms of therapy is chemotherapy. Because the predominant cell is lymphoid, most agents known to have an effect on lymphoid tumors have been tried. Chlorambucil, 2 to 6 mg per day orally, is one of the most effective. Initial priming doses of 6 to 12 mg a day have been used (Bayrd, 1961). Good sustained responses to maintenance therapy have been reported, with remissions lasting between 1½ to 5 years. Symptoms improve, abnormal protein diminishes in most and hemoglobin rises. Interrupted treatment usually results in a relapse (Bayrd, Hagedorn, and McGuckin, 1965). If the cells resemble plasma cells, the patient might be treated as a patient with multiple myeloma, using L-phenylalanine mustard (see Multiple Myeloma). There is evidence from turnover studies of $^{131}$I-labelled autologous macroglobulin that L-phenylalanine mustard acts by depressing synthesis of the macroglobulin, not by decreasing catabolism (Wilkinson, Davidson, and Sommaripa, 1966).

Triethylene melamine (Cohen, Bohannon, and Wallerstein, 1966) and Cytoxan® (Waldenström, 1952) have been reported to induce remissions. Local irradiation may also be useful, either for local lesions or for its general effect on the lymphomatous disease. Cortisone is sometimes very useful not only for the feeling of well-being that it gives the patient but also for its effect on hemolysis, capillary fragility, and on the tumor cells themselves. In the rare case of uncontrollable hemolysis, splenectomy may be indicated.

## H-CHAIN DISEASE

H-chain disease is a recently recognized paraimmunoglobulinopathy similar to multiple myeloma and Waldenström's macroglobulinemia, but in which the paraimmunoglobulin in the blood and urine is either a heavy chain of the immunoglobulins or a portion of the heavy chain. Because there are four kinds of heavy chains, there are four possible kinds of this disease. Until recently, only the heavy chain disease of IgG, involving the γ chain, has been recognized. The cell types involved are the lymphocyte and lymphoid plasma cell. In many respects this is a subcategory of multiple myeloma. It is separated here because the five cases studied thus far suggest that it is a recognizable clinical syndrome (Osserman and Takatsuki, 1964; Franklin *et al.*, 1964). Recently a patient with heavy chain disease of IgA, involving the α chain, has been described (Seligmann and Basch, 1968).

### Pathology

Two of the patients with H-chain disease came to autopsy (Osserman and Takatsuki, 1964). In both cases the salient features were generalized lymphadenopathy, hepatosplenomegaly, and diffuse infiltrations of these organs, of the bone marrow, and of the adrenals by large, immature "reticuloendothelial cells," immature plasmacytic and lymphocytic elements, and eosinophils. Biopsies of lymph nodes and, in one case, of a skin lesion revealed infiltration with similar immature cells. The focal reticulum cell infiltrates, plasmacytosis, lymphocytosis, and eosinophilia combine to form a picture sometimes indistinguishable from Hodgkin's disease; however, giant cells and necrosis are absent.

Zucker-Franklin (1964) has studied the cells from these patients and concluded that they are lymphocytes, lymphoid plasma cells, and plasma cells, essentially similar to the cells seen in Waldenström's macroglobulinemia.

### Clinical Manifestations

The clinical picture of this syndrome resembles that of malignant lymphoma or Hodgkin's disease with several variations. The generalized, often painful and tender lymphadenopathy appears suddenly and may wax and wane spontaneously. Splenomegaly is consistently present; hepatomegaly occurs in most patients.

The peculiar edema and erythema of the palate and uvula may occasionally cause transient respiratory difficulty. There is marked susceptibility to recurrent bacterial infections, especially pneumonia. Fever is common even in the absence of overt infection. Only in one case did x-ray studies reveal moderate osteoporosis. No osteolytic lesions were found.

### Laboratory Findings

Moderate anemia, leukopenia with relative lymphocytosis, eosinophilia, and immature lymphocytes and/or plasma cells are found in the peripheral blood. The bone marrow contains the characteristic lymphoid and plasma cells and increased numbers of eosinophils.

Urinalysis reveals massive proteinuria which is negative with the Bence Jones heat test. A homogeneous $beta_2$ peak is seen upon electrophoresis of the urine. The serum globulins are elevated and upon electrophoresis there is a paraimmunoglobulin peak of the same mobility as the urinary peak. This is at variance with the classic findings in multiple myeloma, where the urinary peak usually has a faster mobility than the serum peak when both are present. There is a marked decrease of all other immunoglobulin components. Immunologic studies are required to demonstrate that both the urinary protein and the abnormal serum protein are heavy chains or heavy-chain fragments. The molecular weight of this protein has been found to be 53,000. The serum uric acid is usually elevated. However, renal function is normal.

### Differential Diagnosis

This condition often has the clinical picture of lymphosarcoma or Hodgkin's disease. Finding the characteristic protein in the blood or urine should distinguish them.

### Prognosis

Since only five cases have been reported, it is difficult to speculate on prognosis. The survival has been from three months to three years, and two patients were still alive at the time of reporting after two and three years' survival (Osserman and Takatsuki, 1964). It is quite possible that the prognosis in this disease will be similar to that of Waldenström's macroglobulinemia.

### Complications and Mode of Death

These are probably similar to what would be expected in lymphoma. Infection, particularly pneumonitis, was a frequent complication in the cases reported (Osserman and Takatsuki, 1964).

### Treatment

There are insufficient data to make a definitive statement. Nitrogen mustards and x-ray therapy to nodes and spleen have been used with some success. Cellular infiltrates appear to be relatively radiosensitive. Other agents effective against the specific cell type, such as chlorambucil or even L-phenylalanine mustard, may be indicated. Prophylactic gamma globulin is useful in the cases in which there is an enhanced susceptibility to recurrent bacterial infections.

## PARAIMMUNOGLOBULINOPATHIES ASSOCIATED WITH OTHER DISEASES

### Chronic Lymphocytic Leukemia, Lymphosarcoma, Reticulum Cell Sarcoma, and Hodgkin's Disease

Paraimmunoglobulins may be seen in some patients with any of these diseases (Krauss and Sokal, 1966). These situations are sometimes considered variants of multiple myeloma with involvement of unusual cell types. Some of them are actually Waldenström's macroglobulinemia or H-chain disease. In other instances, it has been thought that the lymphoma or Hodgkin's disease has occurred in association with an unrelated multiple myeloma (see Interrelationships of the Paraimmunoglobulinopathies). It is felt that *de novo* appearance of a paraimmunoglobulin during the clinical course of lymphoma indicates a relatively poor prognosis (Krauss and Sokal, 1966).

### Other Malignancies

Paraimmunoglobulins may be found in some patients with myelogenous leukemia as well as monocytic leukemia (Osserman, 1967). Since the clinical picture may be that of multiple myeloma coexisting with the leukemia, it has been postulated that the association results from proliferative abnormalities of more than one cell type.

Many patients with various malignancies show plasmacytosis, hypergammaglobulinemia (usually of the diffuse variety, occasionally of the electrophoretically homogeneous myeloma or macroglobulin variety) (Osserman, 1958), and sometimes cryoglobulinemia (Bohrod, 1957). Osserman and Takatsuki (1963a) collected thirty-one patients with homogeneous immunoglobulin peaks associated with neoplasm. These were neoplasms of the rectosigmoid (9), prostate (5), breast (4), oropharynx (4), liver (2), stomach, jejunum, pancreas, uterus, and bladder. Association with chronic myelogenous leukemia has also been described (Osserman and Takatsuki, 1963a; Ritzmann *et al.*, 1966). Anderson and Vye (1967) reported the only case of paraimmunoglobulinopathy associated with thymoma and reviewed fifty-three previously reported associations between paraimmunoglobulinopathy and neoplasms. Absence of a single case of bronchogenic carcinoma was considered striking by Osserman and Takatsuki (1965).

In some instances, the presence of two malignancies, one of them myeloma or macroglobulinemia, in the same patient has been considered as the best explanation. However, in most instances, the diagnosis of myeloma or Waldenström's macroglobulinemia could not be made. A possibility exists that the protein abnormality is related to the neoplasm in each case. Relationship of this paraimmunoglobulinemia and associated blood, bone marrow, and tissue plasmacytosis to immunity to cancer has been considered (Bohrod, 1957).

## Nonneoplastic Conditions Usually Characterized by Diffuse Hyperimmunoglobulinemia

In rare instances of virtually any condition usually associated with a diffuse hyperimmunoglobulinemia, there may be a spike or multiple spikes in the electrophoretic pattern superimposed on a normal or slightly elevated, or, rarely, diminished gamma globulin. The spike is often best seen when electrophoresis is performed in starch gels and may be indistinguishable from a myeloma spike. These conditions include long-standing and protracted chronic inflammatory processes, especially chronic granulomatous pulmonary disease, osteomyelitis, chronic genitourinary infections, and chronic biliary disease; also liver disease, sarcoidosis, cold agglutinin disease, cold allergy, lupus erythematosus, rheumatoid arthritis, Gaucher's disease (Osserman and Takatsuki, 1963a), and papular mucinosis (Osserman and Takatsuki, 1963b). In a series studied at The New York Hospital (Engle *et al.*, 1961), the following heterogeneous cases were found: one patient with hypersensitivity to cold without cold agglutinins or cryoglobulins; another patient with emphysema and gastrointestinal bleeding; another with periodic hypervolemic shock (reported by Clarkson and others [Clarkson *et al.*, 1960]); still another with diabetes, hypertensive cardiovascular disease, and goiter; another with coronary occlusion and bleeding tendency; and finally, one with the hypercorticism syndrome.

It is usually possible to make a primary diagnosis but sometimes it is difficult to decide whether the patient has multiple myeloma or Waldenström's macroglobulinemia with the picture of the other disease, or whether the entire symptom complex results from the other nonmalignant disease. It is interesting to speculate on the possibility that massive benign stimulation of the immune system with proliferation of immunocytes leads to increased susceptibility to malignant change through somatic mutation and that the superimposed spikes seen in the electrophoretic pattern are a manifestation of such clonal proliferation. The chronic antigenic stimulation may be analogous to the intraperitoneal adjuvant in BALB/c mice which over prolonged administration leads first to diffuse hyperimmunoglobulinemia, then finally to paraimmunoglobulinemia (Osserman and Takatsuki, 1965). The electrophoretic pattern may be an indication of somatic mutation among the immunocytes.

## PARAIMMUNOGLOBULINOPATHIES OF UNKNOWN ETIOLOGY

### Idiopathic Paraimmunoglobulinemia

When electrophoretic studies are done routinely on sera of individuals in large unselected population surveys, instances are found with homogeneous peaks characteristic of multiple myeloma (Engle *et al.*, 1961; Osserman, 1958; Waldenström, 1961). A recent report describes the finding of sixty-four instances of abnormal spikes in the paper electrophoretic pattern of almost 7,000 sera from persons over twenty-five screened in a mass health control program in the district of Värmland in Sweden (1%). It was estimated that only two or three of these patients would be expected to have multiple myeloma. The concentration of the abnormal components was usually low, under 1 gm per 100 ml. The incidence of the abnormal components increased with age and was highest (5.7%) in the age class eighty to eighty-nine years (Axelsson, Bachmann, and Hällen, 1966). In other series, about 3 per cent of persons over seventy years of age were found to have such peaks (Hällen, 1963; Fine *et al.*, 1964).

While the above instances can be classified as *Asymptomatic Idiopathic Paraimmunoglobulinemia,* another group of *Symptomatic Idiopathic Paraimmunoglobulinemia* has become apparent where symptoms are related to the effects of the abnormal protein alone, but not to any immunocyte proliferation or to any other underlying condition. Hammack, Bolding and Frommeyer (1959), Smith (1957), and Owen and Rider (1957) reported a total of twenty-one patients with homogeneous serum gamma globulin peaks and/or homogeneous proteinuria; none had skeletal lesions or bone marrow abnormality. They called the condition "dysgammaglobulinemia syndrome" and "nonmyelomatous paraproteinemia" and noted the unusual incidence of recurrent pneumonia and chronic pulmonary disease. Synthesis of normal immunoglobulin was apparently suppressed by the abnormal component.

Zawadski and Edwards (1967) studied eighteen similar patients; in four cases there were morphologic changes of the bone marrow supporting the diagnosis of multiple myeloma; three patients presented with isolated Bence Jones proteinuria; in nine cases the paraimmunoglobulinemia was the only pathological finding; one patient had asymptomatic macroglobulinemia. Wysocki and Mackiewicz (1965) reported homogeneous IgA paraimmunoglobulinemia occurring in three members of one Polish family. The abnormal findings included a bleeding disorder characterized by prolonged clotting time, abnormal prothrombin consumption and pathological thromboplastin generation test in all three patients; some improvement resulted from steroid therapy. The authors postulated activity of the abnormal protein as an anticoagulant. The increase in IgA-globulin was associated with the deficiency in normal IgG-globulin. High sedimentation rate and hypochromic anemia were also present in the propositus.

In other patients idiopathic paraimmunoglobulinemia may be just a stage in the natural history of myeloma. Osserman initially reported on twenty-four (1958) and later on forty (Osserman and Takatsuki, 1963a) asymptomatic patients who had a homogeneous globulin peak on serum electrophoresis. Patients were followed up to nine years. In two patients myeloma developed within a year of the discovery of the serum protein peak. Two additional patients had diffuse plasma cell infiltration of the marrow at autopsy. Kyle and Bayrd (1966) reported a patient in whom clinical myeloma developed sixteen years after hyperglobulinemia and elevated sedimentation rate were discovered. Similar cases have been reported with the interval between discovery of paraimmunoglobulinemia and the onset of clinical multiple myeloma being four years (Baker and Martin, 1959), six years (Stevens, 1965), twelve years (Norgaard, 1964), sixteen years (Bichel and Kirketerp, 1938), and seventeen years (Bloom, Shulman, and Witebsky, 1958).

Some authors emphasize the benign nature of the isolated paraimmunoglobulinemia and call it "benign monoclonal gammopathy" (Waldenström, 1964b). Others (Hällen, 1963) feel that the development of clinical myeloma is a real possibility even after many years of asymptomatic "benign" monoclonal gammopathy and that it is not safe to assume that these patients have a benign condition even after years of observation. These two opposing viewpoints are expressed in the two commonly used terms for this condition: *benign monoclonal gammopathy* on one hand and *premyeloma* on the other. There are valid objections to either appellation. We prefer the terms *asymptomatic paraimmunoglobulinemia* and *asymptomatic paraimmuno-*

*globulinuria* for the instances of those abnormal protein spikes unassociated with any symptoms whatsoever. *Symptomatic idiopathic paraimmunoglobulinemia* is the term we use for cases where abnormal protein spikes are present and may *per se* be responsible for the symptoms, but no underlying cellular pathology can be found. We prefer these terms because they do not imply a benign or a malignant nature of the observed abnormality. While certain of the patients ultimately develop signs and symptoms of overt paraimmunoglobulinopathy such as multiple myeloma, Waldenström's macroglobulinemia, and paraamyloidosis (Osserman and Takatsuki, 1965) after asymptomatic periods of up to seventeen years, it is becoming apparent with increasing laboratory and follow-up experience that overt myeloma and symptomatic macroglobulinemia may not be an invariable development, at least within the life span of these patients. This is especially true of the cases found during surveys of "normal" populations.

Increase in incidence of asymptomatic paraimmunoglobulinemia with age (Hällen, 1963) leads to the postulation of somatic mutation. On the other hand, occurrence of various paraimmunoglobulinemias, symptomatic and asymptomatic, in several members of one family (Wysocki and Mackiewicz, 1965; Seligmann, Danon, and Mihaesco, 1965; Williams *et al.*, 1967) indicates a genetic disorder.

### Idiopathic or Essential Cryoglobulinemia

The great majority of patients with cryoglobulinemia (cold precipitable or cold gelling proteins in blood) have evidence of a primary disease, often multiple myeloma or Waldenström's macroglobulinemia (Hill, Dunlop and Mulligan, 1949; Mackay *et al.*, 1956). In rare instances no primary diagnosis can be made, usually because there is no evidence of plasma cell or lymphocyte infiltration in the marrow or other tissues (Gaddy and Powell, 1958; Volpé *et al.*, 1956; Farmer, Cooper and Pascuzzi, 1960). In one patient studied at The New York Hospital (Barr, Engle, and Russ, 1957), large reticulum-like cells with unusual cytoplasmic characteristics (possibly because of cryoglobulin deposits) and plasma cells were found in appreciable numbers in the bone marrow during life, whereas at autopsy none could be found. If not frankly multiple myeloma or Waldenström's macroglobulinemia, some of these conditions are at least closely related to them. Clinically, they are similar to the syndrome of cryoglobulinemia described in the section on multiple myeloma.

### Idiopathic Pyroglobulinemia

Pyroglobulinemia or the appearance of heat precipitable or gelling proteins in the blood has been described in the section on multiple myeloma, with which it is usually associated. Rarely, no primary disease may be found.

Pyroglobulinemia may be accidentally detected when a routine Wassermann test is performed on the patient's serum and the serum gels upon heating (Lipman, 1964).

## PARAAMYLOIDOSIS

*Definition.* Paraamyloidosis is the term used to designate mesenchymatous amyloidosis seen in association with paraimmunoglobulinopathies such as multiple myeloma and Waldenström's macroglobulinemia. It has been estimated that 10 to 20 per cent of patients with myeloma also have amyloidosis (Bayrd and Bennett, 1950; Magnus-Levy, 1931). Only fourteen patients with Waldenström's macroglobulinemia and paraamyloidosis are on record (Forget, Squires and Sheldon, 1966).

In organ and tissue distribution, in histochemical characteristics of the deposited amyloid and in clinical symptomatology, paraamyloidosis is similar to the other forms of mesenchymatous amyloidosis (old terminology: "primary" amyloidosis) of which it is but one subdivision; the other subdivisions are familial mesenchymatous amyloidosis, idiopathic mesenchymatous amyloidosis, and mesenchymatous amyloidoses of other etiology (drug sensitivity, myxedema, senility, tumors) (Engle and Wallis, 1966). Apitz (1940) found increased numbers of plasma cells in the bone marrow of all his several patients with mesenchymatous amyloidosis. He concluded that most, if not all, cases of mesenchymatous amyloidosis are due to occult or "burned out" myeloma. Indeed, myeloma is frequently the basis of mesenchymatous amyloidosis and should be searched for in every case, even though the bones may appear normal on x-ray examination or even grossly normal at autopsy. When the manifestations of immunocyte dyscrasia (multiple myeloma, macroglobulinemia) are searched for, they are frequently found. Rarely, after careful study no diagnosis other than idiopathic mesenchymatous amyloidosis can be made.

### Pathogenesis

Amyloid is a homogeneous eosinophilic substance, predominantly protein, usually found in the extracellular tissue spaces unassociated with any apparent inflammatory reaction. There is also a carbohydrate component, which consists of glucosamine, galactose, mannose, and fucose (Calkins, Cohen, and Larsen, 1960). It is not a uniform chemical substance but a group of substances which are closely related and which may vary from one patient to another.

Amyloid stains pink with hematoxylin and eosin stain. In the mesenchymatous form of the disease, including paraamyloidosis, it may fail to give the typical staining reactions such as staining brown with iodine, red with Congo red, metachromatically with methyl violet and crystal violet, yellow with van Gieson stain. But in both forms of the disease, amyloid stains with thioflavin T, is birefringent and appears green in sections stained with Congo red and observed under the polarizing microscope.

Whether the protein moiety of amyloid is related to immunoglobulins, as only recently believed, or whether it is a modified fibrous protein either related or unrelated to collagen, has not yet been clarified. It has been suggested (Osserman, 1959) that in immunocyte dyscrasias, microglobulins (proteins of low molecular weight produced by abnormal plasma cells) are capable of diffusing through the capillary beds and that these microglobulins find complementary polysaccharides in only certain tissue sites; microglobulins become bound to these tissue sites in the form of insoluble complexes recognized as amyloid.

The most convincing evidence that amyloid is related to the immunoglobulins or antibodies is the ability of amyloid deposits to stain with fluorescent antibodies against gamma globulin (Vazquez and Dixon, 1956; Mellors *et al.*, 1961; Lachmann *et al.*, 1962; Mellors and Ortega, 1956) and against certain components of complement, particularly $beta_{1c}$ globulin (Lachmann *et al.*, 1962). The fact that a component of complement is also present in amyloid gives support to the thesis that amyloid deposits are insoluble antigen-antibody complexes (Latvalahti, 1953) as does the demonstration of both 19S rheumatoid factor and 7S gamma globulin in the amyloid of patients with rheumatoid arthritis (Mellors *et al.*, 1961). However, careful studies by Calkins, Cohen, and Gitlin (1958) using other immunologic techniques failed to demonstrate appreciable gamma globulin in amyloid deposits of patients with either mesenchymatous or parenchymatous amyloidosis. More recent studies (Paul and Cohen, 1963) using the electron microscope to localize the deposition of ferritin-conjugated antibody have also failed to demonstrate gamma globulin in amyloid fibrils. Likewise, Cathcart and associates find the amyloid fibrils of both mesenchymatous and parenchymatous forms to be related immunologically to a minor circulating $alpha_1$ globulin (P component) found even in normal serum (Cathcart, Comerford, and Cohen, 1965). All of their attempts to relate the amyloid fibrils to gamma globulin have been unsuccessful. However, it is quite possible that portions of the amyloid are lost in the isolation of the fibrils.

The electron microscope studies reveal that the amyloid, a fibrous protein, has a 75 ängstrom periodicity compared to 640 ängstrom periodicity of collagen. Frequently a helical arrangement is formed by two amyloid fibrils twisted together (Sorenson, 1966). In addition, amyloid exhibits a high degree of resistance to collagen-destroying enzymes (Windrum and Kramer, 1957) and to proteolytic enzymes such as pepsin (McAlpine, Radcliffe, and Friedmann, 1963). These observations are inconsistent with a collagen hypothesis.

It seems very likely now that amyloid is a scleroprotein originating from histocytes or reticuloendothelial cells (Gueft and Ghidoni, 1963; Cohen, Gross and Shirahama, 1964). Amyloid fibrils are probably formed at the surface of reticuloendothelial cells just as it is thought that collagen fibrils are formed at the surface of fibroblasts (Sorenson, Heefner, and Kirkpatrick, 1964).

There are two schools of thought concerning the way in which the amyloid is deposited; some favor a cellular origin with local deposition and others favor a humoral mechanism. The cellular theory is favored by Teilum (1956, 1964), who showed that amyloid deposition in the various organs was preceded by a marked proliferation of reticuloendothelial cells. These cells later develop intracytoplasmic periodic acid-Schiff positive granules. The periodic acid-Schiff positive material is then deposited locally as amyloid when the cells degenerate.

Proponents of the humoral theory point out the difficulty of finding any evidence of cellular reaction near deposits of amyloid and hold that the amyloid must arrive at the site of deposition through the bloodstream, although admittedly the amyloid is probably a cellular product. This thesis is strengthened by the observation that in many cases of paraamyloidosis early in the disease the globulin level is high but as the amyloid develops the globulin level may drop to normal or low levels (Eisen, 1946). Osserman, Takatsuki, and Talal (1964) studied the tissue-binding affinities of fluorescein-labeled Bence Jones proteins from patients with and without amyloidosis and were able to demonstrate a greater tissue-binding affinity in those patients with amyloidosis, suggesting that certain Bence Jones proteins have a greater propensity than others for deposition in the tissues in the form of amyloid. Almost all patients with multiple myeloma and amyloidosis have Bence Jones protein in the urine.

Thus, whether a cellular or a humoral theory is favored, it seems likely that amyloid is closely related to the immune response and may or may not involve the immunoglobulins. Osserman (1961) has postulated that the cellular theory is probably best in parenchymatous amyloidosis while the humoral theory may hold for mesenchymatous amyloidoses and especially in paraamyloidosis. That both mechanisms may act in the same patient is also possible, since amyloid deposits may be found in plasmacytomas and amyloid has on occasion been found in plasma cells of patients with multiple myeloma (Dahlin and Dockerty, 1950).

## Pathology

In paraamyloidosis amyloid deposits are usually found in many organs throughout the body, although in some cases only a single organ (e.g., the heart) may be involved. Characteristically the lesions are found in the heart, alimentary tract, tongue, spleen, liver, kidneys, lungs, adrenals, lymph nodes, and skeletal muscle. It is not unusual also to find involvement of the skin, endocrine glands, bone marrow, bones, joints, ligaments, adipose tissue, and nervous system including the choroid plexus, pia mater, meningeal vessels, dorsal root and sympathetic ganglia and perineurium and epineurium of peripherial nerves.

Actually, almost any organ or tissue may be involved. When a single organ is involved it is likely to be the skin, the conjunctiva, an organ in the respiratory system such as the nose, sinuses, mouth, larynx, trachea, bronchi, or lungs, or an organ in the genitourinary tract such as the bladder, urethra, or vagina. In many instances careful search will reveal more generalized amyloidosis than is at first evident.

The amyloid deposits occur in the walls of blood vessels, arteries, arterioles, and around capillaries, and spread to adjacent areas. The vessel walls may be completely replaced by the amyloid, forming rigid tubes. Heller, Missmahl, Sohar, and Gafni (1964) have pointed out that the initial deposits of amyloid in this type of amyloidosis occur adjacent to collagen fibers in the adventitia and media of arteries and in the adventitia of veins. The endothelium and lumen usually remain intact. Thrombosis as a result of amyloid is uncommon. Amyloid deposition results in compression atrophy of parenchymatous cells and ischemia of the normal tissues. There may be giant cell reaction. The amyloid involvement of the parenchyma may be so extensive in some organs as to be indistinguishable from the lesions of classic parenchymatous amyloidosis. Sometimes amyloid nodules, which may have a laminated appearance, are seen with little or no cellularity.

## Clinical Manifestations

Paraamyloidosis may involve any organ or system. It is a polysystemic disease. The most common presenting symptoms are weakness, edema, and purpura. Macroglossia and bilateral paresthesias of the hands are next most common.

### Skin Involvement

In 25 to 40 per cent of patients, classic nodular amyloid infiltrations are present in the skin and mucous membranes. Clinically, the lesions are waxy, shiny, smooth, yellow papules which look like translucent vesicles but feel solid. They are usually 1 mm to 2 cm in diameter but larger nodules, tumors, and plaques have been described. A slight erythematous halo may appear at the base of the papules. The lesions occur most commonly in skin folds, on eyelids, in circumoral areas, on the side of the nose, over the axillae, in antecubital spaces, and on fingers, palms, neck, and the anogenital area. They are seen not infrequently in the mucous membrane of lips and tongue. Amyloid deposits over the cervix have also been reported (Ware and Silverman, 1961).

Scleroderma-like lesions are present in about 10 per cent of cases (Rukavina *et al.*, 1956) with extensive thickening and hardening of the skin on the face, scalp, chin, neck, and hands. Almost complete occlusion of the external auditory canals by scleroderma-like deposits has been described. Pigmentary cutaneous changes have been described in 13 per cent of cases. Pruritus may be prominent. Painless ulceration of these lesions is uncommon but has been described (Rukavina *et al.*, 1956). Alopecia may occur.

In a third of the patients with amyloidosis, purpura and ecchymoses occur, usually on the face and neck but also over the legs and other areas. These bleeding phenomena are due to vascular changes. Skin biopsy in these cases reveals amyloid in the walls of the cutaneous blood vessels. No defects of the coagulation mechanism have been found (Propp *et al.*, 1954). The papules and petechiae are likely to occur in the same areas of the skin.

Any form of local trauma such as stroking, rubbing, or compression may result in development of immediate intralesional bleeding, with the surrounding normal skin remaining free of purpuric change (Hurley and Weinberg, 1964).

A bleeding tendency may also manifest itself in hematemesis, hemoptysis, recurrent epistaxis, gross rectal bleeding, and melena. These bleeding episodes are not associated with demonstrable clotting defects or thrombocytopenia.

Localized amyloidosis of the skin or lichen amyloidosis is relatively rare. The lesion consists of aggregates of intensely pruritic, small, lichenoid papules usually occurring on the anterior and lateral aspects of the legs and sometimes on the lateral surfaces of the forearms; rarely it is seen on other parts of the body. The intracutaneous test with 1.5 per cent solution of Congo red is usually positive (Nomland, 1936). Another skin condition which is probably related to paraamyloidosis in some cases is papular mucinosis or lichen myxedematosus (see Clinical Manifestations of Multiple Myeloma).

### Cardiac Involvement

The heart is involved in a third to a half of patients with paraamyloidosis (Cassidy, 1961). Progressive intractable heart failure is the most common manifestation. It is usually refractory to digitalis and other standard treatment. Digitalis sensitivity has been reported in cardiac amyloidosis (Cassidy, 1961). About 60 per cent of patients with mesenchymatous amyloidosis die of cardiac involvement. The symptoms in cardiac amyloidosis depend on extent and distribution of the amyloid. Involvement of the coronary arteries may lead to angina and congestive heart failure. Endocardial deposits present in half the patients with cardiac amyloidosis may occasionally cause severe valvular deformity resulting in stenosis or insufficiency. Signs and symptoms of mitral, aortic, pulmonary, and tricuspid stenosis have been observed (van Buchem, Mandema, and Arends, 1962). Verrucous valvular lesions have been described (Gonzales-Angulo, Greenberg, and Wallace, 1963). These valvular vegetations may produce embolic phenomena similar to those in subacute bacterial endocarditis. Epicardial and pericardial deposits, although extensive, may not interfere with cardiac function. Amyloid deposits between the muscle bundles in the myocardium do not always disturb cardiac function. Cardiac manifestations may be absent if the infiltration of the heart is minimal. With more extensive involvement the myocardial fibers are subject to compression by the amyloid and both the contractile power and the dilatation ability of the heart are impeded. Symptoms consist of exertional dyspnea, often without orthopnea. Patients may complain of bloating and right upper quadrant or epigastric fullness with nausea and vomiting as a result of hepatic congestion. Dependent edema may be present. Angina may result from interference by the amyloid with the coronary circulation through deposition within coronary vessels. Tachycardia, pulsus alternans, premature contractions, and atrial fibrillation are not rare. Syncope of the Stokes-Adams type has been described in these patients.

Amyloid may completely replace areas of muscle tissue. The clinical picture may closely simulate that of constrictive pericarditis (van Buchem, Mandema and Arends, 1962; Von Hoyningen-Huene, 1964). Blood pressure and pulse pressure may be decreased, venous pressure is elevated, and neck veins are distended. Leg and presacral edema may be followed by anasarca with ascites and hydrothorax; hydrothorax is often unilateral only. The heart is often not enlarged or it may appear spherical on x-ray films. The heart sounds may be unremarkable, but murmurs of various valvular involvement may be present. $S_3$ gallop may be heard.

The electrocardiogram frequently shows a decrease in amplitudes of P waves and QRS complexes (van Buchem, Mandema, and Arends, 1962; Farrokh, Walsh, and Massie, 1964). The T waves are flat or negative; the ST segments may be depressed. The ST segments in the precordial leads may be elevated and have an arcuate configuration reminiscent of myocardial infarction. An atrioventricular block, Wenckebach's phenomenon, bundle-branch block, or atrial fibrillation may be present. Vectorcardiograms usually show a posterior and superior orientation of the QRS loop with marked loss of anterior forces, suggesting a pattern of anteroseptal or anterior myocardial infarction (Farrokh, Walsh, and Massie, 1964).

The right ventricular pressure curves reveal the early diastolic dip followed by a rapid rise of the diastolic pressure as a result of the rapid filling of the right ventricle by the high venous pressure and the limited capacity of the ventricle. This picture is also seen in constrictive pericarditis and endocardial fibroelastosis. These patients respond little or not at all to digitalis preparations.

In summary, the salient features frequently seen in cardiac amyloidosis are intractable heart failure, constrictive pericarditis-like syndrome, nonspecific electrocardiographic abnormalities, refractoriness to digitalis, and sometimes digitalis sensitivity (Cassidy, 1961).

### Gastrointestinal Tract Involvement

The gastrointestinal tract is the second most common site of involvement in paraamyloidosis. Symptoms include macroglossia, xerostomia, dysphagia, epigastric distress, belching, postprandial burning, nausea, vomiting, anorexia, hematemesis, diarrhea, constipation and melena. One of the most striking findings, macroglossia, is present in a third of the patients. The entire tongue may be diffusely enlarged or a tumor mass may protrude from it. The tongue may appear dry, firm, rubbery, hard, nodular, smooth, purpuric, ecchymotic, indented, and occasionally ulcerated and discharging pus. Macroglossia is usually painless but causes dysphagia, dysphonia, and hoarseness; sometimes there is mouth pain and xerostomia. These symptoms may be so disabling that inanition results; subtotal glossectomy has occasionally been resorted to with variable success.

Salivary gland infiltration with complaint of a dry mouth is not uncommon. Gingival involvement may appear as painful blood blisters which break and leave small ulcerations. These may be mistaken for canker sores. Diffuse swelling of gingiva and face as well as localized adenopathy may follow.

Involvement of the esophagus occurs in about 23 per cent of the cases and may result in ulcerations, tumor masses, rigidity, stenosis, or a scleroderma-like picture. Vomiting is common. A case of massive esophageal involvement with hematemesis, melena, and esophageal perforation has been reported (Heitzman, Heitzman, and Elliott, 1962). Perforation of the stomach has been described.

Diffuse deposition of amyloid in the wall of the intestine may result in a fragile, somewhat rigid and poorly distensible viscus. The amyloid may interfere with the peristaltic activity of the intestine and with its absorptive functions. A sudden distention, vigorous peristalsis, or external trauma may cause rupture of the viscus.

Persistent, severe, refractory diarrhea may be a manifestation of autonomic neuropathy comparable to that sometimes seen in diabetes mellitus. The presence of diarrhea sometimes correlates with the finding of amyloid within the sympathetic-parasympathetic ganglia and the splanchnic nerves (Liske, Chou, and Thompson, 1963; Brody, Wertlake, and Laster, 1964; French *et al.*, 1965). Diarrhea is often associated with steatorrhea of 15 to 89 gm of fat excreted a day (Green *et al.*, 1961) and other manifestations of malabsorption. These symptoms are probably due to amyloid infiltration of the intestinal submucosa causing a mechanical interference. Steatorrhea may also result from amyloid infiltration of the pancreas (French *et al.*,

1965). Mild, severe, or disturbing constipation is suffered by 10 to 15 per cent of these patients (Rukavina *et al.*, 1956). Sometimes patients complain of alternating constipation and diarrhea. The occasional finding of a bezoar may be due to the abnormal motility of the stomach from autonomic dysfunction as well as lack of proper secretions. Massive gastrointestinal bleeding has been reported.

### Involvement of Liver, Spleen, and Lymph Nodes

In 30 to 45 per cent of patients with paraamyloidosis hepatomegaly is present (Kyle and Bayrd, 1961). However, only a few of these patients reveal laboratory evidence of hepatic impairment. The amyloid infiltration of the liver alters structure but does not profoundly affect function. With extensive liver amyloidosis, the pattern of the liver function tests may include a high serum alkaline phosphatase, a high bromsulphalein retention, a high cholesterol level, and a normal thymol turbidity. Jaundice occurred in four of twenty patients reported by Briggs (1961). Ascites may be present (Gregg, Herskovic, and Bartholomew, 1965). Dysfunction of liver, heart, and kidneys appeared to be the essential factor in the formation of ascites.

Splenomegaly is noted in about 10 per cent of the patients and usually is slight (Kyle and Bayrd, 1961). Four cases of acute splenic rupture due to amyloid have been recorded (Kyle and Bayrd, 1961). Lymphadenopathy is described in about 10 per cent (Eisen, 1946; Rukavina *et al.*, 1956) but usually is not prominent. However, with macroglossia, submaxillary nodes may be enlarged. Amyloid deposits in intrathoracic peritoneal nodes are common.

### Neurologic Involvement

Neurologic manifestations of amyloidosis are varied (Andrade, 1952; Kernohan and Woltman, 1942; Liske, Chow, and Thompson, 1963; Kantarjian and DeJong, 1953; Munsat and Poussaint, 1962). The bilateral carpal tunnel syndrome, seen in about 5 per cent of these patients, is initially manifested as paresthesias of both hands followed by weakness (Kyle and Bayrd, 1961; Rukavina *et al.*, 1956; Grokoest and Demartini, 1954). Symptoms in the upper extremities consist of hand pain, pain in the fingertips, numbness of the fingers with paresthesias, swelling and burning of the fingers and hands, incoordination, disturbances in grasping, and abnormal hand movements. Symptoms in the lower extremities are weakness, a "furry" feeling, difficulty in walking, painful feet, numbness, burning pain, calf pain, and marked hypersensitivity to touch (Kernohan and Woltman, 1942). Other neurologic symptoms are insomnia, unusual drowsiness leading to sleep during conversation, paranoia, agitation, depression, syncope, anisocoria, impotence, loss of libido, and urinary dysfunction.

Increased weakness and fatigability are an integral part of the clinical picture of amyloidosis. Symmetric wasting of somatic muscles with muscular weakness is also common; as the disease progresses, the gait becomes abnormal; the patients become unable to rise to a sitting position unaided and become bedridden. Sensorimotor neuropathy develops in some patients, leading to delayed pain conduction and absent deep tendon reflexes, especially in the lower extremities. Paresthesias of the extremities of the trunk can occur (Briggs, 1964) as well as striking hyperesthesia, anesthesia, and diminished position sense. Peripheral neuropathy is sometimes associated with autonomic neuropathy and severe refractory diarrhea. These clinical findings may in some cases correlate with the presence of massive amyloid deposits in spinal ganglia, spinal nerves, splanchnic nerves, sympathetic ganglia, and parasympathetic ganglia (Liske, Chou, and Thompson, 1963). In other cases amyloid deposits are not found. Episodes of transient mental confusion and hemiplegia may occur in this disease (Heitzman, Heitzman, and Elliott, 1962) and may be related to the amyloid involvement of cerebral vessels. The cerebrospinal fluid protein becomes moderately elevated in two thirds of the cases of amyloidosis with neurologic involvement.

### Involvement of the Respiratory Tract

Involvement of nose and nasopharynx may give rise to nasal twang. Amyloid involvement of the larynx may cause hoarseness, dyspnea, vocal cord paralysis, and unintelligible, thick, and slurred speech. Dyspnea may also result from amyloid deposits in the walls of the pulmonary alveoli (Groen, quoted by van Buchem, Mandema, and Arends, 1962), in the mucosa of the bronchial tree, or in the mediastinum. Amyloid deposits in the pulmonary arterioles may lead to an increased pulmonary vascular resistance, pulmonary hypertension, and cor pulmonale.

Diffuse submucosal deposition of amyloid in the bronchi may lead to stenosis and atelectasis and may be confused with bronchogenic carcinoma (Domm, Vassallo, and Adams, 1965).

### Urinary Tract Involvement

Almost all patients with paraamyloidosis have Bence Jones proteinuria. About 90 per cent of patients develop albuminuria, usually late in the disease. This is frequently massive and is accompanied by edema of legs and face, anasarca, hypoalbuminemia, and hypercholesterolemia sometimes above 500 mg%. These findings, coupled with a normal blood pressure and normal blood urea nitrogen, are in keeping with the nephrotic syndrome that 10 per cent of these patients present. Hematuria and persistent hyposthenuria may also be present. Renal symptoms are less common in paraamyloidosis than they are in the parenchymatous form.

## Miscellaneous Manifestations

Weakness, fatigability, and anorexia are common complaints in mesenchymatous amyloidosis. Weight loss is complained of by three fourths of patients with amyloidosis (Kyle and Bayrd, 1961); it may amount to as much as sixty pounds and be associated with extreme emaciation.

Amyloid infiltration of the adrenals may lead to adrenal insufficiency. The early complaints of weakness, nausea, abdominal pain, and diarrhea are suggestive of adrenal cortical failure. Absence of hypertension with renal amyloidosis may be due to an associated hypoadrenalism. Although often suspected clinically and found at postmortem, the diagnosis of adrenal involvement by amyloid is not substantiated by endocrine assays. Hypotension is a common finding and is present in 10 to 40 per cent of patients (Kyle and Bayrd, 1961; Rukavina *et al.*, 1956). Orthostatic hypotension is present in about 8 per cent of these patients (Kyle, Kottke, and Schirger, 1966).

Muscle and joint complaints (arthralgias) occur occasionally, and in some patients (van Buchem, Mandema, and Arends, 1962) signs and symptoms of rheumatoid arthritis are present as well. Muscle involvement is sometimes seen on biopsy (Warren, 1930). Pathologic fracture of the femur due to amyloid infiltration has been described (Koletzky and Stecher, 1939). Intermittent claudication and aching in the lower extremities after walking have been reported.

## Laboratory Findings

Mild to moderate anemia is usually present. Persistent anemia unresponsive to iron and vitamin $B_{12}$ may require frequent blood transfusions. Polycythemia has been reported in three patients (Bero, 1957). The possibility was suggested that amyloid involvement of the bone marrow can result in anoxia and lead to polycythemia. The white blood cell count is usually normal. The sedimentation rate may be normal or raised.

Coagulation studies are normal in the majority of patients. However, mild thrombocytopenia, a decrease in prothrombin and fibrinogen levels, and the presence of circulating fibrinolysin have occasionally been observed (Fisher and Preuss, 1951; Orloff and Felder, 1946; Findley and Adams, 1948; Conn and Sundberg, 1961). Factor X (Stuart-Prower) deficiency has been reported in paraamyloidosis with liver involvement (Howell, 1963; Pechet and Kastrul, 1964). The possibility that the involved liver is unable to form factor X is unlikely, as the liver function tests are usually unaltered (Howell, 1963). Factor X is probably formed in these patients but it is taken up selectively by the amyloid deposits. The possibility of neutralization of factor X by abnormal circulating protein has been considered, but ruled out in Pechet and Kastrul's case (Pechet and Kastrul, 1964).

Serum proteins may be significantly altered and their levels diagnostically helpful. The serum albumin is usually low and ranges from 1.4 to 4.5 gm per cent; serum globulin may be low or elevated and ranges from 1.3 to 7.0 gm per cent. Serum electrophoresis frequently reveals a homogeneous peak within the gamma globulin mobility such as would be seen in uncomplicated multiple myeloma. However, in some patients with multiple myeloma and paraamyloidosis, the peak is missing and in these cases gamma globulin tends to be low. Indeed, if there is a diffuse gamma globulin elevation associated with plasmacytosis and amyloidosis but no myeloma peak, this suggests that some cause other than multiple myeloma is responsible.

Serum uric acid may be elevated. Elevation of acid phosphatase has been reported in a patient with mesenchymatous amyloidosis and circulating fibrinolysin in the absence of prostatic malignancy (Realeaf *et al.*, 1963). Serum complement is normal in patients with mesenchymatous amyloidosis without plasmacytosis as it is in patients with parenchymatous amyloidosis secondary to leprosy. It is decreased in paraamyloidosis (Williams and Law, 1960), while it is normal in idiopathic mesenchymatous and in parenchymatous amyloidoses.

Proteinuria is present in three fourths of the cases and the blood urea nitrogen is elevated in most patients. Bence Jones proteinuria is seen in most patients with paraamyloidosis. Occasionally, all serum proteins are found in the urine. Hematuria occurs in 5 per cent of cases. Cylindruria and hyposthenuria are not uncommon.

With malabsorption due to intestinal involvement, fat in the stool may be increased to 15 to 30 gm per day. About 10 per cent of patients are found to have melena. BUN may be normal or increased. Bromsulphalein retention is usually elevated in patients with hepatomegaly but that may be due to associated congestive heart failure. Serum cholesterol is either normal or elevated.

The study of marrow biopsy sections may reveal amyloid deposits in the walls of small medullary vessels (Conn and Sundberg, 1961; Kyle *et al.*, 1966). The amyloid may also spread into adjacent hematopoietic tissue, replacing much of the marrow. Amyloid particles have been observed in the polymorphonuclear leukocytes in the bone marrow of patients with paraamyloidosis (Trubowitz, 1950). The polymorphonuclear leukocytes probably play a role in the removal of amyloid deposits.

## Prognosis

Patients seldom live longer than three years following onset of the disease. The average duration from onset of symptoms until death is estimated as twenty-eight months. There is no regression in paraamyloidosis. The course of the disease varies, depending on the involvement. Congestive heart failure is a serious prognostic sign.

## Complications and Mode of Death

Patients usually die as a result of sepsis, severe anemia, severe diarrhea, pulmonary infection, congestive heart failure, or uremia.

## Diagnosis

Paraamyloidosis should be suspected in patients with paraimmuno-globulinopathy with associated obscure heart disease, gastrointestinal symptoms, skin lesions, and/or neurological symptoms. In addition, amyloidosis should be suspected in any polysystemic involvement with or without overt paraimmunoglobulinopathy.

The Congo red test, the radioiodinated Congo red test, and the Evans blue-radioiodinated albumin test are rarely positive in paraamyloidosis.

Biopsy of grossly normal-appearing gingiva has been reported to be positive for amyloid in patients with generalized disease. This is not a good test. Biopsies of the gingiva and especially of the tongue may be too superficial and miss the underlying deposit.

Peroral intubation biopsy of the small intestine is satisfactory, safe, and reliable. It is positive in the majority of the cases (Green *et al.,* 1961) .

When the liver is involved in amyloidosis, a needle biopsy of this organ will give positive results. However, severe and sometimes fatal hemorrhage has been described (Green *et al.,* 1961) . The mortality rate is below 1 per cent. Renal biopsy is somewhat less dangerous than liver biopsy in this disease; however, bleeding is not infrequent in this procedure.

Gafni and Sohar (1960) reported positive results of biopsy of the rectum in amyloidosis. At the time of sigmoidoscopy, punch biopsy is obtained at two or three different levels. The posterior wall of the rectosigmoid at the level of the upper valve of Houston is the site preferred by Kyle and associates (Kyle, Spencer and Dahlin, 1966) . The biopsy site is cauterized by the local application of 20 per cent silver nitrate solution. Biopsy specimens are fixed in formalin. Paraffin sections are stained with Congo red and examined microscopically. Red-stained amyloid is seen as a thin layer surrounding arterial structures in the submucosa. The importance of including submucosal tissue in the specimen cannot be overemphasized (Kyle, Spencer and Dahlin, 1966) . In a review of diagnostic procedures in 200 cases of known amyloidosis (Blum and Sohar, 1962), the proportion of positive results with rectal biopsy was 75 per cent; gingival biopsy, 19 per cent; liver biopsy, less than 50 per cent; renal biopsy, 87 per cent. Rectal biopsy is relatively easy, painless, and practically devoid of danger. Blum feels it should be performed first; if negative, kidney biopsy may be justifiable (Editorial, 1963) .

When skin and muscle are grossly involved, biopsy of these tissues is recommended. Inducement of intralesional hemorrhage by local pressure while normal skin remains free of purpura is a helpful diagnostic sign (Hurley and Weinberg, 1964; Editorial, 1964).

The routine study of bone marrow biopsy for amyloid deposits may further help in early diagnosis of this disease (Conn and Sundberg, 1961). Amyloid deposits can be found in the walls of small medullary vessels, sometimes partially occluding the lumen, or as extramural deposits. Giant cell foreign body reaction may occasionally be observed around the amyloid (Kyle *et al.*, 1966).

In summary, because of the accessibility of the rectum, skin, bone marrow, and muscle for biopsy purposes, biopsies of these organs are probably the safest and preferred methods for histologic confirmation of the diagnosis. If these are negative in the face of suspected amyloidosis, renal biopsy may be helpful.

Antemortem diagnosis of isolated cardiac amyloidosis is difficult. It is pertinent that hypertension and angina are rare and that the patient is malnourished. A helpful diagnostic finding has been an electrocardiographic abnormality consisting of left axis deviation, low QRS voltage in the limb leads, a QS configuration and/or small R waves in $V_1$ to $V_3$ with or without atrial fibrillation.

## Treatment

Treatment of paraamyloidosis is limited to surgical extirpation of a localized, strategically situated deposit and to chemotherapy of the associated paraimmunoglobulinopathy: L-phenylalanine mustard in case of multiple myeloma and chlorambucil in case of macroglobulinemia. There is controversy concerning the benefit and possible harm of corticosteroid administration. Attention must be directed toward treatment of complications of paraamyloidosis, such as congestive heart failure, diarrhea, malabsorption, and renal failure.

# REFERENCES

A case of plasma-cell leukemia demonstrated at the Postgraduate Medical School of London. *Brit Med J, 5272:*169–177, 1962.

ABERG, H., and CRAIG, D.: Blau's lines in a case of myelomatosis. *Lancet, 86:*503, 1966.

ACKERMAN, A. L.: The ocular manifestations of Waldenström's macroglobulinemia and its treatment. *Arch Ophthal, 67:*701–707, 1962.

ADAMS, D. A.; GOLDMAN, R.; MAXWELL, M. H., and LATTA, H.: Nephrotic syndrome associated with penicillamine therapy of Wilson's disease. *Amer J Med, 36:*330–336, 1964.

ALDRICH, R. A.; STEINBERG, A. G., and CAMPBELL, D. C.: Pedigree demonstrating a sex-linked recessive condition characterized by draining ears, eczematoid dermatitis and bloody diarrhea. *Pediatrics, 13:*133, 1954.

ALEXANDER, J.: Some intracellular aspects of life and disease. *Protoplasma, 14:*296–306, 1931.

ALLEN, A. C.: *The Kidney.* London, Churchill, 1951, p. 277.

ALLEN, J. C., and KUNKEL, H. G.: Antibodies to genetic types of gamma globulin after multiple transfusions. *Science, 139:*418, 1963.

ALLEN, J. C.; KUNKEL, H. G., and KABAT, E. A.: Studies on human antibodies. II. Distribution of genetic factors. *J Exp Med, 119:*453–465, 1964.

ALLEN, R. A., and STRAATSMA, B. R.: Ocular involvement in leukemia and allied disorders. *Arch Ophthal, 66:*490–508, 1961.

ALLIBONE, E. C.; GOLDIE, W., and MARMION, B. P.: Pneumocystis carinii pneumonia and progressive vaccinia in siblings. *Arch Dis Child, 39:*26–34, 1964.

ANDERSEN, S. B.: *Metabolism of Human Gamma Globulin ($\gamma_{ss}$-Globulin)*. Philadelphia, Davis, 1964.

ANDERSON, E. T., and VYE, M. V.: Dysproteinemia of the myeloma type associated with a thymoma. *Ann Intern Med, 66:*141–149, 1967.

ANDRADE, C.: A peculiar form of peripheral neuropathy: Familiar atypical generalized amyloidosis with special involvement of the peripheral nerves. *Brain, 75:*408–427, 1952.

ANFINSEN, C. B.: The formation of the tertiary structure of proteins. *Harvey Lectures, Series 61:*95–116, 1967.

APITZ, K. Die Paraproteinosen; Über die Störung des Eiweisstoffwechsels beim Plasmacytom. *Virch Arch Path Anat, 306:*631–699, 1940.

ARENDS, T.; COONRAD, E. V., and RUNDLES, R. W.: Serum proteins in Hodgkin's disease and malignant lymphoma. *Amer J Med, 16:*833, 1954.

ARGAGNI, I., and KIPKIE, G. F.: Macroglobulinemic nephropathy. Acute renal failure in macroglobulinemia of Waldenström. *Amer J Med, 36:*151–159, 1964.

ARON, E.; VARGUES, R.; CHARMOT, G.; DEU, J.; FOUCHET, M., and RIGAUD, R.: Les macroglobulinémies. Étude sur 30 cas confirmés par ultracentrifugation. *Presse Med, 70:*1071–1074, 1962.

ASKONAS, B. A., and FAHEY, J. L.: Enzymatically produced subunits of proteins formed by plasma cells in mice. II. $\beta_{2a}$-Myeloma protein and Bence Jones protein. *J Exp Med,* *115*:641–653, 1962.

ASKONAS, B. A., and WILLIAMSON, A. R.: Biosynthesis of immunoglobulins on polyribosomes and assembly of the IgG molecule. *Proc Roy Soc Biol, 166*:232–243, 1966a.

ASKONAS, B. A., and WILLIAMSON, A. R.: Biosynthesis of immunoglobulins. Free light chain as an intermediate in the assembly of γG-molecules. *Nature, 211*:369–372, 1966b.

AXELSSON, U.; BACHMANN, R., and HÄLLEN, J.: Frequency of pathological proteins (M-component) in 6,995 sera from an adult population. *Acta Med Scand, 179*:235–247, 1966.

BACHMANN, R.: Studies on the serum γA-globulin levels. III. The frequency of a γA-globulinemia. *Scand J Clin Lab Invest, 17*:316, 1965.

BAGLIONI, C.; ALESCIO ZONTA, L.; CIOLI, D., and CARBONARA, A.: Allelic antigenic factor Inv (a) of the light chains of human immunoglobulins: Chemical basis. *Science, 152*:1517–1519, 1966.

BAITZ, T., and KYLE, R. A.: Solitary myeloma in chronic osteomyelitis: report of a case. *Arch Intern Med, 113*:872–875, 1964.

BAKEMEIER, R. F., and LEDDY, J. P.: Structural aspects of human antierythrocyte antibodies: light and heavy chain determinants (Abstract). *J Clin Invest; 45*:984, 1966.

BAKER, G. P., and MARTIN, N. H.: Symptomless myelomatosis. *Brit Med J, 1*:953, 1959.

BALLIEUX, R. E.; BERNIER, G. M.; TOMINAGA, K., and PUTNAM, F. W.: Gamma globulin antigenic types defined by heavy chain determinants. *Science, 145*:168–170, 1964.

BARANDUN, S.; COTTIER, H., and HASSIG, A.: New aspects of agammaglobulinemia and antibody deficiency syndrome. In *Immunopathology, 1st International Symposium.* Basel, Benno Schwabe Co, 1958, p. 60.

BARNETT, E. V.; CONDEMI, J. J.; LEDDY, J. P., and VAUGHN, J. J.: Gamma$_2$, gamma$_{1a}$ and gamma$_{1m}$ antinuclear factors in human sera. *J Clin Invest, 43*:1104–1115, 1964.

BARR, D. P.; ENGLE, R. L., JR., and RUSS, E. M.: Cryoglobulinemia: a case report. *Ann Intern Med, 47*:1225–1234, 1957.

BARRON, K. D.; ROWLAND, L. P., and ZIMMERMAN, H. M.: Neuropathy with malignant tumor metastases. *J Nerv Ment Dis, 131*:10–31, 1960.

BARTH, W. F.; ASOFSKY, R.; LIDDY, T. J.; TANAKO, Y.; ROWE, D. S., and FAHEY, J. L.: An antibody deficiency syndrome selective immunoglobulin deficiency with reduced synthesis of γ and α immunoglobulin polypeptide chains. *Amer J Med, 39*:319–334, 1965.

BARTH. W. F.; WOCHNER, R. D.; WALDMANN, T. A., and FAHEY, J. L.: Metabolism of human gamma macroglobulins. *J Clin Invest, 43*:1036–1048, 1964.

BAYBUTT, J. E.: Hypersensitivity to immune serum globulin. *JAMA, 171*:415–416, 1959.

BAYRD, E. D.: News and views: sustained remission in multiple myeloma. *Blood, 10*:662, 1955.

BAYRD, E. D.: Continuous chlorambucil therapy in primary macroglobulinemia of Waldenström: report of four cases. *Proc Mayo Clin, 36*:135–147, 1961.

BAYRD, E. D., and BENNETT, W. A.: Amyloidosis complicating myeloma. *Med Clin N Amer, 34*:1151–1164, 1950.

BAYRD, E. D.; HAGEDORN, A. B., and McGUCKIN, W. F.: Macroglobulinemia; its recognition and treatment. *JAMA, 193*:724–726, 1965.

BELFRAGE, S.: Plasma protein pattern in course of acute infectious disease. *Acta Med Scand, (Suppl) 395*:1–169, 1963.

BENACERRAF, B.; SEBESTYEN, M., and COOPER, N. S.: The clearance of antigen antibody complexes from the blood by the reticuloendothelial system. *J Immunol, 82*:131–137, 1959.

BEN-BASSAT, I.; FRAND, U. I.; ISERSKY, C., and RAMOT, B.: Plasma cell leukemia with IgD paraprotein. *Arch Int Med, 121*:361–364, 1968.

BERENBAUM, M. C.: The antibody content of single cells. *J Clin Path, 11*:543–547, 1958.

BERGSAGEL, D. E.: Phase II trials of mitomycin C, AB-100, NSC-1026, L-sarcolysin, and meta-sarcolysin in the treatment of multiple myeloma. *Cancer Chemother Rep, 16*:261–266, 1962.

BERNARD, J.; SELIGMANN, M., and DANON, F.: Attempt at treatment of 21 patients with myeloma and macroglobulinemia with p-di-2-chlorethylamino-1-phenylalanine (melphalan). *Nouv Rev Franc Hemat, 2*:611–616, 1962.

BERNARD, J. G.; LAVERDANT, C.; NICHOLAS, M., and BONNET, D.: Apropos of a case of Waldenström's macroglobulinemia *Bull Soc Med Hop Paris, 77*:1007–1016, 1961.

BERNIER, G. M., CEBRA, J. J.: Polypeptide chains of human gamma globulin: cellular localization by fluorescent antibody. *Science, 144*:1590–1591, 1964.

BERNIER, G. M., and PUTNAM, F. W.: Polymerism, polymorphism, and impurities in Bence Jones proteins. *Biochim Biophys Acta, 86*:295–308, 1964a.

BERNIER, G. M., and PUTNAM, F. W.: Myeloma proteins and macroglobulins; hallmarks of disease and models of antibodies. In MOORE, C. C., and BROWN, B. B. (Eds.) : *Progress in Hematology*. New York, Grune, 1964b, vol. IV, pp. 160–186.

BERO, G. L.: Amyloidosis: its clinical and pathologic manifestations with a report of 12 cases. *Ann Intern Med, 46*:931–955, 1957.

BESSIS, M. C.: Ultrastructure of lymphoid and plasma cells in relation to globulin and antibody formation. *Lab Invest, 10*:1040–1067, 1961.

BETHLEM, J.; VAN GOOL, J., and DEN HARTOG JAGER, W. A.: Progressive multifocal leukoencephalopathy associated with multiple myeloma. *Acta Neuropath (Berlin), 3*:525–528, 1964.

BICHEL, J.; EFFERSOE, P.; GORMSEN, H., and HARBOE, N.: Leukemic myelomatosis (plasma cell leukemia) : review with report of 4 cases. *Acta Radiol, 37*:196–207, 1952.

BICHEL, J., and KIRKETERP, P.: Notes on myeloma. *Acta Radiol, 19*:487, 1938.

BING, J., and NEEL, A.: Two cases of hyperglobulinemia with affection of central nervous system on toxic infectious basis (myelitis, polyradiculitis, spinal fluid changes). *Acta Med Scand, 88*:492–506, 1936.

BIRCH, C. A.; COOKE, K. B.; DREW, C. E.; MACKENZIE, D. H.; LONDON, D. R., and MILNE, M. D.: Hyperglobulinemic purpura due to a thymic tumor. *Lancet, 1*:693–697, 1964.

BIRO, I.: Kryoglobulinaemia és makrokryogelglobulinaemia előfordulása testvéreken. *Orv Hetil, 103*:1709–1712, 1962.

BJÖRNBERG, J.: Extramedullary plasmocytoma in the orbit. *Acta Ophthal (Kobenhavn) 40*:330–335, 1962.

BLACKMAN, S. S., JR.; BARKER, W. H.; BUELL, M. V., and DAVIS, M. V.: On pathogenesis of renal failure associated with multiple myeloma: electrophoretic and chemical analysis of protein in urine and blood serum. *J Clin Invest, 23*:163–166, 1944.

BLAINEY, J. D.; BREWER, D. B.; HARDWICKE, J., and SOOTHILL, J. F.: The nephrotic syndrome; diagnosis by renal biopsy and biochemical and immunological analyses related to response to steroid therapy. *Quart J Med, 29*:235–256, 1960.

BLANCHARD, A. J., and OLIN, J. S.: Histoplasmosis with sarcoid-like lesions occurring in multiple myeloma. *Canad Med Ass J, 85*:307–311, 1961.

BLATTNER, R. J.: Pneumocystis carinii infection: treatment with pentamidine isothionate. *J Pediat, 67*:332–335, 1965.

BLOKHIN, N.; LARIONOV, L.; PEREVODCHIKOVA, N.; CHEBOTAREVA, L., and MERKULOVA, N.:

Clinical experiences with sarcolysin in neoplastic diseases. *Ann NY Acad Sci, 68*:1128–1132, 1958.

BLOOM, M. L.; SHULMAN, S., and WITEBSKY, E.: Anticomplimentary activity of multiple myeloma (Abstract). *Clin Res, 6*:206, 1958.

BLUM, A., and SOHAR, E.: The diagnosis of amyloidosis; ancillary procedures. *Lancet, 1*:721–724, 1962.

BOCCIARELLI, S. D., and VIOLENTE, A.: Morphological modifications of the characteristic pathological cells of the Oberling, Guerin and Guerin myeloma in rats treated with bis (β-chloroethyl)-p-aminophenylalanine. *Rendic 1st Super Sanit, 23*:111, 1960.

BOHROD, M. G.: Plasmacytosis and cryoglobulinemia in cancer. *JAMA, 164*:18–21, 1957.

BRACHET, J.: Protein synthesis in the absence of the nucleus. *Nature, 213*:650–655, 1967.

BREINL, F., HAUROWITZ, F.: Chemische Untersuchung des Präzipitates aus Hämoglobin und Anti-Hämoglobin-Serum und Bemerkungen über die Natur der Antikorper. *Hoppe-Seyler Z Physiol Chem, 192*:45–57, 1930.

BRENNER, S., and MILSTEIN, C.: Origin of antibody variation. *Nature, 211*:242–243, 1966.

BRIGGS, G. W.; Amyloidosis. *Ann Intern Med, 55*:943–957, 1961.

BRIGGS, G. W.: Diagnosis of primary amyloidosis. *Geriatrics, 19*:290–294, 1964.

BRODY, J. I., and BEIZER, L. H.: Immunologic incompetence of the neoplastic lymphocyte. in chronic lymphocytic leukemia. *Ann Intern Med, 64*:1237–1245, 1966.

BRODY, J. I.; BEIZER, L. H., and SCHWARTZ, S.: Multiple myeloma and the myeloproliferative syndromes. *Amer J Med, 36*:315–319, 1964.

BRODY, I. A.; WERTLAKE, P. T., and LASTER, L.: Causes of intestinal symptoms in primary amyloidosis. *Arch Intern Med, 113*:512–518, 1964.

BROMLEY, J. F.: Myelomatosis and the radiotherapist. *Clin Radiol, 12*:8–16, 1961.

BRONSKY, D., and DUNN, Y. O. L.: Sarcoidosis with hypogammaglobulinemia. *Amer J Med Sci, 250*:11–18, 1965.

BRUTON, O. C.: Agammaglobulinemia. *Pediatrics, 9*:722, 1952.

BRYAN, C. W., and HEALY, J. K.: Acute renal failure in multiple myeloma. *Amer J Med, 44*:128–133, 1968.

BUCKLEY, C. E., III, and NAGAZA, H.: Immunologic alterations in lymphocytes, complement, and immunoglobulins in sarcoid (Abstract). *Clin Res, 13*:285, 1965.

BURNET, F. M.: A modification of Jerne's theory of antibody production, using the concept of clonal selection. *Aust J Sci, 20*:67–69, 1957.

BURNET, SIR MACFARLANE: A possible genetic basis for specific pattern in antibody. *Nature, 210*:1308–1310, 1966.

CALKINS, E.; COHEN, A. S., and GITLIN, D.: Immunochemical determinations of gamma globulin content of amyloid (Abstract). *Fed Proc, 17*:431, 1958.

CALKINS, E.; COHEN, A. S., and LARSEN, B.: Amyloidosis: preliminary clinical, chemical, and experimental observations. *Ann NY Acad Sci, 86*:1033–1042, 1960.

CARBONE, P. P.; ZIPKIN, I.; SOKOLOFF, L.; FRAZIER, P.; COOK, P., and MULLINS, F.: Fluoride effect on bone in plasma cell myeloma. *Arch Int Med, 121*:130–140, 1968.

CARSON, C. P.; ACKERMAN, L. V., and MALTBY, J. D.: Plasma cell myeloma. *Amer J Clin Path, 25*:849–888, 1955.

CARTER, R. L.: Antibody formation in infectious mononucleosis. I. Some immunochemical properties of the Paul-Bunnell Antibody. *Brit J Haemat, 12*:259–267, 1966a.

CARTER, R. L.: Antibody formation in infectious mononucleosis. II. Other 19S antibodies and false-positive serology. *Brit J Haemat, 12*:268–275, 1966b.

Case records of the Massachusetts General Hospital—Case 46522. Weekly Clinicopathological Exercises. *New Eng J Med, 263*:1368–1371, 1960.

CASSIDY, J. T.: Cardiac amyloidosis. Two cases with digitalis sensitivity. *Ann Intern Med, 55*:989–994, 1961.

CATHCART, E. S., and COHEN, A. S.: The identification of two new components common to a variety of amyloid tissues. (Abstract) *J Clin Invest, 45*:995, 1966.

CATHCART, E. S.; COMERFORD, F. R., and COHEN, A. S.: Immunologic studies on a protein extracted from human secondary amyloid. *New Eng J Med, 273*:143–146, 1965.

CEBRA, J. J.; COLBERG, J. E., and DRAY, S.: Rabbit lymphoid cells differentiated with respect to, $\alpha$-, $\gamma$-, and $\mu$-heavy polypeptide chains and to allotypic markers A$_A$1 and A$_A$2. *J Exp Med, 123*:547–557, 1966.

CHARMOT, G., and ANDRÉ, L. J.: Essai d'interprétation des macroglobulinémies. *Sem Hop Paris, 40*:2779–2782, 1964.

CHESTERMAN, J. T.: Solitary plasmacytoma of the long bones. *Brit J Surg, 35*:440, 1948.

CHINI, V.: Un nouveau chapitre de la pathologie articulaire: les arthropathies dysprotidémiques: rapport d'un cas personnel. *Rev Rhum, 17*:335–354, 1950.

CHOJNACKI, P.: Ein Beitrag zur Kenntnis der plasmozytären Granulome (Plasmomata conjunctivae). *Klin Monatsbl Augenh, 95*:470–478, 1935.

CHRISTIAN, C. L.: *Rheumatoid Arthritis in Immunological Diseases*. Boston, Little, Brown 1965, p. 725–736.

CHRISTOPHERSON, W. M., and MILLER, A. J.: A re-evaluation of solitary plasma-cell myeloma of bone. *Cancer, 3*:240, 1950.

CIOLI, D., and BAGLIONI, C.: Origin of structural variation in Bence-Jones proteins. *J Mol Biol, 15*:385–388, 1966.

CITRIN, Y.; STERLING, K., and HALSTED, J. A.: The mechanism of hypoproteinemia associated with giant hypertrophy of the gastric mucosa. *New Eng J Med, 257*:906, 1957.

CLAMAN, H. N., and MERRILL, D.: Serum immunoglobulins in rheumatoid arthritis. *J Lab Clin Med, 67*:850–854, 1966.

CLARK, R.; TORNYOS, K.; HERBERT, V., and TWOMEY, J.: Studies on two patients with concomitant pernicious anemia and immunoglobulin deficiency. *Ann Int Med, 67*:403–410, 1967.

CLARKE, E.: Peripheral neuropathy associated with multiple myelomatosis. *Neurology, 6*:146–151, 1956.

CLARKSON, B.; THOMPSON, D.; HORWITH, M., and LUCKEY, E. H.: Cyclical edema and shock due to increased capillary permeability. *Amer J Med, 29*:193, 1960.

CLAUSEN, J.; RASK-NIELSEN, R.; CHRISTENSEN, H. E.; LONTIE, R., and HEREMANS, J.: Macroglobulinemia in a transplantable mouse leukemia. *Proc Soc Exper Biol Med, 103*:802–804, 1960.

CLINE, M. J., and BERLIN, N. I.: Studies of the anemia of multiple myeloma. *Amer J Med, 33*:510, 1962.

CLINE, M. J., and FUDENBERG, H. H.: Defective RNA synthesis in lymphocytes from patients with primary agammaglobulinemia. *Science, 150*:1311–1312, 1965.

CLINE, M. J.; SOLOMON, A.; BERLIN, N. I., and FAHEY, J. L.: Anemia in macroglobulinemia. *Amer J Med, 34*:213, 1963.

Clinicopathological Conference. A case of plasma-cell leukaemia. *Brit Med J, 1*:169–177, 1962.

COHEN, A. S.; GROSS, E. S., and SHIRAHAMA, T.: Production of amyloid by tissue explants. *Arthritis Rheum 7*:301, 1964.

COHEN, D. M.: SVIEN, H. J., and DAHLIN, D. C.: Long-term survival of patients with myeloma of the vertebral column. *JAMA, 187*:914–917, 1964.

COHEN, L.; BLAISDELL, R. K.; DJORDJEVICH, J.; ORMISTE, V., and DOBRILOVIC, L.: Familial xanthomatosis and hyperlipidemia, and myelomatosis. *Amer J Med, 40*:299, 1966.

COHEN, R. J.; BOHANNON, R. A., and WALLERSTEIN, R. O.: Waldenström's macroglobulinemia. A study of ten cases. *Amer J Med, 41*:274–284, 1966.

COHEN, S., and FREEMAN, T.: Metabolic heterogeneity of human gamma globulin. *Biochem J, 76*:475–487, 1960.

COHEN, S., and GORDON, S.: Dissociation of κ- and λ-chains from reduced human immunoglobulins. *Biochem J, 97*:460–465, 1965.

COHEN, S., and MCGREGOR, I. A.: Gamma globulin and acquired immunity to malaria. In *Immunity to Protozoa: A Symposium of British Soc Immunol*, Ed. by Garnham, P. C. C., Pierce, A. E., and Riott, I., Philadelphia, F. A. Davis Co., 1963, pp. 123–159.

COHEN, S., and PORTER, R. R.: Heterogeneity of the peptide chains of gamma globulin. *Biochem J, 90*:278–284, 1964.

COLLINS, J. R., and ELLIS, D. S.: Agammaglobulinemia, malabsorption and rheumatoid-like arthritis. *Amer J Med, 39*:476–482, 1965.

COLTMAN, C. A., JR.: Multiple myeloma without a paraprotein. Report of a case with observations on chromosomal composition. *Arch Int Med, 120*:687–696, 1967.

CONN, H. O.; BINDER, H., and BURNS, B.: Pernicious anemia and immunologic deficiency. *Ann Int Med, 68*:603–612, 1968.

CONN, H. O., and QUINTILIANI, R.: Severe diarrhea controlled by gamma globulin in a patient with agammaglobulinemia, amyloidosis and thymoma. *Ann Intern Med, 65*:528–541, 1966.

CONN, R. B., and SUNDBERG, R. D.: Amyloid disease of the bone marrow. *Amer J Path, 38*:61–72, 1961.

COONS, A. H.; LEDUC, E. H., and CONNOLLY, J. M.: Studies on antibody production. I. A method for the histochemical demonstration of specific antibody and its application to a study of the hyperimmune rabbit. *J Exp Med, 102*:49, 1955.

COOPER, M. D.; CHASE, H. P.; LOWMAN, J. T.; KRIVIT, W., and GOOD, R. A.: Wiskott-Aldrich syndrome. An immunologic deficiency disease involving the afferent limb of immunity. *Amer J Med, 44*:499–513, 1968.

COOPERBAND, S. R.; ROSEN, F. S.; KIBRICK, S., and JANEWAY, C. A.: Gamma globulin synthesis by lymphocytes from normal and agammaglobulinemic individuals. *J Clin Invest, 45*:998, 1966 (Abstract).

CORCOS, J. M.; SOLER-BECHARA, J.; MAYER, K.; FREYBERG, R. H.; GOLDSTEIN, R., and JAFFE, I.: Neutrophilic agranulocytosis during administration of penicillamine, *JAMA, 189*:265–268, 1964.

CORNELIUS, C. E.; GOODBARY, R. F., and KENNEDY, P. C.: Plasma cell myelomatosis in a horse. *The Cornell Veterinarian. 49*, 478–593, 1959.

COSTA, G.; CARBONE, P. P.; GOLD, G. I.; OWENS, A. H., JR.; MILLER, S. P.; KRANT, M. J., and BONO, V. H., JR.: Clinical trial of vinblastine in multiple myeloma. *Cancer Chemother Rep, 27*:87–89, 1963.

COSTANZA, D. J., and SMOLLER, M.: Multiple myeloma with the Fanconi syndrome. Study of a case with electron microscopy of the kidney. *Amer J Med, 34*:125–133, 1963.

COTRAN, R. S., and FORTNER, J. G.: Serum-protein abnormality in a transplantable plasmacytoma of the Syrian golden hamster. *J Nat Cancer Inst, 28*:1193–1205, 1962.

COURET, J. S.: Extramedullary plasma cell tumor of the stomach: a case report. *Amer J Clin Path, 16*:213–218, 1946.

CRABBÉ, P. A., and HEREMANS, J. F.: Selective IgA deficiency with steatorrhea. A new syndrome. *Amer J. Med, 42*:319–326, 1967.

CRADDOCK, C. G., JR.; ADAMS, W. S., and FIGUEROA, W. G.: Interference with fibrin formation in multiple myeloma by an unusual protein found in blood and urine. *J Lab Clin Med, 42*:847–859, 1953.

CRUCHAUD, A.; LOPERRANZA, C.; DUMITTAN, S. H., and FERRIER, P. E.: Agammaglobulinemia in one of two identical twins. *Amer J Med, 40*:127–139, 1966.

CRUCHAUD, A.; ROSEN, F. S.; CRAIG, J. M.; JANEWAY, C. A., and GITLIN, D.: The site of synthesis of the 19S gamma globulins in dysgammaglobulinemia. *J Exp Med, 115*:1141–1148, 1962.

CUNNINGHAM, B. A., GOTTLIEB, P. D., KONIGSBERG, W. H., and EDELMAN, G. M.: The covalent structure of a human γG-immunoglobulin. V Partial amino acid sequence of the light chain. Biochem 7:1983–1995, 1968.

CUTLER, C. W., JR.: Plasma-cell tumor of breast with metastases. *Ann Surg, 100*:392–395, 1934.

DACOSTA, S. F. G.; RELVAS, M. E. S. A.; HALPERN, M. J., and DASILVA, J. A. F.: Contribuições para o estudo da patologia química de um caso de mieloma associado ao síndroma de Fanconi. *Gazeta Médica Portuguesa, 13*:583–590, 1960.

DAHLIN, D. C., and DOCKERTY, M. B.: Amyloid and myeloma. *Amer J Path, 26*:581–594, 1950.

DALTON, A. J.; POTTER, M., and MERWIN, R. M.: Some ultrastructural characteristics of a series of primary and transplanted plasma-cell tumors of the mouse. *J Nat Cancer Inst, 26*:1221–1267, 1961.

DAMESHEK, W.: "Immunoblasts" and "immunocytes"—an attempt at a functional nomenclature. Editorial. *Blood, 21*:243, 1963.

DAMMACCO, F., and CLAUSEN, J.: Antibody deficiency in paraproteinemia. *Acta Med Scand, 179*:755–768, 1966.

DAS, K. C.; AIKAT, B. K.: Chromosomal abnormalities in multiple myeloma. *Blood, 30*:738–748, 1967.

DAVIS, J. S., JR.; WEBER, F. C., and BARTFELD, H.: Conditions involving the hemopoietic system resulting in a pseudorheumatoid arthritis; similarity of multiple myeloma and rheumatoid arthritis. *Ann Intern Med, 47*:10–17, 1957.

DEDMON, R. E.; WEST, J. H., and SCHWARTZ, T. B.: The adult Fanconi syndrome. Report of two cases, one with multiple myeloma. *Med Clin N Amer, 47*:191–206, 1963.

DELDUCA, V., JR., and MORNINGSTAR, W. A.: Multiple myeloma associated with progressive multifocal leukoencephalopathy. *JAMA, 199*:671–673, 1967.

DELTA, B. G.; ROTHENBERG, A. M.; AINSWORTH, H. D., and INNELLA, F.: Congenital alymphoplasmacytic agammaglobulinemia with thymic dysplasia. *JAMA, 194*:507–511, 1965.

DENMAN, A. M., and WARD, H. W. C.: Jaundice during treatment of myelomatosis with 4–4′-diamidinodiphenylamine. *Lancet, 1*:419, 1959.

DEUTSCH, S. E., and MORTON, J. I.: Dissociation of human macroglobulin. *Science, 125*:600–601, 1957.

DE VAAL, O. M., and SEYNHAEVE, V.: Reticular dysgenesis. *Lancet, 2*:1123, 1959.

DICH, J.; PAABY, H., and SCHWARTZ, M.: Protein-secreting tumour of stomach. Severe hypoproteinaemia cured by removal of gastric polyp. *Brit Med J, 2*:686, 1961.

DOLIN, S., and DEWAR, J. P.: Extramedullary plasmocytoma. *Amer J Path, 32*:83–103, 1956.

DOMM, B. M.; VASSALLO, C. L., and ADAMS, C. L.: Amyloid deposition localized to the lower respiratory tract. *Amer J Med, 38*:151–155, 1965.

DOMZ, C. A., and DICKSON, D. R.: The agammaglobulinemias: relations and implications. *Amer J Med, 23*:917–927, 1957.

DOOLITTLE, R. F.; SINGER, S. J., and METZGER, H.: Evolution of immunoglobulin polypeptide chains: carboxyl-terminal of an IgM heavy chain. *Science, 154*:1561–1562, 1966.

DORLAND, W. A. N.: *The American Illustrated Medical Dictionary.* Philadelphia, Saunders, 1940.

DRAGSTEDT, P. J., and HJORTH, N.: The association of the Fanconi syndrome with malignant disease. *Danish Med Bull, 3:*177, 1956.

DRAY, S.: Three gamma globulins in normal human serum revealed by monkey precipitins. *Science, 132:*1313–1314, 1960.

DREYER, W. J., and BENNETT, J. C.: The molecular basis of antibody formation: a paradox. *Proc Nat Acad Sci USA, 54:*864–869, 1965.

DREYER, W. J.; GRAY, W. R., and HOOD, L.: The genetic, molecular, and cellular basis of antibody formation: some facts and a unifying hypothesis. In *Cold Spring Harbor Symposia on Quantitative Biology,* vol. 32, Antibodies, 1967, pp. 353–367.

DUMAS, L. W.; RENTSCHLER, E. H., and EARLE, K. M.: Peripheral neuropathy associated with multiple myelomatosis and amyloidosis. Report of a case. *Dis Nerv System, 18:*419–424, 1957.

DUTCHER, T. F., and FAHEY, J. L.: The histopathology of macroglobulinemia of Waldenström. *J Nat Cancer Inst, 22:*887–918, 1959.

DUTCHER, F., and FAHEY, J. L.: Immunocytochemical demonstration of intranuclear localization of 18S gamma macroglobulin in Macroglobulinemia of Waldenström. *Proc Soc Exp Biol Med 103:*452–455, 1960.

EDELMAN, G. M., and BENACERRAF, B.: On structural and functional relations between antibodies and proteins of the gamma system. *Proc Nat Acad Sci USA, 48:*1035–1042, 1962.

EDELMAN, G. M., and GALLEY, J. A.: The nature of Bence-Jones proteins. Chemical similarities to polypeptide chains of myeloma globulins and normal gamma globulins. *J Exp Med, 116:*207–227, 1962.

EDELMAN, G. M., and GALLY, J. A.: Somatic recombination of duplicated genes: an hypothesis on the origin of antibody diversity. *Proc Nat Acad Sci USA, 57:*353–358, 1967.

EDELMAN, G. M., and POULIK, M. D.: Studies on structural units of the gamma globulins. *J Exp Med, 113:*861–884, 1961.

Editorial: Clinical diagnosis of amyloidosis. *JAMA, 183:*1104, 1963.

Editorial: Fingertip diagnosis of amyloidosis. *JAMA, 188:*820–821, 1964.

EDWARDS, G. A., and ZAWADZKI, Z. A.: Extraosseous lesions in plasma cell myeloma. *Amer J Med, 43:*194–205, 1967.

EHRLICH, P.: *Collected Studies on Immunity.* New York, Wiley, 1906, pp. 47–55.

EISEN, H. N.: Primary systemic amyloidosis. *Amer J Med, 1:*144–160, 1946.

EISEN, H. N.; LITTLE, J. R.; OSTERLAND, C. K., and SIMMS, E. S.: A myeloma protein with antibody activity. In *Cold Spring Harbor Symposia on Quantitative Biology,* vol. 32, Antibodies, 1967, pp. 75–81.

EISENMENGER, W. J., and SLATER, R. J.: Distribution and decay of I[131] tagged albumin and gamma globulin in patients with cirrhosis. *J Clin Invest, 32:*564, 1953.

EISENSTEIN, A. B., and SPENCER, S.: Gluconeogenesis in the isolated perfused rat liver: role of the adrenal cortex (Abstract). *J Clin Invest, 45:*1004, 1966.

ELVES, M. W.: Suppression of antibody production by phytohemagglutinin. *Nature, 213:*495–496, 1967.

ENGLE, R. L., JR., and NACHMAN, R. L.: Two Bence Jones proteins of different immunologic types in the same patient with multiple myeloma. *Blood, 27:*74–77, 1966.

ENGLE, R. L., JR., and NACHMAN, R. L.: unpublished information, 1967.

ENGLE, R. L., JR., and WALLIS, L. A.: Multiple myeloma and the adult Fanconi syndrome. I. Report of a case with crystal-like deposits in the tumor cells and in the epithelial cells of the kidney. *Amer J Med, 22:*5–12, 1957.

ENGLE, R. L., JR., and WALLIS, L. A.: Amyloidosis. In *Tice-Harvey Practice of Medicine,* Vol. I, p. 365–394, 1966.

ENGLE, R. L., JR., and WOODS, K. R.: Pyroglobulinemia: A Clinical-Biochemical Study. Proc 7th Int Cong of Int Soc Hematol, Rome, 1958. New York, Grune, 1960, pp. 1496–1498.

ENGLE, R. L., JR.; WOODS, K. R.; CASTILLO, G. B., and PERT, J. H.: Starch gel electrophoresis of serum proteins and urinary proteins from patients with multiple myeloma, macroglobulinemia, and other forms of dysproteinemia. *J Lab Clin Med, 58*:1–22, 1961.

EPSTEIN, W. V., and GROSS, D.: Naturally occurring human antibody reacting with Bence Jones proteins. *J Exp Med, 120*:733–745, 1964.

EPSTEIN, W. V., and TAN, M.: Bence-Jones proteinemia associated with systemic lupus erythematosus (Abstract). *Arthritis Rheum, 7*:733, 1964.

EPSTEIN, W. V.; TAN, M., and GROSS, D.: Blocked antigenic sites on the L-chain of human gamma globulin. *Nature, 202*:1175–1177, 1964.

ESPOSITO, J. J., and STOUT, A. P.: Multiple plasmocytoma of the jejunum. *Amer J Roentgen, 53*:33–39, 1945.

EYSTER, M. E.; NACHMAN, R. L.; CHRISTENSON, W. N., and ENGLE, R. L., JR.: Structural characteristics of red cell autoantibodies. *J Immun, 96*:107, 1966.

FAGRAEUS, A.: Antibody production in relation to the development of plasma cells. *In vivo* and *in vitro* experiments. *Acta Med Scand (Suppl), 204*:1–122, 1948.

FAHEY, J. L.: Structural basis of differences between type I and type II human gamma globulin molecules. *J Immun, 91*:448–459, 1963.

FAHEY, J. L.: Contribution of gamma globulin subunits to electrophoretic heterogeneity: identification of a distinctive group of 6.6S gamma myeloma proteins. *Immunochem, 1*:121–131, 1964.

FAHEY, J. L.: Antibodies and immunoglobulins. I. Structure and function. *JAMA, 194*:71–74, 1965a.

FAHEY, J. L.: Antibodies and immunoglobulins. II. Normal development and changes in disease. *JAMA, 194*:255–258, 1965b.

FAHEY, J. L., and ASKONAS, B. A.: Enzymatically produced subunits of proteins formed by plasma cells in mice. I. gamma globulin and gamma myeloma proteins. *J Exp Med, 115*:623–639, 1962.

FAHEY, J. L.; FINEGOLD, I.; RABSON, A. S., and MANAKER, R. A.: Immunoglobulin synthesis *in vitro* by established human cell lines. *Science, 152*:1259–1261, 1966.

FAHEY, J. L., and ROBINSON, A. G.: Factors controlling serum gamma globulin concentration. *J Exp Med, 118*:845–868, 1963.

FAHEY, J. L.; SCOGGINS, R.; UTZ, J. P., and SZWED, C. F.: Infection, antibody response and gamma globulin components in multiple myeloma and macroglobulinemia. *Amer J Med, 35*:698, 1963.

FAHEY, J. L., and SOLOMON, A.: Two types of gamma myeloma proteins, $B_{2A}$ myeloma proteins, $\gamma_1$ macroglobulins, and Bence Jones proteins identified by two groups of common antigenic determinants. *J Clin Invest, 42*:811–822, 1963.

FARMER, R. G.; COOPER, T., and PASCUZZI, C. A.: Cryoglobulinemia. Report of 12 cases with bone marrow findings. *Arch Intern Med, 106*:483, 1960.

FARROKH, A.; WALSH, T. J., and MASSIE, E.: Amyloid heart disease. *Amer J Cardiol, 13*:750–756, 1964.

FEINLEIB, M., and MACMAHON, B.: Duration of survival in multiple myeloma. *J Nat Cancer Inst, 24*:1259–1269, 1960.

FEKETE, T.; FLORESCU, I., and WEISS, L.: Asocierea a două boli rare: sindrom Sjögren și purpură hiperglobulinemică Waldenström. *Med Intern (Bucur), 18*:231–241, 1966.

FERGUSON, J., and MACKAY, I. R.: Macroglobulinaemia with chromosomal anomaly. *Aust Ann Med, 12*:197–201, 1963.

FIGI, F. A.; BRODERS, A. C., and HAVENS, F. Z.: Plasma cell tumors of the upper part of the respiratory tract. *Ann Otol Rhin Laryng, 54*:283, 1945.

FINDLEY, J. W., JR., and ADAMS, A.: Primary systemic amyloidosis simulating constrictive pericarditis with steatorrhea and hyperesthesias. *Arch Intern Med, 81*:342–351, 1948.

FINE, J. M.; DERYCKE, C.; BILSKI-PASQUIER, and MARCHAL, G.: Dysglobulinémies atypiques et dysglobulinémies essentielles. In *Abstracts of Xth Congress of International Society of Haematology*, Stockholm, 1964, Abstract D:12.

FINKELSTEIN, M. S., and UHR, J. W.: Specific inhibition of antibody formation by passively administered 19S and 7S antibody. *Science, 146*:67–69, 1964.

FIREMAN, P.; BOESMAN, M., and GITLIN, D.: Ataxia telangiectasia; dysgammaglobulinemia with deficient $\gamma_{1A}$ ($\beta_{2A}$) globulin. *Lancet, 1*:1193–1195, 1964.

FIREMAN, P.; VANNIER, W. E., and GOODMAN, H. C.: The association of skin-sensitizing antibody with the $\beta_{2A}$ globulins in sera from ragweed-sensitive patients. *J Exp Med, 117*:603, 1963.

FIRKIN, B. G., and BLACKBURN, C. R. B.: Congenital and acquired agammaglobulinemia. A report of 4 cases. *Quart J Med, 27*:187, 1958.

FISHER, H., and PREUSS, F. S.: Primary systemic amyloidosis with involvement of nervous system. *Amer J Clin Path, 21*:758–763, 1951.

FISHMAN, M., and ADLER, F. L.: Antibody formation initiated *in vitro*. II. Antibody synthesis in x-irradiated recipients of diffusion chambers containing nucleic acid derived from macrophages inoculated with antigen. *J Exp Med, 117*:595–602, 1963.

FISHMAN, M.; HAMMERSTROM, R. A., and BOND, V. P.: *In vitro* transfer of macrophage RNA to lymph node cells. *Nature, 198*:549–551, 1963.

FITCH, F. W., and WISSLER, R. W.: The histology of antibody production. In SAMTER, M., and ALEXANDER, H. L. (Eds.): *Immunologic Diseases*. Boston, Little, 1965, pp. 65–82.

FJELDE, A.; LAVAN, A., and RASK-NIELSEN, R.: The chromosomes of four transplantable murine plasma cell leukemias characterized by varying pathological serum protein changes and/or amyloid formation. *Hereditas, 48*:630–644, 1962.

FORD, C. E., and MICKLEM, H. S.: The thymus and lymph nodes in radiation chimaeras. *Lancet, 1*:359, 1963.

FORGET, B. G.; SQUIRES, J. W., and SHELDON, H.: Waldenström's macroglobulinemia with generalized amyloidosis. *Arch Intern Med, 118*:363–375, 1966.

FORSHAW, J.: Megaloblastic erythropoiesis in multiple myeloma. *Brit Med J, II*:101–102, 1963.

FRAME, B.; PACHTER, M. R., and NIXON, R. K.: Myelomatosis with xanthomatosis. *Ann Intern Med, 54*:134–140, 1961.

FRANGIONE, B.; FRANKLIN, E. C.; FUDENBERG, H. H., and KOSHLAND, M. E.: Structural studies of human $\gamma$G-myeloma proteins of different antigenic subgroups and genetic specificities. *J Exp Med, 124*:715–732, 1966.

FRANKLIN, E. C.; LOWENSTEIN, J.; BIGELOW, B., and MELTZER, M.: Heavy chain disease—a new disorder of serum gamma globulins. Report of the first case. *Amer J Med, 37*:332–350, 1964.

FREEDMAN, M., and SELA, M.: Recovery of specific activity upon reoxidation of completely reduced polyalanyl rabbit antibody. *J Biol Chem, 241*:5225, 1966.

FREEMAN, T.: Gamma globulin metabolism in normal humans and in patients. In *Series Haematologic No. 4 Gamma Globulins*. Copenhagen, Munksgaard, 1965, pp. 76–86.

FRENCH, J. M.; HALL, G.; PARISH, D. J., and SMITH, W. T.: Peripheral and autonomic nerve involvement in primary amyloidosis associated with uncontrollable diarrhea and steatorrhea. *Amer J Med, 39*:277–284, 1965.

FRICK, P. G.: Inhibition of conversion of fibrinogen to fibrin by abnormal proteins in multiple myeloma. *Amer J Clin Path, 25*:1263–1273, 1955.

FRIEDMAN, H. P.; STAVITSKY, A. B., and SOLOMON, J. M.: Induction *in vitro* of antibodies to phage T2: antigens in the RNA extract employed. *Science, 149*:1106–1107, 1965.

FUDENBERG, H. H.: The hereditary human gamma globulin (Gm) groups: interpretations and extensions. *Progr Allerg, 7*:1–31, 1963.

FUDENBERG, H. H.: The immune globulins. *Ann Rev Microbiol, 19*:301–338, 1965.

FUDENBERG, H. H., and FRANKLIN, E. C.: Human gamma globulin: genetic control and its relation to disease. *Ann Intern Med, 58*:171, 1963.

FUDENBERG, H.; GERMAN, J. L. III, and KUNKEL, H. G.: Occurrence of rheumatoid factor and other abnormalities in families of patients with agammaglobulinemia. *Arthritis Rheum, 5*:565–588, 1962.

FUDENBERG, H. H.; HEREMANS, J. F., and FRANKLIN, E. C.: Hypothesis for genetic control of synthesis of gamma globulins. *Ann Inst Pasteur, 104*:155–168, 1963.

FUDENBERG, H. H., and HIRSCHHORN, K.: Agammaglobulinemia: the fundamental defect. *Science, 145*:611–612, 1964.

GABRIELSEN, A. E., and GOOD, R. A.: Thymoma. *Ann Intern Med, 65*:607–611, 1966.

GADDY, C. G., and POWELL, L. W., JR.: Raynaud's syndrome associated with idiopathic cryoglobulinemias and cold agglutinins: report of a case and discussion of classification of cryoglobulinemias. *Arch Intern Med, 102*:468, 1958.

GAFNI, J., and SOHAR, E.: Rectal biopsy for the diagnosis of amyloidosis. *Amer J Med Sci, 240*:332–336, 1960.

GALGANO, A. R.: Unusual features of multiple myeloma. *Amer J Roentgen, 74*:304–314, 1955.

GALLI, J., and CHITI, E.: Rheumatoid arthritis and plasmacytosis. *Ann Rheumat Dis, 14*:271, 1955.

GARDNER, F. H., and COHEN, P.: The function of androgens and fluoride salts in the treatment of multiple myeloma. *Trans Amer Clin Climat Ass, 77*:226–234, 1966.

GELL, P. G. H., and COOMBS, R. R. A. (Eds.): *Clinical Aspects of Immunology*. Philadelphia (Pa.), Davis, 1963.

GERMAN, J. L.; BIRO, C. E., and BEARN, A. G.: Chromosomal abnormalities in Waldenström's macroglobulinaemia. *Lancet, II*:48, 1961.

GESCHIKTER, C. F., and COPELAND, M. M.: Multiple myeloma. *Arch Surg, 16*:807, 1928.

GIEDION, A., and SCHEIDEGGER, J. J.: Kongeintale Immunoporese bei Fehlen spezifischer β-Globuline und quantitative normalen gamma Globulin. *Helv Paediat Acta, 12*:241, 1957.

GILBERT, E. F.; HARLEY, J. B.; ANIDO, V.; MENGOLI, H. F., and HUGHES, J. T.: Thymoma, plasma cell myeloma, red cell aplasia, and malabsorption syndrome. *Am J Med, 44*:820–829, 1968.

GILBERT, G., and HONG, R.: Qualitative and quantitative immunoglobulin deficiency. *Amer J Med, 37*:602–609, 1964.

GINSBERG, D. M.: Circulating plasma cells in multiple myeloma. A method of detection and review of the problem. *Ann Intern Med, 57*:843, 1962.

GITLIN, D., and CRAIG, J. M.: The thymus and other lymphoid tissues in congenital agammaglobulinemia. I. Thymic alymphoplasia and lymphatic hypoplasia and their relation to infection. *Pediatrics, 32*:517–530, 1963.

GITLIN, D.; GROSS, P. A. M., and JANEWAY, C. A.: The gamma globulins and their clinical significance. II. Hypogammaglobulinemia. *New Eng J Med, 260*:72–76, 1959.

GITLIN, D.; VAWTER, G., and CRAIG, J. M.: Thymic alymphoplasia and congenital aleukocytosis. *Pediatrics, 33*:184–192, 1964.

GIVOL, D., and PORTER, R. R.: The C-terminal peptide of the heavy chain of the rabbit immunoglobin IgG. *Biochem J, 97*:32C–34C, 1965.

GJERLOW, J.: Plasmacelleleukemi. *Nord Med, 62:*1774, 1959.

GLASER, J., and WYSS-SOUFFRANT, W. A.: Alleged anaphylactic reactions to human gamma globulin. *Pediatrics, 28:*376, 1961.

GLEICH, G. J.; UHR, J. W.; VAUGHAN, J. H., and SWEDLEIND, H. A.: Antibody formation in dysgammaglobulinemia. *J Clin Invest, 45:*1334–1340, 1966.

GLENCHUR, H.; ZINNEMAN, H. H., and BRIGGS, D. R.: Macroglobulinemia: report of two cases. *Ann Intern Med, 48:*1055, 1958.

GLUECK, H. I.; WAYNE, L., and GOLDSMITH, R.: Abnormal calcium binding associated with hyperglobulinemia, clotting defects, and osteoporosis: a study of this relationship. *J Lab Clin Med, 59:*40–64, 1962.

GOLD, E. R.; MÄRTENSSON, L.; ROPARTZ, C.; RIVAT, L., and ROUSSEAU, P. Y.: Gm (f) —a determinant of human gamma globulin. Preliminary communication. *Vox Sang, 10:*299–302, 1965.

GOLDBERG, A.; BRODSKY, I., and McCARTY, D.: Multiple myeloma with paramyloidosis presenting as rheumatoid disease. *Amer J Med, 37:*653–658, 1964.

GOLDBERG, A. F.; TAKAKURA, K., and ROSENTHAL, R. L.: Electrophoretic separation of serum acid phosphatase isoenzymes in Gaucher's disease, prostatic carcinoma and multiple myeloma. *Nature, 211:*41–43, 1966.

GONZALES-ANGULO, A.; GREENBERG, S. D., and WALLACE, S. A.: Generalized primary amyloidosis. Report of a case with amyloid verrucous valvular lesions and nephrotic syndrome. *Amer Heart J, 65:*110–115, 1963.

GOOD, R. A., and MAZZITELLO, W. F.: Chest disease in patients with agammaglobulinemia. *Dis Chest, 29:*9–35, 1956.

GOOD, R. A.; ZAK, S. J.; CONDIE, R. M., and BRIDGES, R. A.: Clinical investigation in patients with agammaglobulinemia and hypogammaglobulinemia. *Pediat Clin N Amer, 7:*397, 1960.

GRABAR, P., and WILLIAMS, C. A.: Methode permettant l'étude conjugnée des propriétés électrophorétique et immunochimiques d'un mélange de protéines. Application au sérum sanguin. *Biochim Biophys Acta, 10:*193–194, 1953.

GRADER, J., and MOYNIHAN, J. W.: Multiple myeloma and osteogenic sarcoma in a patient with Paget's disease. *JAMA, 176:*685–687, 1961.

GRAS, J., and DALMAU, M.: Antibody inhibition by a minimal dose of antigen and response to a sudden increase of the dose. *Nature, 210:*430–431, 1966.

GRAY, D. F.: A genetic instructive theory of immunity. *J Reticuloendothel Soc, 1:*97–114, 1964.

GRAY, W. R.: Personal communication, 1966.

GRAY, W.; DREYER, W., and HOOD, L.: Mechanism of antibody synthesis; size differences between mouse kappa chains. *Science, 155:*465–467, 1967.

GREEN, I.; LITWIN, S.; ADLERSBERG, R., and RUBIN, I.: Hypogammaglobulinemia with late development of lymphosarcoma. Case report. *Arch Intern Med, 118:*592–602, 1966.

GREEN, I., and SPERBER, R. J.: Hypogammaglobulinemia, arthritis, sprue, and megaloblastic anemia. *New York J Med, 62:*1679, 1962.

GREEN, P. A.; HIGGINS, J. A.; BROWN, A. L.; HOFFMAN, H. N., and SOMMERVILLE, R. L.: Amyloidosis: appraisal of intubation biopsy of the small intestine in diagnosis. *Gastroenterology, 41:*452–456, 1961.

GREENE, R.; MORGAN, D. C., and BIRD, R.: The plasma proteins in thyroid disorders. *J Clin Endocr, 18:*99–108, 1958.

GREGG, J. A.; HERSKOVIC, T., and BARTHOLOMEW, L. G.: Ascites in systemic amyloidosis. *Arch Int Med, 116:*605–610, 1965.

GREY, H. M., and KUNKEL, H. G.: H-chain subgroups of myeloma proteins and normal 7S gamma globulin. *J Exp Med, 120:*253–266, 1964.

GREY, H. M., and MANNIK, M.: Specificity of recombination of H and L chains from human gamma G-myeloma proteins. *J Exp Med, 122*:619–632, 1965.

GROKOEST, A. W., and DEMARTINI, F. E.: Systemic disease and the carpal tunnel syndrome. *JAMA, 155*:635–637, 1954.

GROSS, D., and EPSTEIN, W. V.: Macroglobulinemia with Bence Jones proteinuria: comparison of urinary protein and L chain of serum proteins. *J Clin Invest, 43*:83–93, 1964.

GRUBB, R.: The Gm groups and their relation to rheumatoid arthritis serology. *Arthritis Rheum, 4*:195–202, 1961.

GRUBB, R., and LAURELL, A.-B.: Hereditary serological human serum groups. *Acta Path Microbiol Scand, 39*:390–398, 1956.

GUEFT, B., and GHIDONI, J. J.: The site of formation and ultrastructure of amyloid. *Amer J Path, 43*:837–854, 1963.

HAGELSTAM, L.: Solitary vertebral plasmacytoma causing paraplegia; satisfactory results of roentgen treatment on the paraplegia and serum globulins; case report. *Acta Chir Scand, 109*:384–394, 1955.

HÄLLEN, J.: Frequency of "abnormal" serum globulin (M-components) in the aged. *Acta Med Scand, 173*:737, 1963.

HAMMACK, W. J.; BOLDING, F. E., and FROMMEYER, W. B.: Dysgammaglobulinemic syndrome. *Ann Intern Med, 50*:288–299, 1959.

HARBOE, M.: Biologically active "monoclonal" γM-globulins. In *Series Haematologica No. 4 Gamma Globulins.* Copenhagen, Munksgaard, 1965, pp. 65–75.

HARBOE, M.; DEVERILL, J., and GODAL, H. C.: Antigenic heterogeneity of Waldenström type γM-globulins. *Scand J Haemat, 2*:137–147, 1965.

HARBOE, M., and LUNDEVALL, J.: A new type in the Gm system. *Acta Path Microbiol Scand, 45*:357–370, 1959.

HARGRAVES, M. M., and OPFELL, R. W.: Systemic lupus erythematosus and the blood. *Progr Hemat, 1*:249, 1956.

HARRINGTON, W. J., and MOLONEY, W. C.: The treatment of multiple myeloma with urethane. *Cancer, 3*:253, 1950.

HARZHEIM, J. V.; STECHELE, U., and KÜNZER, W.: Zur Frage der disymptomatischen Form des Wiskott-Aldrich-Syndroms. *Deutsche Med Wchschr, 90*:2047–2050, 1965.

HASTRUP, J., and GRAHL-MADSEN, R.: Wiskott-Aldrich's syndrome: thrombocytopenia, eczema and recurrent infection. *Danish Med Bull, 12*:99–102, 1965.

HAUROWITZ, F.: Antibody formation and the coding problem. *Nature, 205*:847–851, 1965.

HAUROWITZ, F.: *Immunochemistry and the Biosynthesis of Antibodies.* New York, Interscience Publishers, 1968.

HAVENS, W. P., JR.; DICKENSHEETS, J.; BIERLY, J. A., and EBERHARD, T. P.: The half-life of normal human gamma globulin in patients with hepatic cirrhosis. *J Clin Invest, 32*:573, 1953.

HAVENS, W. P., JR.; SHAFFER, J. M., and HOPKE, C. J., JR.: The production of antibody by patients with chronic hepatic disease. *J Immun, 67*:347, 1951.

HAYES, D. W.; BENNETT, W. A., and HECK, F. J.: Extramedullary lesions in multiple myeloma. Review of literature and pathologic studies. *Arch Path, 53*:262–272, 1952.

HEALY, J. K.: Acute oliguric renal failure associated with multiple myeloma. Report of three cases. *Brit Med J, 1*:1126–1130, 1963.

HEINIVAARA, O., and EISALD, A.: Multiple myeloma. A study of 34 cases with special reference to alpha myeloma. *Acta Med Scand, 168*:211–218, 1960.

HEINLE, E. W.; SARASTI, H. O.; GARCIA, D.; KENNY, J., and WESTERMAN, M. P.: Polycythemia vera associated with lymphomatous diseases and myeloma. *Arch Intern Med, 118*:351–355, 1966.

HEITZMAN, E. J.; HEITZMAN, G. C., and ELLIOTT, C. F.: Primary esophageal amyloidosis. Report of a case with bleeding, perforation, and survival following resection. *Arch Intern Med, 109*:595–600, 1962.

HELLER, H.; MISSMAHL, H.-P.; SOHAR, E., and GAFNI, J.: Amyloidosis: its differentiation into perireticulin and pericollagen types. *J Path Bact, 88*:15, 1964.

HELLWIG, C. A.: Extramedullary plasma cell tumors as observed in various locations. *Arch Path, 36*:95–111, 1943.

HENNEY, C. S., and STANWORTH, D. R.: Reaction of rheumatoid factor with the isolated polypeptide chains of human 7S gamma globulin. *Nature, 201*:511–512, 1964.

HENSTELL, H. H., and KLIGERMAN, M.: A new theory of interference with the clotting mechanism: the complexing of euglobulin with Factor V, Factor VII and prothrombin. *Ann Intern Med, 49*:371, 1958.

HERBERT, V.: Personal communication, 1967.

HEREMANS, J. F.: Immunochemical studies on protein pathology. The immunoglobulin concept. *Clin Chim Acta, 4*:639, 1959.

HEREMANS, J. F.: Les globulines seriques du systeme gamma. Leur nature et leur pathologie. Editions Arsia S. A., Brussels, 1960.

HEREMANS, J. F.: Gamma-1a-globulin in health and disease. In *Series Haematologica No. 4 Gamma Globulins*. Copenhagen, Munksgaard, 1965, pp. 17–27.

HEREMANS, J. F., and VAERMAN, J. P.: B₂A-globulin as a possible carrier of allergic reaginic activity. *Nature, 193*:1091, 1962.

HEREMANS, J. F.; VAERMAN, J. P., and VAERMAN, C.: Studies on the immune globulins of human serum. II. A study of the distribution of anti-Brucella and anti-diphtheria antibody activities among gamma-SS, gamma-1M, and gamma-1A globulin fractions. *J Immun, 91*:11–17, 1963.

HERMANS, P. E.; HUIZENGA, K. A.; HOFFMAN, H. N. II; BROWN, A. L., and MARKOWITZ, H.: Dysgammaglobulinemia associated with nodular lymphoid hyperplasia of the small intestine. *Amer J Med, 40*:78–89, 1966.

HILL, R. L.; DELANEY, R.; FELLOWS, R. E., and LEBOVITZ, H. E.: The evolutionary origins of the immunoglobulins. *Proc Nat Acad Sci USA, 56*:1762–1769, 1966.

HILL, R. M.; DUNLOP, S. G., and MULLIGAN, R. M.: A cryoglobulin present in high concentration in the plasma of a case of multiple myeloma. *J Lab Clin Med, 34*:1057, 1949.

HILSCHMANN, N.: Die chemische Structur von zwei Bence-Jones-Proteinen (Roy und Cum.) vom κ-Typ. Hoppe-Seyler's Z Physiol Chem, *348*:1077–1080, 1967a.

HILSCHMANN, N.: Die vollständige Aminosäuresequenz des Bence-Jones-Protsins Cum (κ-Type) Hoppe-Seyler's Z Physiol Chem, *348*:1718–1722, 1967b.

HINZ, C. F., JR., and BOYER, J. T.: Dysgammaglobulinemia in adult manifested as autoimmune hemolytic anemia: Serologic and immunochemical characterization of antibody of unusual specificity. *New Eng J Med, 269*:1329–1335, 1963.

HIRSCHHORN, K., and RIPPS, C. S.: Immunoglobulin and antibody production by human peripheral lymphocytes *in vitro*. *J Clin Invest, 45*:1023, 1966.

HITZIG, W. H.; KAY, H. E. M., and COTTIER, H.: Familial lymphopenia with agammaglobulinemia. *Lancet, 2*:151, 1965.

HOLLAND, J. F.; HOSLEY, H.; SCHARLAW, C.; CARBONE, P. P.; FREI, E. III; BRINDLEY, C. O.; HALL, T. C.; SHNIDER, B. I.; GOLD, G. L.; LASAGNA, L.; OWENS, A. H., JR., and MILLER, S. P.: A controlled trial of urethane treatment in multiple myeloma. *Blood, 27*:328–342, 1966.

HOLMAN, H. R.: Systemic Lupus Erythematosus. In Samler, M., and Alexander, H. L. (Eds.): *Immunological Diseases*. Boston, Little, 1965, p. 737–748.

HOLMAN, H.; NICKEL, W. F., JR.; SLEISENGER, M. H.: Hypoproteinemia antedating intestinal lesions and possibly due to excessive serum protein loss into the intestine. *Amer J Med, 27:*963–975, 1959.

HOMBURGER, F., and PETERMANN, M. L.: Studies on hypoproteinemia. II. Familial idiopathic dysproteinemia. *Blood, 4:*1085–1108, 1949.

HONG, R.; SCHUBERT, W. K.; PERRIN, E. V., and WEST, C. D.: Antibody deficiency syndrome associated with beta₂-macroglobulinemia. *J Pediat, 61:*831–842, 1962.

HONG, R., and WEST, C. D.: Gamma-1 globulin levels in rheumatic fever. *Arthritis Rheum, 7:*128, 1964.

HOOD, L.; GRAY, W., and DREYER, W.: On the mechanism of antibody synthesis: a species comparison of L-chains. *Proc Nat Acad Sci USA, 55:*826–832, 1966.

HOWELL, M.: Acquired factor X deficiency associated with systematized amyloidosis: a report of a case. *Blood, 21:*739–744, 1963.

HUHNSTOCK, K., and DISTLER, A.: On the urethane gel reaction of paraproteins. *Klin Wschr, 41:*246–248, 1963.

HUIZENGA, K. A.; WOLLAEGER, E. E.; GREEN, P. A., and McKENZIE, B. F.: Serum globulin deficiencies in nontropical sprue with report of two cases of acquired agammaglobulinemia. *Amer J Med, 31:*572, 1961.

HUMPHREY, J. H., and FAHEY, J. L.: The metabolism of normal plasma proteins and gamma-myeloma protein in mice bearing plasma-cell tumors. *J Clin Invest, 40:*1696–1705, 1961.

HUMPHREY, J. H., and McFARLANE, A. S.: Rate of elimination of homologous globulins (including antibody) from the circulation. *Biochem J, 57:*186–191, 1954.

HUNTLEY, C. C.; LAFFERTY, J. W., and LYERLY, A.: Antibody deficiency syndrome with increased $\gamma_{1M}$ ($\beta_{2M}$)-globulins and absent $\gamma_{1A}$ ($\beta_{2A}$)-globulins and $\gamma_2$(G)-globulins. *Pediatrics, 32:*407–415, 1963.

HURLEY, H. J., and WEINBERG, R.: Induced intralesional hemorrhage in primary systemic amyloidosis. *Arch Derm, 89:*678–681, 1964.

HYMAN, A. B., and LEIDER, M.: Erythroplasia of the female genitalia. Report of two cases of a benign form (plasmacytosis pudendi). *Arch Derm, 84:*71–385, 1961.

HYMAN, G. A.; GELLHORN, A., and HARVEY, J. L.: Studies on the anemia of disseminated malignant neoplastic disease. II. Study of the life span of the erythrocyte. *Blood, 11:*618–631, 1956.

INNES, J., and NEWALL, J.: Myelomatosis. *Lancet, 1:*239–245, 1961.

ISHIZAKA, K.; ISHIZAKA, T., and HORNBROOK, M.: Physicochemical properties of reaginic antibody. V. Correlation of reaginic activity with γE antibody. *J Immun, 97:*840–853, 1966.

JAGER, B. V.: Intravenous administration of modified gamma globulin. Several studies on a patient with agammaglobulinemia. *Arch Intern Med, 119:*60–64, 1967.

JARNUM, S., and SCHWARTZ, M.: Hypoalbuminemia in gastric carcinoma. *Gastroenterology, 38:*769, 1960.

JEFFRIES, G. H.; HOLMAN, H. R., and SLEISENGER, M. H.: Plasma proteins and the gastrointestinal tract. *New Eng J Med, 266:*652, 1962.

JEFFRIES, G. H.; WESER, E., and SLEISENGER, M. H.: Malabsorption. *Gastroenterology, 46:*434, 1964.

JERNE, N. K.: The natural selection theory of antibody formation. *Proc Nat Acad Sci USA, 41:*849–857, 1955.

JERNE, N. K.: Immunologic speculations. *Ann Rev Microbiol, 14:*341–358, 1960.

JIM, R. T. S., and REINHARD, E. H.: Agammaglobulinemia and chronic lymphocytic leukemia. *Ann Intern Med, 44:*790, 1956.

KABAT, E. A.: The paucity of species-specific amino acid residues in the variable regions of human and mouse Bence Jones proteins and its evolutionary and genetic implications. *Proc Nat Acad Sci, 57*:1345–1349, 1967.

KAMME, C.; CÖSTER, C.; HAGELQUIST, E.; KALEN, N.; LINDHOLM, H., and GRUBB, R.: Side effects of treatment of hypogammaglobulinaemia with gammaglobulin. *Acta Med Scand, 179*:679–690, 1966.

KANTARJIAN, A. D., and DEJONG, R. N.: Familial primary amyloidosis with nervous system involvement. *Neurology, 3*:399–409, 1953.

KANZOW, U.: Untersuchungen über Serumlipoide bei Paraproteinämien. *European Soc Haemat Trans 6th Cong, 1957, Copenhagen.* Basel, S. Karger, 1958, Part 2, p. 103.

KARUSH, F., and EISEN, H. N.: A theory of delayed hypersensitivity. *Science, 136*:1032–1039, 1962.

KATCHALSKY, A., and OPLATKA, A.: Hysteresis and macromolecular memory. *Neurosciences Res Prog Bull, 4 (Suppl)*:71–93, 1966.

KAYE, R. L.; MARTIN, W. J.; CAMPBELL, D. C., and LIPSCOMB, R. R.: Long survival in disseminated myeloma with onset as solitary lesion: two cases. *Ann Intern Med, 54*:535–544, 1961.

KENNY, J. J., and MALONEY, W. C.: Multiple myeloma: diagnosis and management in a series of 57 cases. *Ann Intern Med, 46*:1079, 1957.

KERNOHAN, J. W., and WOLTMAN, H. W.: Amyloid neuritis. *Arch Neurol, 47*:132, 1942.

KILLMANN, S. A.; CRONKITE, E. P.; FLIEDNER, T. M., and BOND, V. P.: Cell proliferation in multiple myeloma studied with tritiated thymidine *in vivo. Lab Invest, 11*:845–853, 1962.

KILLMANN, S. A.; GJÖRUP, S., and THAYSEN, J. H.: Fatal acute renal failure following intravenous pyelography in a patient with multiple myeloma. *Acta Med Scand, 158*:43–46, 1957.

KIRKPATRICK, C. H., and RUTH, W. E.: Chronic pulmonary disease and immunologic deficiency. *Amer J Med, 41*:427–439, 1966.

KIRKPATRICK, C. H., and SCHINIKE, R. N.: Paternal immunoglobulin abnormalities in congenital hypogammaglobulinemia. *JAMA, 200*:105–110, 1967.

KIRKPATRICK, C. H.; WAXMAN, D.; SMITH, O. D., and SCHIMKE, R. N.: Hypogammaglobulinemia with nodular lymphoid hyperplasia of the small bowel. *Arch Intern Med, 121*:273–277, 1968.

KOHLER, P. F., and FARR, R. S.: Elevation of cord over maternal IgG immunoglobulin: evidence for an active placental IgG transport. *Nature, 210*:1070–1071, 1966.

KOLETZKY, S., and STECHER, R. M.: Primary systemic amyloidosis: involvement of cardiac valves; joints and bones, with pathologic fracture of the femur. *Arch Path, 27*:267–288, 1939.

KORMAN, S.; CORCORAN, C.; FINE, S., and LIPPINCOTT, S. W.: Comparison of labelled beta and gamma globulin metabolism in multiple myeloma. *J Lab Clin Med, 59*:371–380, 1962.

KORNGOLD, L.: Abnormal plasma components and their significance in disease. *Ann NY Acad Sci, 94*:110, 1961.

KORNGOLD, L.: The detection of monoclonal macroglobulinemia with antisera specific for γM-globulins. *Int Arch Allerg, 31*:105–116, 1967.

KORNGOLD, L., and LIPARI, R.: Multiple-myeloma proteins. III. The antigenic relationship of Bence Jones proteins to normal gamma globulin and multiple myeloma serum proteins. *Cancer, 9*:262–272, 1956.

KORNGOLD, L.; VAN LEEUWEN, G., and ENGLE, R. L., JR.: Diagnosis of multiple myeloma and macroglobulinemia by the Ouchterlony gel diffusion technique. *Ann NY Acad Sci, 101*:203–220, 1962.

Kosova, L. A., and Schwartz, S. O.: Multiple myeloma and normal pregnancy. Report of a case. *Blood, 28*:102–111, 1966.

Krainin, P.; D'Angio, C. J., and Smelin, A.: Multiple myeloma with new bone formation. *Arch Intern Med, 84*:976–982, 1949.

Krauss, S., and Sokal, J. E.: Paraproteinemia in the lymphoma. *Amer J. Med, 40*:400–413, 1966.

Krivit, W.: Platelet survival studies in Aldrich syndrome. *Pediatrics, 37*:339–341, 1966.

Krivit, W., and Good, R. A.: Aldrich's syndrome (thrombocytopenia, eczema and infection in infants); studies of the defense mechanisms. *Amer J Dis Child, 97*:137–153, 1959.

Kubota, C.; Schwartz, S. O., and Putnam, F. W.: Multiple myeloma: correlation of the clinical, and marrow and electrophoretic findings. *Acta Haemat, 16*:105–116, 1956.

Kunkel, H. G.; Ahrens, E. H.; Eisenmenger, W. J.; Bongiovanni, A. M., and Slater, R. J.; Extreme hypergammaglobulinemia in young woman with liver disease of unknown etiology. *J Clin Invest, 30*:654, 1951.

Kunkel, H. G.; Müller-Eberhard, H. J.; Fudenberg, H. H., and Tomasi, T. B.: Gamma globulin complexes in rheumatoid arthritis and certain other conditions. *J Clin Invest, 40*:117–129, 1961.

Kunkel, H. G., and Prendergast, R. A.: Subgroups of γA immune globulins. *Proc Soc Exp Biol Med, 122*:910–913, 1966.

Kunkel, H. G.; Yount, W. J., and Litwin, S. D.: Genetically determined antigen of the Ne subgroup of gamma globulin: detection by precipitin analysis. *Science, 154*:1041–1043, 1966.

Kyle, R. A., and Bayrd, E. D.: "Primary" systemic amyloidosis and myeloma. Discussion of relationship and review of 81 cases. *Arch Intern Med, 107*:344–353, 1961.

Kyle, R. A., and Bayrd, E. D.: "Benign" monoclonal gammopathy: a potentially malignant condition? *Amer J Med, 40*:426–430, 1966.

Kyle, R. A.; Kottke, B. A., and Schirger, A.: Orthostatic hypotension as a clue to primary systemic amyloidosis. *Circulation, 34*:883, 1966.

Kyle, R. A., and McGuckin, W. F.: Separation of macroglobulins from myeloma proteins by Sephadex G200 gel filtration. *J Lab Clin Med, 67*:344–354, 1966.

Kyle, R. A.; Spencer, B. J., and Dahlin, D. C.: Value of rectal biopsy in the diagnosis of primary systemic amyloidosis. *Amer J Med Sci, 251*:501–506, 1966.

Kyle, R. A.; Pease, G. L.; Richmond, H., and Sullivan, L.: Bone marrow aspiration in the antemortem diagnosis of primary systemic amyloidosis. *Amer J Clin Path, 45*:252–257, 1966.

Lachmann, P. J.; Müller-Eberhard, H. J.; Kunkel, H. G., and Paronetto, F.: The localization of *in vivo* bound complement in tissue sections. *J Exp Med, 115*:63–82, 1962.

Lamotte, M.; Segrestaa, J. M.; Rousselet, Fr., and Vilde, J. G.: Dysglobulinemic purpura in the course of a severe rheumatoid polyarthritis. *Sem Hop Paris, 41*:2360–2364, 1965.

Lane, S. L.: Plasmocytoma of the mandible. *Oral Surg, 5*:434, 1952.

Langley, G. R.; Sabean, H. B., and Sorger, K.: Sclerotic lesions of bone in myeloma. *Canad Med Assoc J, 94*:940–946, 1966.

Lanzkowsky, P., and Levy, S.: The triad of thrombocytopenia, eczema and infection (Wiskott-Aldrich's syndrome). *S Afr Med J, 39*:280–282, 1965.

Larson, D., and Tomlinson, L.: Quantitative antibody studies in man. II. The relation of the level of serum proteins to antibody production. *J Lab Clin Med, 39*:129, 1952.

Larsson, O., and Leonhardt, T.: Hereditary hypergammaglobulinemia and systemic lupus erythematosus. I. Clinical and electrophoretic studies. *Acta Med Scand, 165*:371–393, 1959.

LATVALAHTI, J.: Experimental studies on the influence of certain hormones on the development of amyloidosis. *Acta Endoc (Suppl) 16*:1–89, 1953.

LAWRENCE, J. H., and WASSERMAN, L. R.: Multiple myeloma: a study of 24 patients treated with radioactive isotopes ($P^{32}$ and $Sr^{69}$). *Ann Intern Med, 33*:41, 1950.

LAWSON, H. A.; STUART, C. A.; PAULL, A. M.; PHILLIPS, A. M., and PHILLIPS, R. W.: Observations on the antibody content of the blood in the patients with multiple myeloma. *New Eng J Med, 252*:13–18, 1955.

LAZOR, M. A., and ROSENBERG, L. E.: Mechanism of adrenal-steroid reversal of hypercalcemia in multiple myeloma. *New Eng J Med, 270*:749, 1964.

LEDDY, J. P., and BAKEMEIER, R. F.: Structural aspects of human erythrocyte autoantibodies. I. L chain types and electrophoretic dispersion. *J Exp Med, 121*:1–17, 1965.

LEHNER, T.; ROSENOER, V. M., and TOPPING, N. E.: Amyloidosis in mice with a transplantable plasma cell tumour. *Nature, 209*:930–931, 1966.

LENNARD-JONES, J. E.: Myelomatosis with lipaemia and xanthomata. *Brit Med J, 1*:781, 1960.

LENNOX, E. S., and COHN, M.: Immunoglobulins. *Ann Rev Biochem, 36*:365–406, 1967.

LEONCINI, D. L., and KORNGOLD, L.: Multiple myeloma in 2 sisters. An immunochemical study. *Cancer, 17*:733–737, 1964.

LERNER, R. G., and PARKER, J. W.: Dysglobulinemia and iron in plasma cells. *Arch Int Med, 121*:284–287, 1968.

LEVEY, R. H.; TRAININ, N., and LAW, L. W.: Evidence for function of thymic tissue in diffusion chambers implanted in neonatally thymectomized mice. *J Nat Cancer Inst, 31*:199, 1963.

LEVIN, W. C.; ABOUMRAD, M. H.; RITZMAN, S. E., and BRANTLY, C.: Gamma-Type I myeloma and xanthomatosis. *Arch Intern Med, 114*:688–692, 1964.

LEVIN, W. C.; RITZMAN, S. E.; HAGGARD, M. E.; GREGORY, R. F., and REINARZ, J. A.: Selective, A-Beta-2A-globulinemia (Abstract). *Clin Res, 11*:294, 1963.

LEVINE, M. A.; HAMMACK, W. J., and FROMMEYER, W. B.: Treatment of macroglobulinemia with penicillamine. *Clin Res, 8*:54, 1960.

LEWIN, H., and STEIN, J. M.: Solitary plasma cell myeloma with new bone formation. *Amer J Roentgen, 79*:630–637, 1958.

LEWIS, E. B.: Leukemia, multiple myeloma, and aplastic anemia in American radiologists. *Science, 142*:1492, 1963.

LEWIS, F. J. W.; MacTAGGART, M.; CROW, R. S., and WILLS, M. R.: Chromosomal abnormalities in multiple myeloma. *Lancet, I*:1183–1184, 1963.

LEWIS, L. A., and PAGE, I. H.: Serum proteins and lipoproteins in multiple myelomatosis. *Amer J Med, 17*:670, 1954.

LICHTENSTEIN, L., and JAFFE, H. L.: Multiple myeloma; survey based on 35 cases, 18 of which came to autopsy. *Arch Path, 44*:207–246, 1947.

LIGHTSTONE, A. C., and COHEN, H. J.: Plasmocytic mucosal infiltrates in multiple myeloma. *Arch Derm, 82*:921–923, 1960.

LINNET-JEPSEN, P.; GALATIUS-JENSEN, G., and HAUGE, M.: On the inheritance of the Gm serum group. *Acta Genet (Basel), 8*:164–196, 1958.

LINTON, A. L.; and DUNNIGAN, M. G., and THOMSON, J. A.: Immune responses in myeloma. *Brit Med J, II*:86–89, 1963.

LIPMAN, I. J.: Pyroglobulinemia. An unusual presenting sign in multiple myeloma. *JAMA, 188*:1002–1004, 1964.

LIPPINCOTT, S. W.; KORMAN, S.; FONG, C.; STICKLEY, E.; WOLINS, W., and HUGHES,

W. L.: Turnover of labeled normal gamma globulin in multiple myeloma. *J Clin Invest, 39:*565–572, 1960.

Liske, E.; Chou, S. M., and Thompson, H. G.: Peripheral and autonomic neuropathy in amyloidosis. A case report. *JAMA, 186:*432–434, 1963.

Litwin, S. D., and Kunkel, H. G.: A gamma globulin genetic factor related to Gm (a) but localized to a different portion of the same heavy chains. *Nature, 210:*866, 1966.

Litwin, S. D., and Kunkel, H. G.: The genetic control of gamma globulin heavy chains. Studies of the major heavy chain subgroup utilizing multiple genetic markers. *J Exp Med, 125:*847–862, 1967.

Logothetis, J.; Silverstein, P., and Coe, J.: Neurologic aspects of Waldenström's macroglobulinemia. *Arch Neurol, 3:*564, 1960.

LoGrippo, G. A.; Hayashi, H.; Sharpless, N.; Wolfram, B., and Jaslow, R.: Effect of infectious hepatitis on the immunoglobulins in mentally retarded children. *JAMA, 195:*939–942, 1966.

Lohss, F., and Hillmann, G.: Myelom-plasma-proteine IV. Mitteilung zur immunochemie der α-und β-Myelomproteine. *Z Naturforsch, 8b:*706–711, 1953.

Lopez, V., and Bütler, R.: The Inv groups in Switzerland with remarks on the methods of detection. *Vox Sang, 10:*314–319, 1965.

Loutsides, E.: Une nouvelle méthode biologique du diagnostic de la myélomatose multiple. La réaction de gel solidification du serum sanguin a l'uréthane. *Presse Méd, 70:*1211, 1962.

Luttgens, W. F., and Bayrd, E. D.: Treatment of multiple myeloma with urethane: experience with sixty-six cases over a two and a half year period. *JAMA, 147:*824, 1951.

Macalister, C. L., and Addison, N. V.: Renal aspects of myelomatosis. *Brit J Urol, 33:*141–148, 1961.

Mackay, I. R., and Burnet, F. M.: *Autoimmune Diseases: Pathogenesis, Chemistry and Therapy.* Springfield (Ill.), Thomas, 1963.

Mackay, I. R.; Eriksen, N.; Motulsky, A. G., and Volwiler, W.: Cryo- and macroglobulinemia: electrophoretic, ultracentrifugal and clinical studies. *Amer J Med, 20:*564, 1956.

Mackay, I. R.; Taft, L. I., and Cowling, D. C.: Lupoid hepatitis and the hepatic lesions of systemic lupus erythematosus. *Lancet, 1:*65, 1959.

MacMahon, B., and Clark, D. W.: The incidence of multiple myeloma. *J Chron Dis, 4:*508–515, 1956.

Magnus-Levy, A.: Bence-Jones-Eiweiss und Amyloid. *Ztschr Klin Med, 116:*510, 1931.

Magnus-Levy, A.: Amyloidosis in multiple myeloma: Progress noted in 50 years of personal observation. *J Mt Sinai Hosp, 19:*8, 1952.

Maldonado, J. E.; Kyle, R. A.; Brown, A. L. Jr., and Bayrd, E. D.: "Intermediate" cell types and mixed cell proliferation in multiple myeloma: electron microscopic observations. *Blood, 27:*212–226, 1966.

Mannik, M., and Kunkel, H. G.: Two major types of normal 7S gamma globulin. *J Exp Med, 117:*213–230, 1963.

Manor, E.: A cryo-precipitating factor. *Ann Intern Med, 57:*810–819, 1962.

Marchioro, T. L; Rowlands, D. T.; Rifkind, D.; Waddell, W. R.; Starzl, T. E., and Fudenberg, H.: Splenic homotransplantation. *Ann NY Acad Sci, 120:*626, 1964.

Marten, R. H.: Xanthomatosis and myelomatosis. *Proc Roy Soc Med, 55:*318, 1963.

Martensson, L.: Genes and immunoglobulins. *Vox Sang, 11:*521–545, 1966.

Martensson, L., and Kunkel, H. G.: Distribution among the gamma globulin molecules of different genetically determined antigenic specificities in the Gm system. *J Exp Med, 122:*799–811, 1965.

MARTENSSON, L.; VAN LOGHEM, E.; MATSUMOTO, H., and NIELSON, J.: Gm (s) and Gm (t) : Genetic determinants of human gamma globulin. *Vox Sang, 11*:393–418, 1966.

MARTIN, N. H.: The incidence of myelomatosis. *Lancet, 1*:237–239, 1961.

MATTHEWS, R. J.: Idiopathic autoimmune hemolytic anemia and idiopathic thrombocytopenic purpura associated with diffuse hypergammaglobulinemia, amyloidosis, hypoalbuminemia and plasmacytosis. *Amer J Med, 39*:972–984, 1965.

McALPINE, J. C.; RADCLIFFE, A., and FRIEDMANN, I.: Primary amyloidosis of the upper air passages. *J Laryng, 77*:1–27, 1963.

McFARLIN, D. E.; STROBER, W.; WOCHNER, R. D., and WALDMANN, T. A.: Immunoglobulin A production in ataxia telangiectasia. *Science, 150*:1175–1177, 1965.

McGUIGAN, J. E.; PURKERSON, M. L.; TRUDEAU, W. L., and PETERSON, M. L.: Studies of the immunologic defects associated with intestinal lymphangiectasia, with some observations on dietary control of chylous ascites. *Amer J Med, 44*:398–404, 1968.

McINTIRE, K. R.; ASOFSKY, R. M.; POTTER, M., and KUFF, E. L.: Macroglobulin-producing plasma-cell tumor in mice: identification of a new light chain. *Science, 150*:361–363, 1965.

MELLORS, R. C., and KORNGOLD, L.: The cellular origin of human immunoglobulins ($\gamma_2,\gamma_{1M},\gamma_{1A}$) . *J Exp Med, 118*:387–396, 1963.

MELLORS, R. C.; NOWOSLAWSKI, A.; KORNGOLD, L., and SENGSON, B. L.: Rheumatoid factor and the pathogenesis of rheumatoid arthritis. *J Exp Med, 113*:475–484, 1961.

MELLORS, R. C., and ORTEGA, L. G.: New observations on the pathogenesis of glomerulonephritis, lipid nephrosis, periarteritis nodosa, and secondary amyloidosis in man. *Amer J Path, 32*:455–500, 1956.

MELTZER, M., and FRANKLIN, E. C.: Cryoglobulinemia—a study of twenty-nine patients. I. IgG and IgM cryoglobulins and factors affecting cryoprecipitability. *Amer J Med, 40*:828–836, 1966.

MELTZER, M.; FRANKLIN, E. C.; ELIAS, K.; McCLUSKEY, R. T., and COOPER, N.: Cryoglobulinemia—a clinical and laboratory study. II. Cryoglobulins with rheumatoid factor activity. *Amer J Med, 40*:837–856, 1966.

MELTZER, M.; FRANKLIN, E. C.; FUDENBERG, H., and FRANGIONE, B.: Single peptide differences between gamma globulins of different genetic (Gm) types. *Proc Nat Acad Sci USA, 51*:1007–1014, 1964.

MERIGAN, T. C. JR., and HAYES, R. E.: Treatment of hypercalcemia in multiple myeloma. *Arch Intern Med, 107*:389–394, 1961.

MERWIN, R. M., and ALGIRE, G. H.: Induction of plasma-cell neoplasms and fibrosarcomas in BALB/c mice carrying diffusion chambers. *Proc Soc Exp Biol Med, 101*:437, 1959.

METZGER, H., and MANNIK, M.: Recombination of antibody polypeptide chains in the presence of antigen. *J Exp Med, 120*:765–782, 1964.

Midwest Cooperative Chemotherapy Group, Study Committee of. Multiple myeloma. General aspects of diagnosis, course, and survival. *JAMA, 188*:741–745, 1964.

MIGITA, S., and PUTNAM, F. W.: Antigenic relationships of Bence Jones proteins, myeloma globulins, and normal human gamma globulin. *J Exp Med, 117*:81–104, 1963.

MILLER, J. F. A. P.: Immunological function of the thymus. *Lancet, 2*:748–749, 1961.

MILLER, J. F. A. P.: Role of the thymus in immunity. *Brit Med J, 2*:459, 1963.

MILSTEIN, C.: Chemical structure of light chains. *Proc Roy Soc (Biol) , 166*:138, 1966.

MILSTEIN, C.: Interchain disulphide bridge in Bence Jones proteins and in gamma globulin B chains. *Nature, 205*:1171–1173, 1965.

MILSTEIN, C.: Comparative peptide sequences of kappa and lambda chains of human immunoglobulins. *J Molec Biol, 21*:203–205, 1966a.

MILSTEIN, C.: Variations in amino-acid sequence near the disulphide bridges of Bence-Jones proteins. *Nature, 209*:370–373, 1966b.

MILSTEIN, C.: Linked groups of residues in immunoglobulin κ chains. *Nature, 216:*330–332, 1967.

MONGAN, E. S.; KERN, W. A., and TERRY, R.: Hypogammaglobulinemia with thymoma, hemolytic anemia, and disseminated infection with cytomegalovirus. *Ann Intern Med, 65:*548–554, 1966.

MUDD, S.: A hypothetical mechanism of antibody formation. *J Immun, 23:*423–427, 1932.

MULLINAX, F.; MULLINAX, G. L., and HIMROD, B.: RNA metabolism and protein synthesis in plasma cell leukemia. *Amer J Med, 42:*302–308, 1967.

MUNSAT, T. L., and POUSSAINT, A. F.: Clinical manifestations and diagnosis of amyloid polyneuropathy. Report of three cases. *Neurology, 12:*413–422, 1962.

MUNTENDAM, H.: Multipele myelomatosis et het syndroom van DeToni-Fanconi. *Nederl Tydschr Geneesk, 102:*1690, 1958.

NACHMAN, R. L.: Personal communication, 1967.

NACHMAN, R. L., and ENGLE, R. L., JR.: Gamma globulin: unmasking of hidden antigenic sites on light chains. *Science, 145:*167–168, 1964.

NACHMAN, R. L.; ENGLE, R. L. JR., and COPELAND, L.: Correlation of immunologic and structural heterogeneity of Bence Jones proteins. *J Immun, 97:*356–362, 1966.

NATVIG, J. B.; KUNKEL, H. G., and GEDDE-DAHL, T., JR.: Genetic studies of the heavy chain subgroups of γG globulin. Recombination between the closely linked cistrons. In Nobel Symposium 3, *Gamma Globulins, Structure and Control of Biosynthesis,* Ed. by J. Killander, New York, Interscience Publishers, 1967, pp. 313–328.

NEUSTADT, D. H.: Agammaglobulinemia and arthritis. *Rheumatism, 21:*45–49, 1965.

Nomenclature for human immunoglobulins. *Bull Wld Hlth Org, 30:*447, 1964.

NOMLAND, R.: Localized (lichen) amyloidosis of skin; report of 2 cases, with vital staining of amyloid nodules by Congo Red injected intracutaneously or subcutaneously. *Arch Derm Syph, 33:*85–98, 1936.

NORGAARD, O.: Recherches sur l'évolution préclinique du myèlome multiple. *Acta Med Scand, 176:*137, 1964.

NOSSAL, G. J. V.: Genetic control of lymphopoiesis, plasma cell proliferation, and antibody production. *Int Rev Exp Path, 1:*1–72, 1962.

NOSSAL, G. J. V., and MÄKELÄ, O.: Autoradiographic studies on the immune response. I. The kinetics of plasma cell proliferation. *J Exp Med, 115:*209, 1962.

NOSSAL, G. J. V.; SZENBERG, A.; ADA, G. L., and AUSTIN, C. M.: Single cell studies on 19S antibody production. *J Exp Med, 119:*485–503, 1964.

Notation for genetic factors of human immunoglobulins. *Nature, 209:*653–655, 1966.

NUSSENZWEIG, V., and BENACERRAF, B.: Differences in the electrophoretic mobilities of guinea pig 7S antibodies of different specificities. *J Exp Med, 119:*409–423, 1964.

ODELBERG-JOHNSON, O.: Osteosclerotic changes in myelomatosis. *Acta Radiol, 52:*139, 1959.

OHLER, R. L.; HOUGHTON, J. D., and MOLONEY, W. C.: Urethane toxicity, report of a case of hepatic necrosis apparently due to urethane. *New Eng J Med, 243:*984, 1950.

OLIVER, J., and MacDOWELL, M.: Cellular mechanisms of protein metabolism in the nephron. VII. The characteristics and significance of the protein absorption droplets (hyaline droplets) in epidemic hemorrhagic fever and other renal diseases. *J Exp Med, 107:*731–754, 1958.

ORLOFF, J., and FELDER, L.: Primary systemic amyloidosis. *Amer J Med Sci, 212:*275–279, 1946.

OSGOOD, E. E.: The survival time of patients with plasmocytic myeloma. *Cancer Chemother Rep, 9:*1–10, 1960.

OSSERMAN, E. F.: Natural history of multiple myeloma before radiological evidence of disease. Memorial Fund lecture. *Radiology, 71:*157–174, 1958.

OSSERMAN, E. F.: Plasma cell myeloma. II. Clinical aspects. *New Eng J Med, 261*:952; 1006, 1959.

OSSERMAN, E. F.: Editorial: Amyloidosis: Tissue proteinosis: Gammaloidosis. *Ann Intern Med, 55*:1033–1036, 1961.

OSSERMAN, E. F.: Therapy of plasma cell myeloma with melphalan. *Proc Amer Assn Cancer Res, 2*:50, 1963.

OSSERMAN, E. F.: The association between plasmacytic and monocytic dyscrasias in man: clinical and biochemical studies. In Nobel Symposium 3, *Gamma Globulins, Structure and Control of Biosynthesis,* Killander, J., Ed. New York, Interscience, 1967, pp. 573–583.

OSSERMAN, E. F.; GRAFF, A.; MARSHALL, M.; LAWLOR, D., and GRAFF, S.: Incorporation of $N^{15}$-L Aspartic acid into the abnormal serum and urine proteins of multiple myeloma. (Studies of the inter-relationship of these proteins). *J Clin Invest, 36*:352–360, 1957.

OSSERMAN, E. F., and LAWLOR, D. P.: Abnormal serum and urine proteins in 35 cases of multiple myeloma, as studied by filter paper electrophoresis. *Amer J Med, 18*:462–476, 1955.

OSSERMAN, E. F., and LAWLOR, D.: Immunoelectrophoretic characterization of the serum and urinary proteins in plasma cell myeloma and Waldenström's macroglobulinemia. *Ann NY Acad Sci, 94*:93–109, 1961.

OSSERMAN, E. F., and TAKATSUKI, K.: Plasma cell myeloma: gamma globulin synthesis and structure. A review of biochemical and clinical data with the description of a newly-recognized and related syndrome, "$H^{\gamma-2}$-chain (Franklin's) Disease." *Medicine, 42*:357–384, 1963a.

OSSERMAN, E. F., and TAKATSUKI, K.: Role of an abnormal, myeloma-type serum gamma globulin in the pathogenesis of the skin lesions of papular mucinosis (lichen myxedematosus) (Abstract). *J Clin Invest, 42*:962, 1963b.

OSSERMAN, E. F., and TAKATSUKI, K.: Clinical and immunochemical studies of four cases of heavy ($H^{\gamma2}$) chain disease. *Amer J Med, 37*:351–373, 1964.

OSSERMAN, E. F., and TAKATSUKI, K.: Considerations regarding the pathogenesis of the plasmacytic dyscrasias. In *Series Haematologica No. 4 Gamma Globulin,* Copenhagen, Munksgaard, 1965, pp. 28–49.

OSSERMAN, E. F.; TAKATSUKI, K., and TALAL, N.: The pathogenesis of amyloidosis. *Seminars Hemat, 1*:3–86, 1964.

OSTERLAND, C. K.; MILLER, E. J.; KARAKAWA, W. W., and KRAUSE, R. M.: Characteristics of streptococcal group-specific antibody isolated from hyperimmune rabbits. *J Exp Med, 123*:599–614, 1966.

OVARY, Z.: The structure of various immunoglobulins and their biologic activities. *Ann NY Acad Sci, 129*:776–786, 1966.

OWEN, J. A., and RIDER, W. D.: Electrophoretic analysis of serum and urinary proteins in the diagnosis of myelomatosis. *J Clin Path, 10*:373, 1957.

OWINGS, W. J. B.: Hypersensitivity to gamma globulin. A case report. *J Med Ass Alabama, 23*:74–75, 1953.

PAGE, A. R.; CONDIE, R. M., and GOOD, R. A.: Suppression of plasma cell hepatitis with 6-mercaptopurine. *Amer J Med, 36*:200–213, 1964.

PARASKEVAS, F.; HEREMANS, J., and WALDENSTRÖM, J.: Cytology and electrophoretic pattern in $\gamma_{1A}$ ($\beta_{2A}$) myeloma. *Acta Med Scand, 170*:575–589, 1961.

PARKINS, R. A.: Protein-losing enteropathy in the sprue syndrome. *Lancet, 2*:1366, 1960.

PARSONS, D. F.; DARDEN, E. B., JR.; LINDSLEY, D. L., and PRATT, G. T.: Electron microscopy of plasma-cell tumors of the mouse. I. MPC-1 and X5563 tumors. *J Biophys Biochem Cytol, 9*:353–368, 1961a.

PARSONS, D. F.; BENDER, M. A.; DARDENS, E. B., JR.; PRATT, G. T., and LINDSLEY, D. L.: Electron microscopy of plasma-cell tumors of the mouse. II. Tissue cultures of the X5563 tumor. *J Biophys Biochem Cytol, 9*:369–381, 1961b.

PATTERSON, R.; WEISZER, I.; RAMBACH, W.; ROBERTS, M.; and SUSZKO, I. M. Comparative cellular and immunochemical studies of two cases of pyroglobulinemia. *Amer J Med, 44*:147–153, 1968.

PAUL, W. E., and COHEN, A. S.: Electron microscopic studies of amyloid fibrils with ferritin-conjugated antibody. *Amer J Path, 43*:721–738, 1963.

PAULING, L.: A theory of the structure and process of formation of antibodies. *J Amer Chem Soc, 62*:2643–2657, 1940.

PECHET, L., and KASTRUL, J. J.: Amyloidosis associated with factor X (Stuart) deficiency. *Ann Intern Med, 61*:315–318, 1964.

PEETOOM, F., and VAN LOGHEM-LANGEREIS, E.: IgM-IgG cryoglobulinemia, an autoimmune phenomenon. *Vox Sang, 10*:281–292, 1965.

PELKONEN, R.; SIURALA, M., and VUOPIO, P.: Inherited agammaglobulinemia with malabsorption and marked alterations in the gastrointestinal mucosa. *Acta Med Scand, 173*:549, 1963.

PERL, A. F.: Multiple myeloma simulating rheumatoid arthritis. *Canad Med Ass J, 79*:122–123, 1958.

PERNIS, B.; COHEN, M. W., and THORBECKE, G. J.: Specificity of reaction of antigen stimulation in lymph nodes of immature rabbits. I. Morphological changes and gamma globulin production following stimulation with diphtheria toxoid and silica. *J Immun, 91*:541–552, 1963.

PERRY, H. O., MONTGOMERY, H., and STICKNEY, J. M.: Further observations on lichen myxedematosus. *Ann Intern Med, 53*:955–969, 1960.

PETERSON, R. D. A.; COOPER, M. D., and GOOD, R. A.: The pathogenesis of immunologic deficiency diseases. *Amer J Med, 38*:579–604, 1965.

PETERSON, R. D. A; COOPER, M. D., and GOOD, R. A.: Lymphoid tissue abnormalities associated with ataxia-telangiectasia. *Amer J Med, 41*:342–359, 1966.

PETERSON, R. D. A.; KELLY, W. D., and GOOD, R. A.: Ataxia-telangiectasia. Its association with a defective thymus, immunological deficiency disease, and malignancy. *Lancet, 1*:1189–1193, 1964.

PFEIFFER, R., and MARX: Die Bildungsstätte der Choleraschutzstoffe. *Z Hyg Infektionskrankh, 27*:272–297, 1898.

POE, R. H.; GABLE, C. E., and JARROLD, T.: Hypogammaglobulinemia in Hodgkin's disease treated with nitrogen mustard. *Arch Intern Med, 118*:199–202, 1966.

PORTER, D. D.; DIXON, F. J., and LARSEN, A. E.: The development of a myeloma-like condition in mink with Aleutian disease. *Blood, 25*:736–742, 1965.

PORTER, R. R., and PRESS, E. M.: Immunochemistry. *Ann Rev Biochem, 31*:625, 1962.

POTTER, M.; APPELLA, E., and GEISSER, S.: Variations in the heavy polypeptide chain structure of gamma myeloma immunoglobulins from an inbred strain of mice and a hypothesis as to their origin. *J Molec Biol, 14*:361–372, 1965.

POTTER, M., and BOYCE, C. R.: Induction of plasma-cell neoplasma in strain BALB/c mice with mineral oil and mineral oil adjuvants. *Nature, 193*:1086–1087, 1962.

POTTER, M.; DREYER, W. J.; KUFF, E. L., and MCINTIRE, K. R.: Heritable variation in Bence Jones protein structure in an inbred strain of mice. *J Molec Biol, 8*:814–821, 1964.

POTTER, M., and FAHEY, J. L.: Studies on eight transplantable plasma-cell neoplasms of mice. *J Nat Cancer Inst, 24*:1153–1165, 1960.

POTTER, M., and LEON, M. A.: Three IgA myeloma immunoglobulins from the BALB/c mouse: precipitation with pneumococcal c polysaccharide, *Science, 162*:369–371, 1968.

POTTER, M., and ROBERTSON, C. L.: Development of plasma-cell neoplasms in BALB/c mice after intraperitoneal injection of paraffin-oil adjuvant, heat-killed staphylococcus mixtures. *J Nat Cancer Inst, 25*:847–861, 1960.

POULIK, M. D.: Filter paper electrophoresis of purified diphtheria toxoid. *Canad J Med Sci, 30*:417–419, 1952.

POULIK, M. D.: Heterogeneity of the L(B) chains of gamma globulins. *Nature, 202*:1174–1175, 1964.

POULIK, M. D.: Structure and pathologic variations of immunoglobulins. In *Advances in Immunogenetics*, Greenwalt, T. J., Ed. Philadelphia and Toronto, Lippincott, 1967, pp. 31–73.

POULIK, M. D., and SHUSTER, J.: Heterogeneity of H chains of myeloma proteins: susceptibility to papain and trypsin. *Nature, 204*:577–579, 1964.

POULIK, M. D., and SHUSTER, J.: Role of cysteine in the production of Fc and F'c sub-components of γG myeloma globulins. *Nature, 207*:1092–1093, 1965.

PRESS, E. M.; PIGGOT P. J., and PORTER, R. R.: The N- and C-terminal amino acid sequences of the heavy chain from a pathological human immunoglobulin IgG. *Biochem J, 99*:356–366, 1966.

PROPP, S.; SCHARFMAN, W. B.; BECBE, R. T., and WRIGHT, A. W.: Atypical amyloidosis with non thrombocytopenic purpura and plasmocytic hyperplasia of the bone marrow. *Blood, 9*:125, 1954.

PUTKONEN, T.; JOKINEN, E. J., and MUSTAKALLIO, K. K.: Unusual immunologic alterations in sarcoidosis during repeated Kveim testing. *Amer J Med, 39*:985–993, 1965.

PUTNAM, F. W.: Plasma-cell myeloma and macroglobulinemia. I. Physiocochemical, immunochemical and isotopic turnover studies of the abnormal serum and urinary proteins. *New Eng J Med, 261*:902–908, 1959.

PUTNAM, F. W., and EASLEY, C. W.: Structural studies of the immunoglobulins. I. The tryptic peptides of Bence-Jones proteins. *J Bio Chem, 240*:1626–1638, 1965.

PUTNAM, F. W., and MIYAKE, A.: Proteins in multiple myeloma. VIII. Biosynthesis of abnormal proteins. *J Bio Chem, 231*:671–684, 1958.

PUTNAM, F. W.; TITANI, K., and WHITLEY, E., JR.: Chemical structure of light chains: amino acid sequence of type K Bence-Jones proteins. *Proc Roy Soc (Biol), 166*:124, 1966.

PUTNAM, F. W., TITANI, K., WIKLER, M., and SHINODA, T.: Structure and evolution of kappa and lambda light chains. In *Cold Spring Harbor Symposiaon Quantitative Biology*, vol. 32, Antibodies, 1967, pp. 9–28.

PUTNAM, F. W.; TOMOTAKA, S.; TITANI, K., and WIKLER, M.: Immunoglobulin structure: variation in amino acid sequence and length of human lambda light chains. *Science, 157*:1050–1053, 1967.

RACE, R. R., and SANGER, R.: *Blood Groups in Man*, 4th ed., Oxford, Blackwell, 1962.

RASK-NIELSEN, R.: Evidence of murine, virus-induced, paraprotein-producing leukemia and its relation to other virus-induced leukemias. *Nature, 200*:440, 453, 1963.

RASK-NIELSEN, R., and GORMSEN, H.: On the occurrence of plasma-cell leukemia in various strains of mice. *J Nat Cancer Inst, 16*:1137–1144, 1956.

REALEAF, P. D.; DAVIS, R. B.; KUCINSKI, C.; HOILUND, L., and GANS, H.: Amyloidosis with an unusual bleeding diathesis: observations on the use of epsilon aminocaproic acid. *Ann Intern Med, 58*:347–354, 1963.

REBUCK, J. W.; RIDDLE, J. M.; BROWN, M. G.; JOHNSON, S. A., and MONTO, R. W.: Volumetric and ultrastructural studies of abnormal platelets. In JOHNSON, S. A.; MONTO, R. W.; REBUCK, J. W., and HORN, R. C., JR. (Eds.): *Blood Platelets. Henry Ford International Symposium*. Boston, Little, 1961, pp. 533–552.

RECANT, L., and HARTROFT, S. H.: Clinicopathologic conference; acute renal failure of obscure etiology. *Amer J Med, 30:*464–471, 1961.

RECANT, L., and LACY, P.: Clinicopathologic conference; multiple myeloma. *Amer J Med, 36:*121–134, 1964.

REID, R. T.; MINDEN, P., and FARR, R. S.: Reagin activity associated with IgG immunoglobulin. *J Exp Med, 123:*845–858, 1966.

REISFELD, R. A., and SMALL, P. A., JR.: Electrophoretic heterogeneity of polypeptide chains of specific antibodies. *Science, 152:*1253–1255, 1966.

REJNEK, J.; KOSTKA, J., and KOTYNEK, O.: Electrophoretic behavior of H and L chains of human serum and colostrum gamma globulin. *Nature, 209:*926–928, 1966.

REUTTER, F. W., and SIEBENMANN, R.: Die Wirkung von Natriumfluorid bei metabolischen Knochenerkrankungen bolischen. *Helvet Med Acta, 32:*493–497, 1965.

RICH, C., and IVANOVICH, P.: Response to sodium fluoride in severe primary osteoporosis. *Ann Intern Med, 63:*1069–1074, 1965.

RICHARDS, W. G.; KATZMANN, F. S., and COLEMAN, F. C.: Extramedullary plasmocytoma arising in head of pancreas: report of case. *Cancer, 11:*649–652, 1958.

RICHERSON, H. B., and SEEBOHM, P. M.: Anaphylactoid reaction to human gamma globulin. Report of a case and inquiry into mechanism. *Arch Intern Med, 117:*568–572, 1966.

RIEKE, W. O.: Lymphocytes from thymectomized rats: immunologic, proliferative, and metabolic properties. *Science, 152:*535–538, 1966.

RITZMANN, S. E.; Coleman, S. L., and LEVIN, W. C.: Effect of some mercaptanes upon macrocryogelglobulin: modifications induced by cysteamine, penicillamine and penicillin. *J Clin Invest, 39:*1320–1329, 1960.

RITZMANN, S. E., and LEVIN, W. C.: Cryopathies: a review. Classification; diagnostic and therapeutic considerations. *Arch Intern Med, 107:*754–772, 1961.

RITZMANN, S. E., and LEVIN, W. C.: Differentiation of "true" and "spurious" macroglobulinemias associated with high RA-factor activity (Abstract). *J Lab Clin Med, 62:*1008–1009, 1963.

RITZMANN, S. F.; STOUFFLAT, E. J.; HOUSTON, E. W., and LEVIN, W. C.: Coexistent chronic myelocytic leukemia, monoclonal gammopathy and multiple chromosomal abnormalities. *Amer J Med, 41:*981–989, 1966.

RITZMANN, S. E.; THURM, R. H.; TRUAX, W. E., and LEVIN, W. C.: The syndrome of macroglobulinemia. *Arch Intern Med, 105:*939, 1960.

RIVERS, S. L.; WHITTINGTON, R. M., and PATINO, M. E.: Comparison of effect of cyclophosphamide and a placebo in treatment of multiple myeloma. *Cancer Chemother Rep, 29:*115–119, 1963.

ROBBINS, J. H.: Tissue culture studies of the human leukocyte. *Science, 146:*1648–1654, 1964.

ROBERTS, A. N.: Rapid uptake of tritiated antigen by mouse eosinophils. *Nature, 210:*266–269, 1966.

ROCKEY, J. H.; HANSON, L. A.; HEREMANS, J. F., and KUNKEL, H. G.: Beta-2A-aglobulinemia in two healthy men. *J Lab Clin Med, 63:*205–212, 1964.

ROGENTINE, G. N.; ROWE, D. S.; BRADLEY, J.; WALDMAN, T. A., and FAHEY, J. L.: Metabolism of human immunoglobulin D (IgD). *J Clin Invest, 45:*1467–1478, 1966.

ROGERS, B. H. G.; MANALIGOLD, J. R., and BLAZEK, W. V.: Thymoma associated with pancytopenia and hypogammaglobulinemia. *Amer J Med, 68:*154, 1968.

ROGERS, W. R., and WELCH, J. D.: Purpura hyperglobulinemica terminating in multiple myeloma. *Arch Intern Med, 100:*478, 1957.

ROHOLT, O. A., and PRESSMAN, D.: Antibody molecules: discontinuous heterogeneity of heavy chains. *Science, 153:*1257–1259, 1966.

ROHOLT, O. A.; RADZIMSKI, G., and PRESSMAN, D. Specificity in the combination of Fd fragments with L chains to form hapten-binding sites. *J Exp Med, 123*:921–934, 1966.

ROITT, I. M.; CAMPBELL, P. N., and DONIACH, D.: The nature of the thyroid auto-antibodies present in patients with Hashimoto's thyroiditis (lymphadenoid goitre). *Biochem J, 69*:248–256, 1958.

ROPARTZ, C.; RIVAT, L.; ROUSSEAU, P.-Y.; BAITSCH, H., and VAN LOGHEM, J.: Les systèmes Gm et Inv en Europe. *Acta Genet, 13*:109–123, 1963.

ROPARTZ, C.; RIVAT, L.; ROUSSEAU, P.-Y., and LENOIR, J. Les facteurs Gma, Gmb, Gmx, Gm-like et Inv chez les Japonais. *Rev Franc Etud Clin Biol, 6*:813–816, 1961.

ROPARTZ, C.; ROUSSEAU, P.-Y.; RIVAT, L., and LENOIR, J.: Étude génétique du facteur sérique Inv. Fréquence dans certaines populations. *Rev France Etud Clin Biol, 6*:374, 1961.

ROPARTZ, C.; WALTER, H.; ARNDT-HANSER, A.; RIVAT, L.; ROUSSEAU, P.-Y., and BERNARD, W.: On the frequency of the Gm- and Inv-serum groups in South-Western Germany. *Acta Genet, 14*:298, 1964.

ROSEN, F. S., and BOUGAS, J. A.: Acquired dysgammaglobulinemia: elevation of 19S gamma and deficiency of 7S gammaglobulin in woman with chronic progressive bronchiectasis. *New Eng J Med, 269*:1336–1340, 1963.

ROSEN, F. S.; GITLIN, D., and JANEWAY, C. A.: Alymphocytosis, agammaglobulinemia, homograft and delayed hypersensitivity: study of a case. *Lancet, 2*:380–381, 1962.

ROSEN, F. S.; KEVY, S. V.; MERLER, E.; JANEWAY, C. A., and GITLIN, D.: Recurrent bacterial infections and dysgammaglobulinemia; deficiency of 7S gamma globulins in presence of elevated 19S gamma globulins; report of two cases. *Pediatrics, 28*:182–195, 1961.

ROSENBERG, B.; ATTIE, J. N., and MANDELBAUM, H. L.: Breast tumor as the presenting sign of multiple myeloma. *New Eng J Med, 269*:359–361, 1963.

ROSENKRANTZ, J. A., and GLUCKMAN, E. C.: Coexistence of Paget's disease of bone and multiple myeloma: case reports of two patients. *Amer J Roentgen, 78*:30–38, 1957.

ROSEVEAR, J. W., and SMITH, E. L.: Glycopeptides. I. Isolation and properties of glycopeptides from a fraction of human gamma globulin. *J Biol Chem, 236*:425–435, 1961.

ROTSTEIN, J., and GOOD, R. A.: The significance of the simultaneous occurrence of connective tissues disease and the agammaglobulinemic state. *Arthritis Rheum, 4*:436, 1961 (Abstract).

ROWE, D. S., and FAHEY, J. L.; New class of human immunoglobulin: II. Normal serum IgD. *J Exp Med, 121*:185–199, 1965.

RUKAVINA, J. G.; BLOCK, W. D.; JACKSON, C. E.; FALLS, H. F.; CAREY, J. H., and CURTIS, A. C.: Primary systemic amyloidosis: a review and an experimental, genetic, and clinical study of 29 cases with particular emphasis on the familial form. *Medicine 35*:239–334, 1956.

RUNDLES, R. W.; DILLON, M. L., and DILLON, E. S.: Multiple myeloma. III. Effect of urethane therapy on plasma cell growth, abnormal serum components and Bence-Jones proteinuria. *J Clin Invest, 29*:1243, 1950.

RUNDLES, R. W., and REEVES, R. J.: Multiple myeloma. II. Variability of roentgen appearance and effect of urethane therapy on skeletal disease. *Amer J Roentgen, 64*:799–809, 1950.

RUSSO, P. E., and BROWN, B. H.: Solitary myeloma of bone; case report. *Amer J Roentgen, 76*:972–976, 1956.

SABIN, F. R.: Cellular reactions to a dye-protein with a concept of the mechanism of antibody formation. *J Exp Med, 70*:67–82, 1939.

SACHS, V.: Die Häufigkeit der Serumgruppe Inv (a+) (Gm-like?) in Schleswig-Holstein. *Z Immun Forsch, 123*:284, 1962.

SACREZ, R., WILLARD, D.; BEAUVAIS, P., and KORN, R.: Étude des troubles digestifs et respiratoires dans un cas de lymphocytophtisie du nourrisson. *Arch Franc Pédiat, 20:*401, 1963.

SAMTER, M., and ALEXANDER, H. L.: *Immunological Diseases.* Boston, Little, 1965.

SANCHEZ, L. M., and DOMZ, C. A.: Renal patterns in myeloma. *Ann Intern Med, 52:*44–54, 1960.

SANFORD, J. P.; FAVOUR, C. B., and TRIBEMAN, M. S.: Absence of serum gamma globulins in adults. *New Eng J Med, 250:*1027, 1954.

SAUERBRUNN, B. J. L.; RYAN, C. M., and SHAW, J. F.: Chronic fluoride intoxication with fluorotic radiculomyelopathy. *Ann Intern Med, 63:*1074–1078, 1965.

SCHALLER, J.; DAVIS, S. D., and WEDGWOOD, R. J.: Failure of development of the thymus, lymphopenia and hypogammaglobulinemia. An atypical case. *Amer J Med, 41:*462–472, 1966.

SCHEINBERG, I. H., and STERNLIEB, I.: The long term management of hepatolenticular degeneration (Wilson's disease). *Amer J Med, 29:*316, 1960.

SCHINZ, H. R.; BAENSCH, W. E.; FRIEDL, E., and UEHLINGER, E.: In CASE, J. T. (Ed.): *Roentgen-Diagnostics.* New York, Grune, 1952a, vol. 2, p. 947–955.

SCHINZ, H. R.; BAENSCH, W. E.; FRIEDL, E., and UEHLINGER, E.: In CASE, J. T. (Ed.): *Roentgen-Diagnostics,* New York, Grune, 1952b, vol. 2, p. 957.

SCHMITT, F. O., and DAVISON, P. F.: Role of protein in neural function. *Neurosciences Res Prog Bull, 3:*55–76, 1965.

SCHULTZE, H., and HEREMANS, J. F.: *Molecular Biology of Human Proteins with Special Reference to Plasma Proteins.* Vol. 1, *Nature and Metabolism of Extracellular Proteins;* Vol. 2, *Physiology and Pathology of Plasma Proteins.* New York and Amsterdam, Elsevier, 1966.

SCHWARTZ, J. H., and EDELMAN, G. M.: Comparisons of Bence Jones proteins and L polypeptide chains of myeloma globulins after hydrolysis with trypsin. *J Exp Med, 118:*41–54, 1963.

SCHWARTZ, H. J., and FREDD, S. B.: The benign purpuric hyperglobulinemia of Waldenström. *JAMA, 187:*230–232, 1964.

SCHWARTZ, M., and JARNUM, S.: Gastrointestinal protein loss in idiopathic (hypercatabolic) hypoproteinemia. *Lancet, 1:*327, 1959.

SCHWEET, R., and HEINTZ, R.: Protein synthesis. *Ann Rev Biochem, 35:*723–758, 1966.

SEIDEN, G. E., and KRAMER, M.: Idiopathic benign hyperglobulinemic purpura. *NY J Med, 58:*3848–3851, 1958.

SELIGMANN, M.: Personal communication to Barth, *et al.,* 1965.

SELIGMANN, M., and BASCH, A.: The clinical significance of pathological immunoglobulins. Plenary Session Papers, XII Congress, Internat. Soc. Hemat., New York, 1968, pp. 21–31.

SELIGMANN, M.; DANON, F., and FINE, J. M.: Immunological studies in familial $\beta$2-macroglobulinemias. *Proc Soc Exp Biol Med, 114:*482–486, 1963.

SELIGMANN, M.; DANON, F., and MIHAESCO, C.: Family studies in Waldenström's macroglobulinemia. In *Series Haematologica No. 4 Gamma Globulins,* Copenhagen, Munksgaard, 1965, pp. 50–64.

SELIGMANN, M.; DANON, F.; MIHAESCO, C., and FUDENBERG, H. H.: Immunoglobulin abnormalities in families of patients with Waldenström's macroglobulinemia. *Amer J Med, 43:*66–83, 1967.

SELL, S.: Gamma globulin metabolism in germfree guinea pigs. *J Immun. 92:*559–564, 1964.

SERRE, H., and SIMON, L.: Paget's disease of bone and plasmocytic multiple myeloma. *Rev Rhum, 26:*347–353, 1959.

SHAPIRO, A. L.; SCHARFF, M. D.; MAIZEL, J. V., and UHR, J. W.: Synthesis of excess light chains of gamma globulin by rabbit lymph node cells. *Nature, 211*:243–245, 1966.

SHARP, J. T.; CALKINS, E.; COHEN, A. S.; SCHUBERT, A. F., and CALABRO, J. J.: Observations on the clinical, chemical and serological manifestations of rheumatoid arthritis, based on the course of 154 cases. *Medicine, 43*:41, 1964.

SHEON, R. P., LEWIS, L. L., and BATTLE, J. D.: Late occurrence of plasmocytoma of the tongue in "benign" hyperglobulinemic purpura of Waldenström. Twenty year progress report. *Ann Intern Med, 64*:386–390, 1966.

SHORT, I. A., and SMITH, J. P.: Myelomatosis associated with glycosuria and aminoaciduria. *Scot Med J, 4*:89, 1959.

SHUSTER, S.; JONES, J. H., and FLYNN, G.: Renal tubular secretion of human plasma proteins and Bence Jones protein. *Brit J Exp Path, 44*:145–150, 1963.

SICKEL, G. W.: Crystalline glomerular deposits in multiple myeloma. *Amer J Med, 27*:354–356, 1959.

SIEGEL, M.; LEE, S. L.; GINSBERG, V.; SCHULTZ, F., and WONG, W.: Racial differences in serum gamma globulin levels: comparative data for Negroes, Puerto Ricans, and other caucasians. *J Lab Clin Med, 66*:715–720, 1965.

SILVER, R. T.: Infections, fever, and host resistance in neoplastic diseases. *J Chron Dis, 16*:677–701, 1963.

SILVER, R. T.: Personal communication, 1965.

SILVER, R. T.; PEDREIRA, L.; KORNGOLD, L., and ENGLE, R. L., JR.: Studies of serum protein abnormalities in kala azar. *Proc Soc Exp Biol Med, 106*:365–368, 1961.

SINGER, M. F., and LEDER, P.: Messenger RNA: an evaluation. *Ann Rev Biochem, 35*:195–230, 1966.

SINGH, A.; JOLLY, S. S.; BANSAL, B. C., and MARTHUR, C. C.: Endemic fluorosis. Epidemiological, clinical and biochemical study of chronic fluorine intoxation in Panjab (India). *Medicine, 42*:229, 1963.

SIROTA, J. H., and HAMERMAN, D.: Renal function studies in an adult subject with the Fanconi syndrome. *Amer J Med, 16*:138–152, 1954.

SIRRIDGE, M. S.; BOWMAN, K. S., and GARBER, P. E.: Fibrinolysis and changes in fibrinogen in multiple myeloma. *Arch Intern Med, 101*:630–635, 1958.

SITOMER, G.; BLUM, J. J., and SLAVIN, R. E.: Cryoglobulinemia: an inherited molecular disease. *Amer J Med, 34*:565, 1963.

SJÖQUIST, J.: Heterogeneity of heavy (γ) chain preparations from human γG-immunoglobulins. *Nature, 210*:1182–1183, 1966.

SJÖQUIST, J., and VAUGHAN, M. H., JR.: Heterogeneity of H and L chains of normal and myeloma γG-globulin. *J Molec Biol, 20*:527–536, 1966.

SKINNER, W.; BERGSAGEL, D. E., and TRUAX, W.: Evaluation of new chemotherapeutic agents in treatment of multiple myeloma. VII. M and B 938. *Cancer Chemother Rep, 28*:13–15, 1963.

SKOOG, W. A.: Personal communication, 1965.

SKOOG, W. A., and ADAMS, W. S.: Metabolic balance study of a patient with multiple myeloma treated with dexamethasone. Dexamethasone-induced fatal necrotizing polyarteritis of coronary vessels and kidneys. *Amer J Med, 34*:417, 1963.

SKOOG, W. A., and ADAMS, W. S.: Clinical and metabolic investigations of eight cases of multiple myeloma during prolonged cyclophosphamide administration. *Amer J Med, 41*:76–95, 1966.

SKOOG, W. A.; ADAMS, W. S., and COBURN, J. W.: Metabolic balance study of plasmapheresis in a case of Waldenström's macroglobulinemia. *Blood, 19*:425–438, 1962.

SLATER, R. J.: The serum gamma globulins defined by electrophoretic and immunologic analyses. *Arch Biochem Biophys, 59*:33–44, 1955.

SLATER, R. J.; WARD, S. M., and KUNKEL, H. G.: Immunologic relationships among the myeloma proteins. *J Exp Med, 101:*85–108, 1955.

SMITH, E. W.: Non-myelomatous paraproteinemia. *Clin Res Proc, 5:*158, 1957.

SMITH, E.; KOCHWA, S., and WASSERMAN, L. R.: Aggregation of IgG globulin *in vivo.* I. The hyperviscosity syndrome in multiple myeloma. *Amer J Med, 39:*35–48, 1965.

SMITHIES, O.: Gamma globulin variability: a genetic hypothesis. *Nature, 199:*1231–1236, 1963.

SMITHIES, O.: Antibody variability. Somatic recombination between the elements of "antibody gene pairs" may explain antibody variability. *Science, 157:*267–273, 1967.

SMITHIES, R.; WALKER, P.; TARGETT, G., and FREEMAN, T.: Quoted in Freeman, T. (1965).

SNAPPER, I.; TURNER, L. B., and MOSCOVITZ, H. L.: *Multiple Myeloma.* New York, Grune, 1953.

SOLOMON, J.; ALEXANDER, M. J., and STEINFELD, J. L.: Cyclophosphamide. A Clinical Study. *JAMA, 183:*165–170, 1963.

SOLOMON, A., and FAHEY, J. L.: Plasmapheresis therapy in macroglobulinemia. *Ann Intern Med, 58:*789, 1963.

SOLOMON, A., and FAHEY, J. L.: Bence Jones Proteinemia. *Amer J Med, 37:*206–222, 1964.

SOLOMON, A.; FAHEY, J. L., and MALMGREN, R. A.: Immunohistologic localization of gamma-1-macroglobulins, beta-2A-myeloma proteins, 6.6S gamma-myeloma proteins and Bence Jones proteins. *Blood, 21:*403–423, 1963.

SOLOMON, A.; KILLANDER, J.; GREY, H. M., and KUNKEL, H. G.: Low molecular weight proteins related to Bence Jones proteins in multiple myeloma. *Science, 151:*1237–1239, 1966.

SOLOMON, A., and TOMASI, T. B., JR.: Metabolism of IgA ($\beta_{2A}$) globulin (Abstract). *Clin Res, 12:*452, 1964.

SOLOMON, A.; WALDMANN, T. A., and FAHEY, J. L.: Clinical and experimental metabolism of normal 6.6S gamma globulin in normal subjects and in patients with macroglobulinemia and multiple myeloma. *J Lab Clin Med, 62:*1–17, 1963.

SOOTHILL, J. F.: The concentration of $\gamma_1$, macroglobulin (Iota) in the serum of patients with hypogammaglobulinemia. *Clin Sci, 23:*27–38, 1962.

SORENSON, G. D.: Electron microscopic observations of viral particles within myeloma cells of man. *Exp Cell Res, 25:*219–221, 1961.

SORENSON, G.: Clinicopathologic conference; amyloidosis. *Amer J Med, 40:*603–617, 1966.

SORENSON, G. D.; HEEFNER, W. A., and KIRKPATRICK, J. B.: Experimental amyloidosis; II. Light and electron microscopic observations of liver. *Amer J Path, 44:*629–644, 1964.

SOUTH, M. A.; COOPER, M. D.; WOLLHEIM, F. A.; HONG, R., and GOOD, R. A.: The IgA system. I. Studies of the transport and immunochemistry of IgA in the saliva. *J Exp Med, 123:*615–627, 1966.

SPAIN, D. M.; GREENBLATT, I. J.; SNAPPER, I., and COHN, T.: Degree of coronary and aortic atherosclerosis in necropsied cases of multiple myeloma. *Amer J Med Sci, 231:*165, 1956.

SPEIRS, R. S., and SPEIRS, E. E.: Cellular reactions to reinjection of antigen. *J Immun, 92:*540–549, 1964.

STARCICH, R.: Histopathological and microradiological observations on myelomatous osteopathy. *Acta Haemat, 18:*113–125, 1957.

STASTNY, P., and ZIFF, M.: Responsiveness of lymphoid cells to phytohemagglutinin: unresponsiveness of thymus cells. *J Clin Invest, 45:*1076, 1966 (Abstract).

STEIN, S.; NACHMAN, R. L., and ENGLE, R. L., JR.: Individual and sub-group antigenic specificity of Bence Jones protein. *Nature, 200:*1180–1181, 1963.

STEINBERG, A. G.: Progress in the study of genetically determined human gamma globulin types (The Gm and Inv groups). In STEINBERG, A. G., and BEARN, A. G. (Eds.) : Progress in Medical Genetics, vol. II, New York and London, Grune, 1962, pp. 1–33.

STEINBERG, A. G.: Comparison of Gm (f) with Gm (b²) [Gm (bʷ)] and a discussion of their genetics. *Amer J Hum Genet, 17*:311–319, 1965.

STEINBERG, A. G.: Genetic variations in human immunoglobulins: the Gm and Inv types. In *Advances in Immunogenetics,* Ed. by T. J. Greenwalt. Philadelphia and Toronto, J. B. Lippincott Company, 1967, pp. 75–98.

STEINBERG, A. G.; GILES, B. D., and STAUFFER, R.: A Gm-like factor present in negroes and rare or absent in whites: its relation to Gmᵃ and Gmˣ. *Amer J Hum Genet, 12*:44–51, 1960.

STEINBERG, A. G., and GOLDBLUM, R.: A genetic study of the antigens associated with the Gm (b) factor of human gamma globulin. *Amer J Hum Genet, 17*:133–147, 1965.

STEINBERG, A. G., and POLMAR, S. H.: The relation of the S and F fragments and the H and L chains of gamma globulin to the Gm groups. *Vox Sang, 10*:369–370, 1965.

STEINBERG, A. G.; WILSON, J., and LANSET, S.: A new human gamma globulin factor determined by an allele at the Inv locus. *Vox Sang, 7*:151–156, 1962.

STEINFELD, J. L.; Davidson, J. D.; GORDON, R. S., JR., and GREENE, F. E.: The mechanism of hypoproteinemia in patients with regional enteritis and ulcerative colitis. *Amer J Med, 29*:405, 1960.

STERZL, J.; KOSTKA, J.; MANDEL, L.; RIHA, I., and HOLUB, M.: Development of the formation of gamma globulin and of normal and immune antibodies in piglets reared without colostrum. In HOLUB, M., and JAROSKOVA, L. (Eds.) : *Mechanisms of Antibody Formation.* New York and London, Academic, 1962, p. 130.

STEVENS, A. R.: Evolution of multiple myeloma. *Arch Intern Med, 115*:90, 1965.

ST. GEME, J. W., JR.; PRINCE, J. T.; BURKE, B. A.; GOOD, R. A., and KRIVIT, W.: Impaired cellular resistance to herpes-simplex virus in Wiskott-Aldrich syndrome. *New Eng J Med, 273*:229–234, 1965.

STIEHM, E. R., and FUDENBERG, H. H.: Antibodies to gamma globulin in infants and children exposed to isologous gamma globulin. *Pediatrics, 35*:229–235, 1965.

STIEHM, E. R., and FUDENBERG, H. H.: Serum levels of immune globulins in health and disease: a survey. *Pediatrics, 37*:715–727, 1966a.

STIEHM, E. R., and FUDENBERG, H. H.: Clinical and immunologic features of dysgammaglobulinemia Type I. Report of a case diagnosed in the first year of life. *Amer J Med, 40*:805–815, 1966b.

STRAUSS, W. G.: Purpura hyperglobulinemia of Waldenström. Report of a case and review of the literature. *New Eng J Med, 260*:857–860, 1959.

STROBER, W.; WOCHNER, R. D., CARBONE, P. D. and WALDMANN, T. A.: Intestinal lymphangiectasia: a protein-losing enteropathy with hypogammaglobulinemia, lymphocytopenia and impaired homograft rejection. *J. Clin Invest, 45*:1077, 1966 (Abstract).

Study Committee of the Midwest Cooperative Chemotherapy Group. Multiple myeloma: general aspects of diagnosis, course and survival. *JAMA 188*:741–745, 1964.

SUISSA, L.; LAROSA, J., and LINN, B.: Plasmacytoma of lymph node. *JAMA, 197*:294–296, 1966.

SVEHAG, S.-E.; CHESEBRO, B., and BLOTH, B.: Ultrastructure of gamma M immunoglobulin and alpha M macroglobulin: electron microscope study. *Science, 158*:33–36, 1967.

SWAN, A.: *Proceedings of Eighth Congress of European Society of Hematology, Vienna, 1961, Part I.* Basle and New York, Karger, 1961, p. 162.

TAKATSUKI, K., and OSSERMAN, E. F.: Structural differences between two types of "heavy chain" disease proteins and myeloma globulins of corresponding types. *Science, 145*:499–500, 1964a.

TAKATSUKI, K., and OSSERMAN, E. F.: Demonstration of two types of low molecular weight gamma globulins in normal human urine. *J Immun, 92*:100–107, 1964b.

TALAL, N., and BARTH, W.: Macroglobulinemia in Sjögren's syndrome (Abstract). *J Clin Invest, 45*:1079, 1966.

TALBOTT, J. H.: Gout and dyscrasias. *Medicine, 38*:173–205, 1959.

TALMAGE, D. W.: Allergy and immunology. *Ann Rev Med, 8*:239–256, 1957.

TALMAGE, D. W., and PEARLMAN, D. S.: The antibody response: a model based on antagonistic actions of antigen. *J Theoret Biol, 5*:321–339, 1963.

TEILUM, G.: Periodic acid-Schiff-positive reticulo-endothelial cells producing glycoprotein. Functional significance during formation of amyloid. *Amer J Path, 32*:945–960, 1956.

TEILUM, G.: Pathogenesis of amyloidosis. The two-phase cellular theory of local secretion. *Acta Path Microbiol Scand, 61*:21, 1964.

TERRY, W. D., and FAHEY, J. L.: Subclasses of human $\gamma_2$-globulin based on differences in the heavy polypeptide chains. *Science, 146*:400–401, 1964.

TERRY, W. D.; FAHEY, J. L., and STEINBERG, A. G.: Gm and Inv factors in subclasses of human IgG. *J Exp Med, 122*:1087–1102, 1965.

TERRY, W. D., and ROBERTS, M. S.: Antigenic heterogeneity of human immunoglobulin A proteins. *Science, 153*:1007–1008, 1966.

TERRY, W. D.; SMALL, P. A., JR., and REISFELD, R. A.: Electrophoretic heterogeneity of the polypeptide chains of human G-myeloma proteins. *Science, 152*:1628–1630, 1966.

teVELDE, K.; HUBER, J., and VAN DER SLIKKE, L. B.: Primary acquired hypogamma-globulinemia, myasthenia and thymoma. *Ann Intern Med 65*:554–559, 1966.

THEOLOGIDES, A.; OSTERBERG, K., and KENNEDY, B. J.: Cerebral toxoplasmosis in multiple myeloma. *Ann Intern Med, 64*:1071–1074, 1966.

THOMAS, T. F.: Multiple myeloma in siblings. *New York J Med, 64*:2096–2099, 1964.

THORBECKE, G. J., and KEUNING, F. J.: Antibody and gamma globulin formation *in vitro* in haemopoetic organs. *J Infect Dis, 98*:157–171, 1956.

THORLING, E. B.: Leukemic myelomatosis (Plasma-cell leukemia). *Acta Haemat 28*:222–229, 1962.

TIDSTROM, B.: A case of $\alpha_2$-myelomatosis. *Acta Med Scand, 173*:281–284, 1962.

TISELIUS, A., and KABAT, E. A.: An electrophoretic study of immune sera and purified antibody preparations. *J Exp Med, 69*:119, 1939.

TITANI, K.; WHITLEY, E., JR., and PUTNAM, F. W.: Immunoglobulin structure: variation in the sequence of Bence Jones proteins. *Science, 152*:1513–1516, 1966.

TITANI, K.; WIKLER, M., and PUTNAM, F. W.: Evolution of immunoglobulins: structural homology of kappa and lambda Bence Jones proteins. *Science, 155*:828–835, 1967.

TOMASI, T. B., JR.: Human gamma globulin. *Blood, 25*:382–403, 1965.

TOMASI, T. B., JR.; TAN, E. M.; SOLOMON, A., and PRENDERGAST, R. A.: Characteristics of an immune system common to certain external secretions. *J Exp Med, 121*:101–124, 1965.

TOMASI, T. B., and ZIGEBAUM, S.: The selective occurrence of $\gamma_{1A}$ globulins in certain body fluids. *J Clin Invest, 42*:1552–1560, 1963.

TOURTELLOTTE, C. R., and CALL, M. K.: Prolonged remission of myeloma with cyclophosphamide. *Arch Intern Med, 113*:758–763, 1964.

TRUBOWITZ, S.: The sternal marrow aspiration of amyloid in multiple myeloma. *Blood, 5*:581, 1950.

TURKINGTON, R. W., and BUCKLEY, C. E.: Macroglobulinemia and sarcoidosis. *Amer J Med, 40*:156–164, 1966.

UCLA Interdepartmental Conference. Opportunistic pulmonary infections. *Ann Intern Med, 65*:566–594, 1966.

VAERMAN, J.-P., and HEREMANS, J. F.: Subclasses of human immunoglobulin A based on differences in the alpha polypeptide chains. *Science, 153:*647–649, 1966.

VALENTINE, R. C.: Electron microscopy of IgG immunoglobulins. In Nobel Symposium 3, *Gamma Globulins. Structure and Control of Biosynthesis.* J. Killander, Ed. New York, Interscience, 1967, pp. 251–258.

VAN BUCHEM, F. S. P.; MANDEMA, E., and ARENDS, A.: Amyloidosis of the heart. *Acta Med Scand, 171:*159–172, 1962.

VARRIALE, P.; GINSBERG, D. M., and SASS, M. D.: A urinary cryoprotein in multiple myeloma. *Ann Intern Med, 57:*819–823, 1962.

VASSAR, P. S., and CULLING, C. F. A.: Flourescent amyloid staining of casts in myeloma nephrosis. *Arch Path, 73:*59–63, 1962.

VAUGHAN, J. H.; JACOX, R. F., and GRAY, B. A.: Light and heavy chain components of gamma globulins in urines of normal persons and patients with agammaglobulinemia. *J Clin Invest, 46:*266–279, 1967.

VAZQUEZ, J. T., and DIXON, F. J.: Immunohistochemical analysis of amyloid by the fluorescence technique. *J Exp Med, 104:*727–736, 1956.

VESIN, P.; TROUPEL, S.; ACAR, J.; RENAULT, H.; DESBUQUAIS, G., and CATTAN, R.: Entéropathie avec perte de protéins et stéatorrhée. Étude par le PVP-I$^{131}$ et la trioléine I$^{131}$. Action du regime sans gluten. *Bull Soc Med Hop Paris, 1:*261, 1960.

VICTOR, M.; BANKER, B. Q., and ADAMS, R. D.: Neuropathy of multiple myeloma. *J Neurol Neurosurg Psychiat, 21:*73–88, 1958.

VIDEBAEK, A.: Unusual cases of osteomyelosclerosis. *Acta Med Scand, 153:*459, 1956.

VOLPÉ, R.; BRUCE-ROBERTSON, A.; FLETCHER, A. A., and CHARLES, W. B.: Essential cryoglobulinemia: review of the literature and report of a case treated with ACTH and cortisone. *Amer J Med, 20:*533, 1956.

VON BEHRING and KITASATO: Ueber das Zustandekommen der Diphtherie-Immunität und der Tetanus-Immunität bei Thieren. *Deutsche Med Wschr, 16:*1113–1114, 1890.

VON HOYNINGEN-HUENE, C. B. J.: Systemic amyloidosis presenting as constrictive pericarditis. A case studied with cardiac catheterization. *Amer Heart, J, 67:*290–294, 1964.

WAGER, O.; MUSTAKALLIO, K. K., and RÄSÄNEU, J. A.: Mixed IgA-IgG cryoglobulinemia. Immunological studies and case reports of three patients. *Amer J Med, 44:*179–187, 1968.

WAKSMAN, B. H.; ARNASON, B. G., and JANKOVIC, B. D.: Role of the thymus in immune reactions in rats. III. Changes in the lymphoid organs of thymectomized rats. *J Exp Med, 116:*187–206, 1962.

WALDENSTRÖM, J.: Incipient myelomatosis or "essential" hyperglobulinemia with fibrinopenia—new syndrome? *Acta Med Scand, 117:*216, 1944.

WALDENSTRÖM, J.: Abnormal proteins in multiple myeloma. *Advances Intern Med, 5:*398, 1952.

WALDENSTRÖM, J.: Studies on conditions of disturbed gamma globulin formation (gammopathies). *Harvey Lect, 56:*211–231, 1961.

WALDENSTRÖM, J.: Melphalan therapy in myelomatosis. *Brit Med J, 1:*859–865, 1964a.

WALDENSTRÖM, J.: The occurrence of benign, essential monoclonal (M type), non-macromolecular hyperglobulinemia and its differential diagnosis. IV. Studies in the gammopathies. *Acta Med Scand, 176:*345, 1964b.

WALDMANN, T. A., and SCHWAB, P. J.: IgG (7S gamma globulin) metabolism in hypogammaglobulinemia. Studies in patients with defective gamma globulin synthesis, gastrointestinal loss or both. *J Clin Invest, 44:*1523–1533, 1965.

WALDMANN, T. A.; STEINFELD, J. L., DUTCHER, T. F.; DAVIDSON, J. D., and GORDON, R. S.,

J<small>R</small>.: The role of the gastrointestinal system in "idiopathic hypoproteinemia." *Gastroenterology, 41*:197, 1961.

W<small>ALLIS</small>, L. A.; A<small>SCH</small>, T., and M<small>AISEL</small>, B. W.: Diffuse skeletal hemangiomatosis. Report of two cases and review of literature. *Amer J Med, 37*:545–563, 1964.

W<small>ALLIS</small>, L. A., and E<small>NGLE</small>, R. L., J<small>R</small>.: The adult Fanconi syndrome. II. Review of eighteen cases. *Amer J Med, 22*:13–23, 1957.

W<small>ANEBO</small>, H. J.; G<small>ALLMEIER</small>, W. M.; B<small>OYSE</small>, E. A., and O<small>LD</small>, L. J.: Paraproteinemia and reticulum cell sarcoma in an inbred mouse strain. *Science, 154*:901–903, 1966.

W<small>ARE</small>, W. H., and S<small>ILVERMAN</small>, S.: Primary amyloid disease: review of the literature and report of a case. *J Oral Surg, 19*:140–145, 1961.

W<small>ARREN</small>, S.: Generalized amyloidosis of the muscular system. *Amer J Path, 6*:161–167, 1930.

W<small>ATSON</small>, J. D.: *Molecular Biology of the Gene*. New York, W. A. Benjamin, 1965a p. 415.

W<small>ATSON</small>, J. D.: *Molecular Biology of the Gene*. New York, W. A. Benjamin, 1965b, chaps. 10, 11, 14 and 15.

W<small>ATSON</small>, R. J.; S<small>HAPIRO</small>, H. D.; E<small>LLISON</small>, R. R., and L<small>ICHTMAN</small>, H. C.: Splenic aspiration in clinical and experimental hematology. *Blood, 10*:259–271, 1955.

W<small>EICKER</small>, H., and H<small>UHNSTOCK</small>, K.: Characterization of some urinary protein fractions in patients with multiple myeloma. *Nature, 196*:480–481, 1962.

W<small>EIR</small>, R. C.; P<small>ORTER</small>, R. R., and G<small>IVOL</small>, D.: Comparison of the C-terminal amino-acid sequence of two horse immunoglobulins IgG and IgG (T). *Nature, 212*:205–206, 1966.

W<small>EISS</small>, H. J.; D<small>EMIS</small>, D. J.; E<small>LGART</small>, M. L.; B<small>ROWN</small>, C. S., and C<small>ROSBY</small>, W. H.: Treatment of two cases of hyperglobulinemic purpura with thioguanine. *New Eng J Med, 268*:753–756, 1963.

W<small>EITZEL</small>, R. A.: Carcinoma coexistent with malignant disorders of plasma cells: An autopsy survey. *Cancer, 11*:546–549, 1958.

W<small>ELTON</small>, J.; W<small>ALKER</small>, S. R.; S<small>HARP</small>, G. C.; H<small>ERZENBERG</small>, L. A.; W<small>ISTAR</small>, R., J<small>R</small>., and C<small>REGER</small>, W. P.: Macroglobulinemia with bone destruction. *Amer J Med, 44*:280–288, 1968.

W<small>EST</small>, C. D.; H<small>ONG</small>, R., and H<small>OLLAND</small>, N. H.: Immunoglobulin levels from the newborn period to adulthood and in immunoglobulin deficiency states. *J Clin Invest, 41*:2054, 1962.

W<small>HITEHOUSE</small>, H. L. K.: Crossover model of antibody variability. *Nature, 215*:371–374, 1967.

W<small>HITELAW</small>, D. M.: Pain in multiple myeloma. *Canad Med Ass J, 88*:1242–1243, 1963.

W<small>IENER</small>, A. S.: *Advances in Blood Grouping II*. New York and London, Grune, 1965.

W<small>IGZELL</small>, H.: Antibody synthesis at the cellular level. Antibody-induced suppression of 7S antibody synthesis. *J Exp Med, 124*:953–969, 1966.

W<small>IKLER</small>, M.; T<small>ITANI</small>, K.; S<small>HINODA</small>, T., and P<small>UTNAM</small>, F. W.: The complete amino acid sequence of a lambda type Bence Jones protein. *J Biol Chem, 242*:1668–1670, 1967.

W<small>ILKINSON</small>, P.; D<small>AVIDSON</small>, W., and S<small>OMMARIPA</small>, A.: Turnover of I[131]-labeled autologous macroglobulin in Waldenström's macroglobulinemia. Report of a case studied during treatment with phenylalanine mustard. *Ann Intern Med, 65*:308–316, 1966.

W<small>ILLIAMS</small>, C. A., J<small>R</small>., and G<small>RABAR</small>, P.: Immunoelectrophoretic studies on serum proteins. I. The antigens of human serum. *J Immun, 74*:158–168, 1955.

W<small>ILLIAMS</small>, R. C., J<small>R</small>.: Heterogeneity of L-chain sites on Bence Jones proteins reacting with antiglobulin factors. *Proc Nat Acad Sci USA, 52*:60–64, 1964.

W<small>ILLIAMS</small>, R. C.; B<small>RUNNING</small>, R. D., and W<small>OLLHEIM</small>, F. A.: Light chain disease, an abortive variant of multiple myeloma. *Ann Intern Med, 65*:471–486, 1966.

W<small>ILLIAMS</small>, R. C., J<small>R</small>.; E<small>RICKSON</small>, J. L.; P<small>OLESKY</small>, H. F., and S<small>WAIM</small>, W. R.: Studies of monoclonal immunoglobulins (M-components) in various kindreds. *Ann Int Med,* 67:309–327, 1967.

WILLIAMS, R. C., JR. and LAW, D. H., 4th.: Serum complement in amyloidosis. *J. Lab Clin Med,* 56:629–633, 1960.

WILLIAMS, R. C., JR.; PINNELL, S. R., and BRATT, G. T.: Low molecular weight L-chain components related to Bence Jones proteins. *J Lab Clin Med,* 68:81–89, 1966.

WILSON, I. D.; WILLIAMS, R. C., and TOBIAN, L. JR.: Renal tubular acidosis. Three cases with immunoglobulin abnormalities in the patients and their kindreds. *Amer J Med,* 43:356–370, 1967.

WINDRUM, G. M., and KRAMER, H.: Some observations on the histochemical reactions of amyloid. *Arch Path,* 63:373–378, 1957.

WIRTSCHAFTER, S. K., and RAPAPORT, S. I.: The familial occurrence of chronic lymphocytic leukemia and multiple myeloma. *Calif Med,* 92:165–166, 1960.

WISKOTT, A.: Familiärer angeborener Morbus Werlhoffi. *Mschr Kinderheilk,* 68:212–216, 1937.

WOLLHEIM, F. A., and WILLIAMS, R. C., JR.: Studies on the macroglobulins of human serum. I. Polyclonal immunoglobulin class M (IgM) increase in infectious mononucleosis. *New Eng J Med,* 274:61–67, 1966.

WOODRUFF, M. F. A.: *The Transplantation of Tissues and Organs.* Springfield (Ill.), Thomas, 1960.

World Health Organization. Deaths from multiple myeloma (plasmocytoma) in selected countries. *Epidem Vital Statist Rep,* 8:21–54, 1955.

WOSTMANN, B. S., and OLSON, G. B.: Precipitating antibody production in germfree chickens. *J Immun,* 92:41–48, 1964.

WRIGHT, C. J. E.: Long survival in solitary plasmocytoma of bone. *J Bone Joint Surg,* 43B:767–771, 1961.

WUHRMANN, F., WUNDERLY, C.: *Die Bluteiweisskörper des Menschen.* Basel, Benno Schwabe Co., 1957.

WUKETICH, ST., and MAEHR, G.: Generalisiertes plasmozytom mit ungewöhnlich mächtiger Infiltration des Magens. *Wien Klin Wschr,* 75:232–236, 1963.

WYSOCKI, K., and MACKIEWICZ, S.: Familial anomalous $\beta_{2A}$-globulin accompanied by disorders of blood coagulation and pathologic immune phenomena. *Arch Intern Med,* 116:351–356, 1965.

YAGI, Y.; MAIER, P.; PRESSMAN, D.; ARBESMAN, C. E.; REISMAN, R. E., and LENZNER, A. R.: Multiplicity of insulin binding antibodies in human sera. Presence of antibody activity of $\gamma$, $\beta_{2A}$ and $\beta_{2M}$ globulins. *J Immun,* 90:760, 1963a.

YAGI, Y. P.; MAIER, P.; PRESSMAN, D.; ARBESMAN, C. E., and REISMAN, R. E.: The presence of the ragweek-binding antibodies in the $\beta_{2A}$, $\beta_{2M}$ and gamma globulins of the sensitive individuals. *J Immun,* 91:83, 1963b.

YENTIS, I.: Radiological aspects of myelomatosis. *Clin Radiol,* 12:1–7, 1961.

ZAWADZKI, Z. A., and EDWARDS, G. A.: Dysimmunoglobulinemia in the absence of clinical features of multiple myeloma and macroglobulinemia. *Amer J Med,* 42:67–88, 1967.

ZINNEMAN, H. H.; GLENCHUR, H., and GLEASON, D. F.: The significance of urine electrophoresis in patients with multiple myeloma. *Arch Intern Med,* 106:172–178, 1960.

ZINNEMAN, H., and HALL, W.: Recurrent pneumonia in multiple myeloma and some observations on immunologic response. *Ann Intern Med,* 41:1152, 1954.

ZUCKER-FRANKLIN, D.: Structural features of cells associated with the paraproteinemias. *Seminars Hemat,* 1:165–198, 1964.

# INDEX

## A

Acid phosphatase, serum
  in multiple myeloma, 180
  in paraamyloidosis, 215
Adjuvants to antibody stimulation, 55
Adrenal insufficiency, in paraamyloidosis, 214
Adult Fanconi syndrome
  in multiple myeloma, 138, 148, 156, 179–181
  plasma cells in, 144
Agammaglobulinemia
  See also Hypoimmunoglobulinemia
  congenital, sex-linked, 66, 72–75
  Swiss-type, with lymphopenia, 68–72
Agglutinin reaction, 42
Albumin in infection, 114
Albuminuria in paraamyloidosis, 213, 215
Aldrich syndrome, See Familial hyper-IgA-globulinemia
Aleutian disease of mink, 131
Alkaline phosphatase, serum, in multiple myeloma, 180
Alkeran ®
  in treatment of multiple myeloma, 190–191
α-chain disease, See H-chain disease
Aluminum salts, stimulation of immune response by, 55
Ambiguous reading of code, 57
Amino acid-activating enzymes, 57
Amyloid, 62
  See also Amyloidosis, Paraamyloid, and Paraamyloidosis
  in conjunctival plasmomas, 146
  definition of, 205–206
  electron microscopy of, 206
  formation of, 206–207
  in multiple myeloma, See Paraamyloid
  in myeloma kidney, 138, 148
  in plasma cells, 207
  in polymorphonuclear leukocytes, 215

Amyloid (Continued)
  properties of, 205–206
  relation to collagen, 206
  relation to immunoglobulins, 206
Amyloidosis
  See also Amyloid, Paraamyloid, and Paraamyloidosis
  in Evans-Duane syndrome, 120
  mesenchymatous, See also Paraamyloidosis
  in mouse, 131
  in multiple myeloma, See Paraamyloidosis
  parenchymatous, 207, 215
  with secondary hypoimmunoglobulinemia, 91
  with secondary hypoimmunoglobulinemias associated with hypoalbuminemia, 90
  in selective hypo-IgA and M-globulinemia with slight decrease in IgG, 89
Anamnestic response, 60
Anaphylactic reaction, 43
Androgens in treatment of multiple myeloma, 187, 190
Anemia
  aplastic, in congenital sex-linked agammaglobulinemia, 75
  in H-chain disease, 199
  in macroglobulinemia (Waldenström's), 194
  in multiple myeloma, 168
  in paraimmunoglobulinopathies, pathogenesis of, 132, 138
Antibiotics in treatment of hypoimmunoglobulinopathies, 107
Antibody (ies)
  See also Immunoglobulins
  distribution of, 61
  eluted from red cells, 41
  Gm and Inv factors in, 41
  heterogeneity of, 41
  in IgG, IgM, and IgA, 41

253

Antibody (ies) *(Continued)*
 in multiple myeloma, 136–137
 in paraimmunoglobulinopathies, 136–137
 passive transfer of, 42
 phytohemagglutinin effect on, 54–55
 production of, 46–62
  effect of antigen on, 59
  theories of, 55–60
 relative homogeneity of, 40, 142
 release of, 61
 single species of, 40
 stimulating factors of, 54–55
 suppression of, 54–55
 tertiary structure of, 55
Antigen, definition of, 54
Antigen-antibody reactions, 42
 harmful effects of, 43
Antigen-combining site, 18–19
Antinuclear antibodies in rheumatoid arthritis, 117
Antiosteoporotic regimen in multiple myeloma, 186
Anuria, acute, in multiple myeloma, 157–158
 treatment of, 186
Arthritis, association with hypoimmunoglobulinemia, 103–104
Arthus reaction, 43
Ataxia-telangiectasia, 75–78
 cellular changes in, 75–77
 definition of, 75
 IgA deficiency in, 78
 immunoglobulins in, 76, 78
 intestinal lesions in, 101
 malignancies of reticuloendothelial system in, 106
 mode of inheritance of, 75–76
 organ involvement in, 75–77
 pathogenesis of, 96–97
Atherosclerosis, associated with multiple myeloma, 167
Autoimmune diseases
 complement in, 118–119
 hyperimmunoglobulinemia in, 115–120
 pathogenesis of, 115
 secondary hypoimmunoglobulinemias associated with, 92
Autoimmune hemolytic anemia
 hyperimmunoglobulinemia in, 120
 in macroglobulinemia (Waldenström's), 141

**B**

Bence Jones proteinemia
 in lupus erythematosus, 120
 in multiple myeloma, 173, 175
Bence Jones protein (s)
 amino acid composition of, 22, 30–37

Bence Jones protein (s) *(Continued)*
 amino acid sequence of, 30–37
 comparison of human and mouse, 37–38
 definition of, 28, 179
 disulfide linkages of, 31, 34, 36
 electrophoresis of, 173–176, 178
 electrophoresis-chromatography of tryptic digests of, 30
 Gm and Inv types of, 39–40
 in H-chain disease, 199
 heterogeneity of, 28–29, 31
 in macroglobulinemia (Waldenström's), 192, 194
 of mouse, 36–37, 131
 in multiple myeloma, 137, 156, 173–174, 176, 178–179
 properties of, 28
 in renal lesions, 137–138
 specific antigen-binding site of, 18–19
 structure of, 30–39
 synthesis, 132–133
  in tumor cells, 50–51
 switch peptide of, 31, 34
 tertiary and quaternary structure, 36
 in tumor cells, 50–51, 132, 133
 type K and type L, 28
Bence Jones proteinuria
 determination of, 179
 in Evans-Duane syndrome, 120
 in H-chain disease, 199
 in macroglobulinemia (Waldenström's), 192, 194
 in mink, 131
 in multiple myeloma, 137, 156, 173–174, 176, 178–179
 in paraamyloidosis, 213, 215
 therapy of, 185
Benign hyperglobulinemic purpura (Waldenström's), *See* Hyperglobulinemic purpura, benign (Waldenström)
Benign monoclonal gammopathy, 203
"Benign plasmacytosis pudendi," 153
Benign primary erythroplasia of Queyrat, 153
Bing-Neel syndrome, 193–194
Bleeding manifestations
 in paraamyloidosis, 209
 in paraimmunoglobulinopathies, pathogenesis of, 135–136
Blood examination
 in H-chain disease, 199
 in macroglobulinemia (Waldenström's), 194
 in multiple myeloma, 168–170
 in paraamyloidosis, 214
Blood transfusion in treatment of multiple myeloma, 187

Boeck's sarcoid
  myeloma cells in, 145
  serum immunoglobulin concentration in, 112
Bone formation, new, in multiple myeloma, 165
Bone marrow
  immunocytes in, 52
  in macroglobulinemia (Waldenström's), 194
  in multiple myeloma, 144, 170–171
  role in diagnosis, 107
  transplantation of, 110
Bone marrow biopsy
  in multiple myeloma, 170
  in paraamyloidosis, 215, 217
Bone pain
  in macroglobulinemia (Waldenström's), 149
  in multiple myeloma, 132, 148–149
  pathogenesis of, 132
Bone tenderness, pathogenesis of, 132
Bronchiectasis
  cryoglobulins in, 134
  immunoglobulins in, 114
  with secondary hypoimmunoglobulinemia, 92–93
Brucellosis, immunoglobulins in, 115
Burkitt's lymphoma, lymphocytes in, 47
Bursa of Fabricius, 53, 100
  embryology of, 96
Bursa-, appendix-, tonsil-dependent lymphoid tissue, 95–96

**C**

Calcium
  in myeloma kidney, 138, 148, 157
  role in bleeding manifestations of paraimmunoglobulinopathies, 135
Calcium, serum, in multiple myeloma, 180
Calf, paraimmunoglobulinopathies in, 131
Carcinoma
  associated with multiple myeloma, 167
  in selective hypo- IgA and M-globulinemia with slight decrease in IgG, 89
  with secondary hypoimmunoglobulinemia associated with hypoalbuminemia, 90, 101
Cardiac involvement
  in multiple myeloma, 158–159
  in paraamyloidosis, 209–211, 217
Cellular theory of amyloid formation, 207
Central lymphoid tissue, 95–96, 102
Charmot's syndrome, 124
Chemicals as etiologic agent of paraimmuno-globulinopathies, 128
Chicken, antibodies in, 53

Chlorambucil
  suppression of immune response by, 55
  in treatment of macroglobulinemia (Waldenström's), 197–198
  in treatment of paraamyloidosis, 217
Cholesterol
  in multiple myeloma, 167
  in paraamyloidosis, 213, 215
Chromosomes
  in macroglobulinemia (Waldenström's), 128–129
  in multiple myeloma, 128–129
Chronic infections with secondary hypoim-munoglobulinemia, 92–93
Cirrhosis
  cryoglobulins in, 119, 134
  rate of immunoglobulin synthesis in, 112
Cirrhosis, Laennec's
  immunoglobulins in, 124, 125
  serum immunoglobulin concentration in, 112
Coccidiomycosis, immunoglobulins in, 115
Cold agglutinin disease
  cold agglutinins in, 41
  cryoglobulins in, 134
  hyperimmunoglobulinemia in, 120
  paraimmunoglobulinemia in, 201
  relation to macroglobulinemia (Walden-ström's), 195–196
Cold agglutinins
  and cryoglobulins, 135
  homogeneity of, 41
  in infectious mononucleosis, 121
Cold hypersensitivity, paraimmunoglobulin-emia in, 201
Collagen disorders
  association with hypoimmunoglobulinemia, 103–104
  rate of immunoglobulin synthesis in, 112
Collagen, relation to amyloid, 206
Complement, 42
  in autoimmune disorders, 118–119
  in multiple myeloma, 137
  in paraamyloidosis, 206, 215
  role in diagnosis, 107
Complement fixation, 13, 19–20
Complex cryoglobulinemia, 134; *See also* "Rheumatoid factor"-hyperglobulinemia, 118–119
Complex macroglobulinemia, 134; *See also* "Rheumatoid factor"-hyperglobulinemia, 118–119
Complexes of immunoglobulins, 118–119
Compression fracture in multiple myeloma, 164–165

Congenital alymphoplasmocytic agammaglobulinemia with thymic dysplasia, *See* Swiss-type agammaglobulinemia with lymphopenia

Congenital sex-linked agammaglobulinemia, 72–75
  arthritis in, 103–104
  cellular changes in, 74
  immunoglobulins in, 73
  infections in, 72–73, 100
  intestinal lesions in, 101
  mode of inheritance, 72
  organ involvement in, 74
  pathogenesis of, 73, 96–99
  *Pneumocystis carinii* pneumonia in, 73
  resistance to viral infections, 73
  treatment of, 75

Congenital thymic alymphoplasia, *See* Reticular dysgenesis

Congo red stain for amyloid, 205, 216

Congo red test for paraamyloidosis, 216

Conjunctival plasmoma, 146, 153

Constrictive pericarditis, *See* Pericarditis, constrictive

"Copy-splice" mechanism, 57

Corticosteroids
  suppression of immune response by, 55
  in treatment of hypoimmunoglobulinopathies, 110
  in treatment of multiple myeloma, 186–187, 191
  in treatment of paraamyloidosis, 217

C-reactive protein in infection, 114

Cryofibrinogens and cryoglobulins, 135

Cryoglobulin (s)
  *See also* Cryoglobulinemia
  in bronchiectasis, 134
  in cirrhosis, 119, 134
  and cold agglutinins, 135
  in cold agglutinin disease, 134
  in complex or mixed cryoglobulinemia, 118
  and cryofibrinogens, 135
  definition of, 118, 133–134
  determination of, 134, 178
  in hyperviscosity syndromes, 135
  in kala-azar, 115, 134
  in leukemia, chronic lymphatic, 118
  in liver disease, 118
  in lupus erythematosus, 134
  in lymphosarcoma, 118
  in macroglobulinemia (Waldenström's), 118, 194–195
  in multiple myeloma, 118, 159, 178
  in polyarteritis nodosa, 134
  in rheumatic fever, 134
  in rheumatoid arthritis, 117, 118, 134

Cryoglobulin (s)  *(Continued)*
  rheumatoid factor activity with, 118–119
  in sarcoidosis, 119
  in Sjögren's syndrome, 118, 134
  in subacute bacterial endocarditis, 134
  in syphilis, 134
  in thyroiditis, 118
  in urine, 29

Cryoglobulinemia, 133–135
  *See also* Cryoglobulin (s)
  definition of, 133–134
  essential, *See* Idiopathic cryoglobulinemia, family studies in, 128
  idiopathic, *See* Idiopathic cryoglobulinemia
  in malignancy, 201
  pathology of, 134–135
  Raynaud's phenomenon in, 134
  in sarcoidosis, 122

Cryoprotein in urine, 179

Crystal violet stain for amyloid, 205

Cyclophosphamide
  suppression of immune response by, 55
  in treatment of multiple myeloma, 189–190

Cytoxan ®
  in treatment of macroglobulinemia (Waldenström's), 198
  in treatment of multiple myeloma, 189–190

**D**

Delayed hypersensitivity reaction (s)
  antibodies in, 61
  antibody levels in, 43
  in congenital sex-linked agammaglobulinemia, 73
  in familial hyper-IgA-globulinemia, 113
  in multiple myeloma, 137
  role in diagnosis, 106–107
  in selective hypo-IgA and M-globulinemia with slight decrease in IgG, 88

Dermatomyositis
  associated with hypoimmunoglobulinemia, 103
  hyperglobulinemia in, 112
  hyperimmunoglobulinemia in, 120

Digitalis
  refractoriness in paraamyloidosis, 210–211
  sensitivity in paraamyloidosis, 209, 211

Dinitrofluorobenzene (DNFB)
  reactivity to
    in ataxia-telangiectasia, 78
    in congenital sex-linked agammaglobulinemia, 73
    in Swiss-type agammaglobulinemia with lymphopenia, 69
  role in diagnosis, 107

Direct template theories, 55
Discoid lupus, hyperglobulinemia in, 112
Disseminated myelomatosis, 154; *See also* Multiple myeloma
DNA, random errors in, 57
Dog, paraimmunoglobulinopathies of, 131
Dysgammaglobulinemia syndrome, 202
Dysgammaglobulinemia, type 1, *See* Selective hypo-IgA- and IgG-globulinemia with increased IgM
Dysproteinemia, *See* Paraimmunoglobulinopathy and Paraimmunoglobulinemia (s)

E

Electrocardiogram in paraamyloidosis, 210, 217
Electron microscopy of immunoglobulins, 20
Electrophoresis
    Fc fragment of immunoglobulins, 18
    heavy chains, 17–18
    immunoglobulins, 11–18
    light chains, 17–19
    role in diagnosis, 107
    of serum proteins
        in macroglobulinemia (Waldenström's), 172, 195
        in multiple myeloma, 171–177
    of urinary proteins in multiple myeloma, 173–176, 178
Embryology
    of immunoglobulin-producing system, 95–96
    of thymus, 95–96
Endoplasmic reticulum, 47–53, 192
Endotoxin, stimulation of immune response by, 55
Enteritis, acute with secondary hypoimmunoglobulinemia associated with hypoalbuminemia, 90, 101
Enzymes, mechanism for specificity of, 60
Eosinophil (s), role in antibody formation, 47
Eosinophilia
    in H-chain disease, 198
    in multiple myeloma, 169
Erythema nodosum, hyperimmunoglobulinemia in, 120
Erythrocyte sedimentation rate in multiple myeloma, 170
Essential cryoglobulinemia, *See* Idiopathic cryoglobulinemia
Evans blue-radioiodinated albumin test in paraamyloidosis, 216
Evans-Duane syndrome, hyperimmunoglobulinemia in, 120
External secretions, IgA in, 42
Extramedullary lesions in multiple myeloma, pathogenesis of, 132

Extramedullary myeloma, *See* Extramedullary plasmacytoma
Extramedullary plasmacytoma, 146, 152–153

F

Factor V, role in bleeding manifestations, paraimmunoglobulinopathies, 135, 194
Factor VII, role in bleeding manifestations, paraimmunoglobulinopathies, 135, 194
Factor X, in paraamyloidosis, 214
Familial hyperglobulinemia, 112–113
Familial hyper-IgA-globulinemia, 113–114
    definition of, 113
    eczema in, 113
    infection in, 101, 113
    isohemagglutinins in, 113
    mode of inheritance, 113
    pathogenesis of, 114
    treatment of, 113
"Familial idiopathic dysproteinemia" of Homburger and Petermann, 89–90
Family studies
    in cryoglobulinemia, 128
    in leukemia, chronic lymphocytic, 128
    in macroglobulinemia (Waldenström's), 128
    in multiple myeloma, 128
    in paraimmunoglobulinemias, asymptomatic, 204
Fanconi syndrome, *See* Adult Fanconi syndrome
Fever, influence on immunoglobulin catabolism, 63
Fibrinogen
    in infection, 114
    role in bleeding manifestations, paraimmunoglobulinopathies, 135, 194
Fibrinolysis
    in multiple myeloma, 136
    in paraamyloidosis, 214, 215
Flame cells in multiple myeloma, 144–145
Fluoride, sodium, *See* Sodium fluoride
Forssman antibody (ies)
    in selective hypo-IgA and G-globulinemia with increased IgM, 184–185
    in serum sickness, 121
Fractional catabolic rate, immunoglobulins, 61, 63, 112
Fracture in multiple myeloma, *See* Compression fracture, Pathologic fracture, and Pseudofracture
Fracture, pathologic, *See* Pathologic fracture
Fragment of immunoglobulins
    Fab fragment
        activity of, 18–19
        definition of, 15–16
F (ab′) $_2$ fragment, definition of, 16–17

Fragment of immunoglobulins (*Continued*)
Fc fragment
  activity of, 19–20
  definition of, 15–16
  electrophoresis-chromatography of pep-
    tides of, 36, 38
  electrophoretic heterogeneity of, 18
  reaction with rheumatoid factor, 117
  in urine, 29
Fd fragment, definition of, 15–16

**G**

γ-chain disease, *See* H-chain disease
Gamma globulin (s)
  *See also* Immunoglobulin (s)
  adverse reactions to, 108–109
  in treatment of
    hypoimmunoglobulinopathies, 107–110
    H-chain disease, 200
    multiple myeloma, 186
Gastric polyps, with secondary hypoimmunoglobulinemia associated with hypoalbuminemia, 90, 101
Gastrointestinal tract
  *See also* Intestinal
  immunoglobulin loss through, 62
  involvement in
    multiple myeloma, 158
    paraamyloidosis, 211, 212
Gaucher's disease
  associated with multiple myeloma, 167
  paraimmunoglobulinemia in, 201
Generalized adult hypoimmunoglobulinemia,
  79–80
  definition of, 79
  immunoglobulins in, 79–80
  intestinal lesions in, 101
Generation time of myeloma cells, 131–132
Germ-free animals, hypoimmunoglobulinemia
  of, 94
Germinal centers
  antibody production in, 54
  spleen and lymph nodes, 54
Giant myeloma cells, 144, 170
Giedion-Scheidegger syndrome, *See* Selective
  hypo-IgA and M-globulinemia with
  normal IgG
Glomerulonephritis in multiple myeloma, 157
Gm factors
  activity of, 22
  antibodies to, 109
  of antibodies, 41
  classification of, 21–22
  genetics of, 23, 26, 27
  incidence in various populations, 22, 23, 25–
    27, 40

Gm factors (*Continued*)
  localization of, 21–22
  method of identification of, 20–21
  of myeloma protein, serum, 39–40
Golgi apparatus, 61
  electron micrograph of, 49–50
Gout, association with multiple myeloma, 166
"Grape" cells, 144
Gum biopsy in paraamyloidosis, 181, 216

**H**

Half-life, biological, immunoglobulins, 61–62
  in ataxia-telangiectasia, 78
Hamster, paraimmunoglobulinopathies of, 131
Haptoglobin in infections, 114
Hashimoto's thyroiditis, hyperimmunoglobulinemia in, 120
H-chain disease, 198–200
  clinical manifestations of, 199
  complications of, 200
  definition of, 198
  differential diagnosis of, 199
  immunoglobulins in, 133
  laboratory findings in, 199
  mode of death, 200
  pathology of, 198–199
  peptide maps of Fc fragments in, 36, 38
  prognosis of, 199–200
  relationship to Hodgkin's disease, 198
  relationship to other paraimmunoglobulin-
    opathies, 140, 200
  treatment of, 200
  with secondary hypoimmunoglobulinemia,
    91
  urinalysis in, 199
Heavy chains
  amino-acid sequences of, 38
  definition of, 14–15
  electrophoresis of, 17–18
  electrophoresis-chromatography of, 38
  heterogeneity of, 17–18
  of horse, 38
  of rabbit, 38
  subclasses of, 17
  synthesis of, 132
Hemolytic anemia, autoimmune
  eluted antibodies, 41
  in selective hypo-IgA and IgG-globulinemia
    with increased IgM, 85–87
Hemorrhagic manifestations, *See* Bleeding
  manifestations
Hepatitis, *See* Infectious or serum hepatitis
Hepatoma, hyperglobulinemic purpura in, 122
Hepatomegaly
  in multiple myeloma, 158
  in paraamyloidosis, 212

Hepatomegaly (*Continued*)
  in paraimmunoglobulinopathy, pathogenesis of, 132
Heredity, role in paraimmunoglobulinopathies, 128
Heterophile antibody (ies)
  in infectious mononucleosis, 121
  in selective hypo-IgA and G-globulinemia with increased IgM, 85
Histamine, 43
Histoplasmosis
  association with multiple myeloma, 167
  immunoglobulins in, 115
Hodgkin's disease
  in ataxia-telangiectasia, 76
  hyperimmunoglobulinemia in, 120–121
  lesions in multiple myeloma, 146, 181
  relationship to H-chain disease, 198, 200
  relationship to paraimmunoglobulinopathies, 139–140, 200
  with secondary hypoimmunoglobulinemia, 92
Homograft rejection
  antibodies in, 61
  in ataxia-telangiectasia, 77, 107
  in congenital sex-linked agammaglobulinemia, 73, 107
  in generalized adult hypoimmunoglobulinemia, 80, 107
  in multiple myeloma, 137
  in selective hypo-IgA and M-globulinemia with slight decrease in IgG, 88
  in Swiss-type agammaglobulinemia with lymphopenia, 69, 107
  role in diagnosis, 107
Horse, paraimmunoglobulinopathies in, 131
Humoral theory of amyloid formation, 207
Hypercalcemia in multiple myeloma, treatment of, 185–187
Hypercalcification in multiple myeloma, 165
Hyperimmunoglobulinemia (s)
  associated with autoimmune diseases, 115–120
  in autoimmune hemolytic anemia, 120
  in cold agglutinin disease, 120
  definition of, 7
  in dermatomyositis, 120
  in erythema nodosum, 120
  in Evans-Duane syndrome, 120
  familial, 112–113
  in Hashimoto's thyroiditis, 120
  in Hodgkin's disease, 120–121
  in infectious mononucleosis, 121–122
  in liver disease, 124–125
  in lupoid hepatitis, 120
  in lupus erythematosus, 119–120

Hyperimmunoglobulinemia (s) (*Continued*)
  associated with malignancies, 120–121
  in periarteritis nodosa, 120
  in reticulum cell sarcoma, 120–121
  in rheumatic fever, 120
  in rheumatoid arthritis, 115–117
  in sarcoidosis, 122
  in scleroderma, 120
  secondary, 114–125
  secondary to infection, 114–115
  in Sjögren's syndrome, 120
Hyperglobulinemic purpura, 122
  differential diagnosis of, 122–123
  in hepatoma, 122
  in lupus erythematosus, 122
  in Mikulicz's syndrome, 122
  in multiple myeloma, 122
  in reticulum cell sarcoma, 122
  in rheumatoid arthritis, 122
  in sarcoidosis, 122
  in Sjögren's syndrome, 122
  in thymoma, 122
  in tuberculosis, 122
Hyperglobulinemic purpura, benign (Waldenström's), 122–124
  infection in, 44
  treatment of, 124
Hyper-IgA-globulinemia, *See* Familial hyper-IgA-globulinemia
Hyperimmunoglobulinopathy (ies), 111–125
  classification of, 111
  definition of, 7
Hyperviscosity syndrome, 118, 135
  in multiple myeloma, 160, 180
Hypoalbuminemia, secondary, hypoimmunoglobulinemias associated with, 90–91
Hypoimmunoglobulinemia (s)
  adult, generalized, 79–80
  adult, selective, 80–89
  associated with arthritis, 103–104
  associated with autoimmune disease, *See* Secondary hypoimmunoglobulinemias
  classification of, 67
  associated with chronic infections, *See* Secondary hypoimmunoglobulinemias
  associated with collagen disorders, 103–104
  definition of, 7
  associated with hypoalbuminemia, *See* Secondary hypoimmunoglobulinemia
  of late onset, 78–90
    definition of, 78
    immunoglobulins in, 78–79
    infections in, 100
    intestinal lesions in, 101
    pathogenesis of, 96–97, 99
  associated with malignancies of the reticulo-

Hypoimmunoglobulinemia (s) *(Continued)*
  endothelial system, *See* Secondary hypo-
    immunoglobulinemias
  in paraimmunoglobulinopathies, 136–137
  associated with pernicious anemia, *See* Sec-
    ondary hypoimmunoglobulinemias
  physiologic, 93–94
  secondary, *See* Secondary hypoimmunoglob-
    ulinemia
  susceptibility to infection in, 44
  treatment of, 107–110
Hypoimmunoglobulinopathy (ies) , 66–94
  cellular abnormalities in, 98
  classification of, 66–67
  definition of, 7, 66
  diagnosis of, 106–107
  etiology of, 95–100
  intestinal lesions in, 101–103
  malignancies of reticuloendothelial system
    in, 91–92, 106
  pathogenesis of, 95–98
  protein abnormalities of, 98–99
  symptoms in common, 100–106
  thymoma in, 104–106
  treatment of, 107–110

**I**

Idiopathic cryoglobulinemia, 204
  immunoglobulins in, 118
  plasma cells in, 144, 204
  reticulum cells in, 144, 204
  relation to multiple myeloma, 134
Idiopathic pyroglobulinemia, 204
Idiopathic thrombocytopenia purpura with
    secondary hypoimmunoglobulinemia, 92
IgA, *See* Immunoglobulins, IgA
IgD, *See* Immunoglobulins, IgD
IgE, *See* Immunoglobulins, IgE
IgG, *See* Immunoglobulins, IgG
IgM, *See* Immunoglobulins, IgM
Immune response
  stimulation of, 54–55
  suppression of, 54–55
Immunity
  cellular type, 43
  role in etiology of paraimmunoglobulin-
    opathies, 129
Immunocyte (s)
  definition of, 5
  in paraimmunoglobulinopathies, 139
Immunoelectrophoresis
  role in diagnosis, 107
  of serum
    in macroglobulinemia (Waldenström's) ,
      195
    in multiple myeloma, 176–177

Immunoglobulin (s)
  activity of, 41–45
  carbohydrate fraction, 20
  catabolism of, 63
  classes of, 11–14
  complexes of, 118–119
  definition of, 5
  denatured, 62
  destruction of, 62
  distribution of, 61
  electron microscopy of, 20
  electrophoretic distribution of, 12
  families of, 11–14
  fragments of, 16–17
  genetic origins of, 38–39
  history of, 3–4
  hypotheses for heterogeneity of, 56–60
  IgA
    absence in jejunal mucosa of patients with
      IgA deficiency, 83
    activities of, 42
    alterations in relatives of patients with
      generalized adult hypoimmunoglobu-
      linemia, 80
    possible relation to reagins, 43
    presence in plasma cells, 83
    properties of, 12–14
    synthesis in gastrointestinal tract, 46
  IgD, properties of, 13–14
  IgE
    possible relation to reagins, 14
    properties of, 13–14
  IgG
    pass placental barrier, 93
    possible relation to reagins, 43
    production late in antibody formation, 46
    properties of, 12–13
    turnover, 48
  IgM
    production early in antibody formation, 46
    properties of, 13–14
  immunologic types K and L, 14
  in germ-free animals, 44
  in infection, 114–115
  in infectious hepatitis, 125
  in infectious mononucleosus, 121–122
  intracellular synthesis of, 47–52
  intravascular distribution of, 61
  in Laennec's cirrhosis, 124–125
  in liver disease, 124–125
  metabolism of, 61–63, 136
    in paraimmunoglobulinopathies, 136
  nomenclature, 6
  nonantibody, 45
  papain digestion of, 16
  pepsin digestion of, 16–17

Immunoglobulin (s)  *(Continued)*
    production of, 46–62
    reductive alkylation of, 14–15
    relation to amyloid, 206
    in serum hepatitis, 125
    serum levels
        determinants of, 63
        normal, 13, 61, 63–65
    site of destruction of, 62
    structure of, 11–41
    synthesis of, 46–55, 112, 132–133
        in macroglobulinemia (Waldenström's),
            132–133
        in multiple myeloma, 132–133
    terminology, *See* Nomenclature
    types K and L, 14–15
Immunoglobulin system, definition of, 5
Immunoglobulinopathy (ies)
    classification of, 8
    definition of, 7
Immunologic paralysis, 54
Immunologic tolerance, 54, 60
Immunology, history of, 3–5
Imuran, suppression of immune response by,
    55
Indirect template theories, 55
Infants, transient physiologic hypogammaglob-
    ulinemia of, 93–94
Infection
    chronic, 44
        myeloma cells in, 145
        paraimmunoglobulinemia in, 201
    in H-chain disease, 199–200
    hyperimmunoglobulinemia in, 114–115
    in macroglobulinemia (Waldenström's),
        194, 196
    in multiple myeloma, 154, 157, 183
        treatment of, 186
    rate of immunoglobulin synthesis in, 112
    role in etiology of paraimmunoglobulin-
        opathies, 129
    susceptibility to, 44; *see also* under specific
        disease
    in hypoimmunoglobulinopathies, 100–101
Infectious hepatitis
    gamma globulin in attenuation of, 108
    immunoglobulins in, 114–115, 125
    serum immunoglobulin concentration in,
        112
Infectious mononucleosis, 121–122
    hyperimmunoglobulinemia in, 121–122
Instructive theories, 55, 59–60
Interferon in familial hyper-IgA-globulinemia,
    113
Intestinal, *See also* Gastrointestinal

Intestinal lesions in hypoimmunoglobulin-
    opathies, 101–103
    pathogenesis of, 101–103
Intestine, small, biopsy of in paraamyloidosis,
    216
Intrachromatid inversion, 56
Intravascular distribution, immunoglobulins,
    61
Intravenous pyelography (IVP) in multiple
    myeloma, 179–180
Inv factors
    activity of, 22
    amino acid substitutions of, 22
    of antibodies, 41
    of Bence Jones proteins, 39–40
    classification of, 21–22
    genetics of, 23, 26, 27
    incidence in various populations, 23–24
    localization of, 21–22
    method of identification of, 20–21
Iron-containing inclusions in myeloma cells,
    144
Irradiation as etiologic agent of paraimmuno-
    globulinopathy, 127
Isohemagglutinins, serum
    in ataxia-telangiectasia, 76
    in congenital sex-linked agammaglobulin-
        emia, 73
    in familial hyper-IgA-globulinemia, 113
    in multiple myeloma, 137
    role in diagnosis, 106
    in selective hypo-IgA and G-globulinemia
        with increased IgM, 84–85, 87
    in selective hypo-IgA and M-globulinemia
        with normal IgG, 88
    in selective hypo-IgA and M-globulinemia
        with slight decrease in IgG, 89

### K

Kala-azar
    cryoglobulins in, 115, 134
    immunoglobulins in, 115
Kidney diseases, immunoglobulin loss in, 62
Kidney lesions, *See* Renal lesions
Kveim antigen in sarcoidosis, 122
Kwashiorkor with secondary hypoimmunoglob-
    ulinemia associated with hypoalbumin-
    emia, 91

### L

Laennec's cirrhosis, *See* Cirrhosis, Laennec's
Laminectomy in treatment of multiple mye-
    loma, 186
Latex fixation test, 116
L E cell preparation
    in lupus erythematosus, 119

L E cell preparation *(Continued)*
  in lupoid hepatitis, 125
  in rheumatoid arthritis, 117
Leishmaniasis, rheumatoid factor in, 117
Leprosy
  immunoglobulins in, 115
  rheumatoid factor in, 117
Leukemia, acute lymphoblastic
  in congenital sex-linked agammaglobulin-
    emia, 74
  with secondary hypoimmunoglobulinemia,
    91
Leukemia, chronic lymphocytic
  abnormal lymphocytes in, 91
  cryoglobulins in, 118
  family studies in, 128
  effect of phytohemagglutinin on lympho-
    cytes in, 54
  with secondary hypoimmunoglobulinemia,
    91
Leukemia, chronic myelocytic with secondary
  hypoimmunoglobulinemia, 91
Leukemia, lymphocytic, relationship to paraimmunoglobulinopathies, 140, 195, 200
Leukemia, monocytic, paraimmunoglobulinemia in, 200
Leukemia, myelogenous
  paraimmunoglobulinemia in, 200–201
  rate of immunoglobulin synthesis in, 112
Leukemia, plasma cell, 147, 169
Leukemoid reaction in multiple myeloma, 169
Leukoencephalopathy, progressive multifocal,
  in multiple myeloma, 155–156
Leukopenia in paraimmunoglobulinopathies,
  pathogenesis of, 132
Lichen amyloidosis, 209
Lichen myxedematosus
  in multiple myeloma, 160–161
  relation to paraamyloidosis, 209
Light chains
  *See also* Bence Jones proteins
  definition of, 14–15
  electrophoresis of, 17–19
  heterogeneity of, 17–18
  synthesis of, 132
  types K and L, 14–15
  in urine, 29
Lipid, in multiple myeloma, 167
Liver
  immunocytes in, 52
  immunoglobulin destruction in, 62
Liver biopsy in paraamyloidosis, 216
Liver disease
  cryoglobulins in, 118
  hyperimmunoglobulinemia in, 124–125
  immunoglobulins in, 124–125

Liver disease *(Continued)*
  infections in, 44
  myeloma cells in, 145
  paraimmunoglobulinemia in, 201
  rheumatoid factor in, 117
L-phenylalanine mustard in treatment of
  macroglobulinemia (Waldenström's), 198
  multiple myeloma, 190–191
  paraamyloidosis, 217
Lung, immunocytes in, 52
Lupoid hepatitis
  hyperimmunoglobulinemia in, 120
  immunoglobulins in, 125
  serum immunoglobulin concentration in,
    112
  treatment of, 125
Lupus erythematosus
  cryoglobulins in, 134
  hyperglobulinemia in, 112
  hyperglobulinemic purpura in, 122
  hyperimmunoglobulinemia in, 119–120
  immunoglobulins in, 119–120
  macroglobulins in, 195
  myeloma cells in, 145
  paraimmunoglobulinemia in, 201
  with secondary hypoimmunoglobulinemia,
    92, 103
  serum immunoglobulin concentration in,
    112
Lymph node (s)
  antibody production in, 54
  immunocytes in, 52
Lymph node biopsy
  in multiple myeloma, 181
  role in diagnosis, 107
Lymphadenopathy
  in multiple myeloma, 158
  paraamyloidosis in, 212
Lymphadenopathy in paraimmunoglobulinopathies, pathogenesis of, 132
Lymphangiectasia of small intestine with secondary hypoimmunoglobulinemia associated with hypoalbuminemia, 90, 101
Lymphocyte (s) , 46
  electron micrograph of, 50
  endoplasmic reticulum of, 47
  in H-chain disease, 199
  in macroglobulinemia (Waldenström's),
    192–194
  in multiple myeloma, 52, 145
  role in antibody formation, 47
Lymphogranuloma venereum, immunoglobulins in, 115
Lymphoid follicles, 47
  in secondary response, 54

Lymphoid plasma cells, 46
  electron micrograph of, 53
  endoplasmic reticulum of, 53
  in H-chain disease, 199
  in macroglobulinemia (Waldenström's)
    192, 194
Lymphomas with secondary hypoimmunoglob-
    ulinemia, 91
Lymphopenic hypogammaglobulinemia, *See*
    Swiss-type agammaglobulinemia with lym-
    phopenia
Lymphosarcoma
  in ataxia-telangiectasia, 76
  cryoglobulins in, 118
  in multiple myeloma, 181, 200
  relationship to paraimmunoglobulin-
    opathies, 140, 195, 200
  with secondary hypoimmunoglobulinemia,
    91
Lytic reaction, 42

**M**

Macroglobulinemia
  in Charmot's syndrome, 124
  in mouse, 131
  in sarcoidosis, 122
Macroglobulinemia (Waldenström's), 192–198
  autoimmune hemolytic anemia in, 141
  bone pain in, 149, 194
  chromosomes in, 128–129
  clinical manifestations of, 193–194
  cold agglutinins in, 44, 195
  complications of, 196
  cryoglobulins in, 118
  definition of, 192
  differential diagnosis of, 195–196
  electron micrograph of lymphoid plasma
    cell in, 53
  etiology of, 127–130
  family studies in, 128
  hyperviscosity syndrome in, 135
  immunoglobulin synthesis in, 132–133
  incidence of, 131
  infection in, 194–196
  laboratory findings in, 194–195
  mode of death in, 196
  neurologic involvement in, 193–194
  pathology of, 192–193
  peripheral blood in, 194
  plasma cells in, 52, 144
  prognosis of, 196
  proteins, serum, in, 195
  relationship to other paraimmunoglobulin-
    opathies, 140, 195, 200
  renal involvement in, 194, 196

Macroglobulinemia (Waldenström's) (*Contin-
    ued*)
  with secondary hypoimmunoglobulinemia, 91
  treatment of, 196–198
  urinalysis in, 194
Macroglossia in paraamyloidosis, 211–212
Macrophages, role in antibody formation, 47
Malaria, immunoglobulins in, 63, 115
Malignancies
  hyperimmunoglobulinemia in, 120–121
  myeloma cells in, 145
Malignancies, other, in multiple myeloma,
    167, 200–201
Malignancies of reticuloendothelial system,
    secondary hypoimmunoglobulinemias as-
    sociated with, 91–92, 106
Marschalko-type plasma cell in multiple mye-
    loma, 143
Mast cells, tissue, in macroglobulinemia,
    (Waldenström's), 194
Measles, gamma globulin therapy in, 107
Megaloblastic marrow
  in multiple myeloma, 139, 171
  in paraimmunoglobulinopathies, 139
Melphalan, in treatment of multiple myeloma,
    190–191
Membrane transmission, 20
Menetrier's disease, with secondary hypoim-
    munoglobulinemias associated with hypo-
    albuminemia, 90, 101
6-Mercaptopurine, suppression of immune re-
    sponse by, 55
Metabolic rate, influence on catabolism of im-
    munoglobulins, 63
Metabolism of immunoglobulins in paraim-
    munoglobulinopathies, 136
Methyl voilet stain for amyloid, 205
Microimmunoglobulin (s), definition of, 7
Microimmunoglobulinemia, definition of, 7
Microimmunoglobulinuria
  definition of, 7
  occurrence of, 29–30
Mikulicz's syndrome, hyperglobulinemic pur-
    pura in, 122
Milkman's fracture in multiple myeloma, *See*
    Pseudofracture
Mineral oil as etiologic agent of paraimmuno-
    globulinopathies, 128
Mink, paraimmunoglobulinopathies of, 131
Mixed cryoglobulinemia, *See* "Rheumatoid
    factor" hyperglobulinemia, 118–119
Monoclonal gammopathy, *See* Paraimmuno-
    globulinopathy
Morula cells, 144
Mott bodies in myeloma cells, 144, 170
Mott cells, 144, 170

Mouse
  Bence Jones proteins of, 36–37
  paraimmunoglobulinopathies in, 128–129,
    131, 202
mRNAs, single-stranded, 59
Multiple germ line genes, 57
Multiple myeloma, 143–191
  adult Fanconi syndrome in, 138, 148, 156
  antibodies in, 136–137
  associated with other diseases, 165–167
  asymptomatic patients, 168
  Bence Jones proteins in, 137, 156, 173–174,
    176, 178–179
  Bence Jones proteinuria in, 137, 156, 173–
    174, 176, 178–179
  biopsy in, 181
  blood chemistry in, 180–181
  blood coagulation in, 180
  bone marrow in, 144, 170–171
  bone pain in, 132, 148–149
  cardiac involvement in, 158–159
  chromosomes in, 128–129
  clinical manifestations of, 148–168
  complement in, 137
  complications of, 183
  cryoglobulins in, 118, 159
  definition of, 143
  delayed hypersensitivity reactions in, 137
  diagnosis of, 184–185
  differential diagnosis of, 184–185
  etiology of, 127–130
  family studies in, 128
  fibrinolysis in, 136
  gastrointestinal involvement in, 158
  hepatomegaly in, 158
  Hodgkin's disease, lesions in, 146, 181
  homograft rejection in, 137
  hyperglobulinemic purpura in, 122
  hyperviscosity syndrome in, 135, 160
  immunoglobulin synthesis in, 132–133
  incidence of, 130
  infection in, 154, 157, 183
  isohemagglutinins, serum, in, 137
  laboratory findings in, 168–181
  lymphadenopathy in, 158
  lymphocytes in, 52
  lymphosarcoma in, 181, 200
  management of, 185–191
  mechanism of protein synthesis in, 59
  megaloblastic marrow in, 139
  mode of death, 183
  myeloid metaplasia in, 138
  neurologic involvement in, 154–156, 183
  pathologic fracture in, 146, 149–150
  pathology of, 143–148
  peripheral blood in, 168–170

Multiple myeloma (*Continued*)
  plasma cells in, 61, 143–146
  prevention of complications of, 185
  prognosis of, 181–183
  pyroglobulinemia in, 135
  radiologic manifestations, 161–165
  relationship to other paraimmunoglobulin-
    opathies, 140, 200
  renal function, tests of, 179–180
  renal involvement in, 156–158, 181, 183
  respiratory tract involvement in, 154, 183
  reticulum cell sarcoma lesions in, 146, 181,
    200
  rheumatoid arthritis in, 141
  with secondary hypoimmunoglobulinemia,
    91
  serum proteins in, 171–178
  skin manifestations in, 160–161
  splenomegaly in, 158
  systemic manifestations of, 161
  thymoma in, 136
  treatment of, 185–191
  tumor formation in, 150–153
  urinalysis in, 178–179
Multiple plasmacytomas, 152
Muscle biopsy in paraamyloidosis, 216–217
Myasthenia gravis in generalized adult hypo-
    immunoglobulinemia, 79, 104, 106
Myelofibrosis associated with multiple mye-
    loma, 167
Myeloid metaplasia
  in multiple myeloma, 138, 168
  in paraimmunoglobulinopathies, 138
Myeloma, extramedullary, *See* Extramedullary
    plasmacytoma
Myeloma, solitary, *See* Solitary plasmacytoma
Myeloma cells
  characteristic for individual patient, 50
  electron micrograph of, 51–52
  morphology of, 143–146
  in multiple myeloma, 143–146
Myeloma kidney
  in macroglobulinemia (Waldenström's),
    196
  in multiple myeloma, 147–148, 156–158
  pathogenesis of, 137–138
Myeloma neuropathy or polyneuropathy, 155
Myeloma proteins, serum
  antibody activity of, 44
  electrophoresis of, 9, 171–178
  Gm and Inv types of, 39–40
  heterogeneity of, 9, 28, 175
  of mouse, 131
  possible qualitative abnormality, 40
  synthesis of, 132–133
    in tumor cells, 50, 132–133

**N**

Negroes, hyperimmunoglobulinemia in, 112
Neoplasms, other, associated with multiple
myeloma, 167, 200–201
Nephrotic syndrome
macroglobulins in, 195
in multiple myeloma, 157
in paraamyloidosis, 213
with secondary hypoimmunoglobulinemia
associated with hypoalbuminemia, 90
secondary to penicillamine therapy, 197
Nerve cells, information storage in, 60
Neuritis, peripheral
in multiple myeloma, 147
in paraimmunoglobulinopathies, 138
Neurologic involvement
in multiple myeloma, 154–156, 183
in paraamyloidosis, 212–213
Neutropenia, cyclic in congenital sex-linked
agammaglobulinemia, 75
Nitrogen mustard (s)
in treatment of H-chain disease, 200
in treatment of macroglobulinemia (Waldenström's) , 198
suppression of immune response by, 55
Nonmyelomatous paraproteinemia, 202
Nutritional hypogammaglobulinemia, 90–91

**O**

Opsonin reaction, 42
Orosomucoid in infection, 114
Osteomalacia in multiple myeloma, 165
Osteomyelitis
association with multiple myeloma, 166–167
paraimmunoglobulinemia in, 201
Osteoporosis
in macroglobulinemia (Waldenström's) , 194
in multiple myeloma, 146, 161–163
treatment of, 186
Ouchterlony plate method
in macroglobulinemia (Waldenström's) , 195
in multiple myeloma, 177–179

**P**

Paget's disease, association with multiple myeloma, 166
Papular mucinosis
in multiple myeloma, 160–161
paraimmunoglobulinemia in, 201
relation to paraamyloidosis, 209
Paraamyloid
See also Amyloid, Amyloidosis and Paraamyloidosis
definition of, 9
in macroglobulinemia (Waldenström's) ,
136, 196

Paraamyloid (*Continued*)
in multiple myeloma, 133, 136
Paraamyloidosis, 205–217
See also Amyloid, Amyloidosis, and Paraamyloid
Bence Jones proteinuria in, 213–215
blood coagulation in, 214
bone marrow in, 215
cardiac involvement in, 209–211, 216
clinical manifestations of, 208–214
complications of, 216
definition of, 9, 205
diagnosis of, 216–217
gastrointestinal tract involvement in, 211–
212, 216
hepatomegaly in, 212
laboratory findings in, 214–215
lymphadenopathy in, 212
in macroglobulinemia (Waldenström's) , 136,
193–194, 205
mode of death in, 216
in multiple myeloma, 136, 147, 157, 180, 205
neurologic involvement in, 212–213
pathogenesis of, 205–207
pathology of, 207–208
plasma cells in, 144
prognosis of, 215
relationship to paraimmunoglobulinopathies,
140, 205
renal involvement in, 213, 216
respiratory tract involvement in, 213, 216
rheumatoid arthritis associated with, 214
serum proteins in, 215
skin involvement in, 208–209
splenomegaly in, 212
treatment of, 217
urinalysis in, 215
Paraimmunoglobulinemia (s)
See also Paraimmunoglobulinopathy (ies)
definition of, 7
idiopathic, 202–204
asymptomatic, 202–204
symptomatic, 202–204
Paraimmunoglobulinopathy (ies)
See also Paraimmunoglobulinemia
in animals, 131
classification of, 8, 126–127
associated with cold agglutinin disease, 201
associated with cold hypersensitivity, 201
definition of, 7, 126–127
etiology of, 127–130
associated with
Gaucher's disease, 201
Hodgkin's disease, 200
hypoimmunoglobulinemia in, 136–137
incidence of, 130–131

Paraimmunoglobulinopathy (ies)    (*Continued*)
    associated with infection, chronic, 201
    interrelationships of, 139–142
    associated with leukemia, chronic lympho-
        cytic, 200
    associated with leukemia, monocytic, 200
    associated with leukemia, myelogenous, 200–
        201
    associated with liver disease, 201
    associated with lymphosarcoma, 200
    associated with lupus erythematosus, 201
    associated with malignancies, 200–201
    megaloblastic marrow in, 139
    myeloid metaplasia in, 138
    neuritis, peripheral, in, 138
    associated with osteomyelitis, 201
    associated with papular mucinosis, 201
    pathogenesis of, 132–139
    pathogenesis of renal lesions in, 137–138
    associated with reticulum cell sarcoma, 200
    associated with rheumatoid arthritis, 201
    associated with sarcoidosis, 201
    associated with thymoma, 201
    uric acid in, 138
Paraimmunoglobulinuria
    asymptomatic, 203
    definition of, 7
Paraplegia in multiple myeloma, pathogenesis
    of, 132
Passive cutaneous anaphylactic reaction, 43
Pathologic fracture
    in multiple myeloma, 146, 149–150, 164–165,
        183
    in paraamyloidosis, 214
    pathogenesis of, 132
Paul-Bunnell antibody in infectious mononu-
    cleosis, 121
Penicillamine in treatment of macroglobulin-
    emia (Waldenström's), 197
Pentamidine isothianate in treatment of Pneu-
    mocystis carinii pneumonia, 73, 107
Periappendiceal tissue, 53–54
Periarteritis nodosa, *See* Polyarteritis
Pericarditis, constrictive, in paraamyloidosis,
    210
Peripheral lymphoid tissue, 95–96
Peripheral neuritis, *See* Neuritis, peripheral
Pernicious anemia
    in selective hypo-IgA and M-globulinemia
        with slight decrease in IgG, 89
    with secondary hypoimmunoglobulinemia,
        92
Peyer's patches, 53, 95–96
Phagocytosis, 42, 62
Phaseolus vulgaris, 54

Phenylalanine mustard in treatment of
    macroglobulinemia (Waldenström's), 198
    multiple myeloma, 190–191
    paraamyloidosis, 217
Phosphorus, radioactive, in treatment of mul-
    tiple myeloma, 189
Physiologic hypoimmunoglobulinemia (s), 93–
    94
    of infants, transient, 93–94
Phytohemagglutinin
    definition of, 54
    effect *in vivo,* 54–55
    effect on lymphocytes, 54, 98
    effect on thymocytes, 52
Pig, paraimmunoglobulinopathies of, 131
Placental transmission, 13, 20
Plasma cell (s), 46
    amyloid in, 207
    antibody content of, 48
    antibody production of, 48
    electron micrograph of, 48–49, 51–52
    endoplasmic reticulum, 47–49, 51–52
    excretory mechanism of, 61
    fragmentation of, 61
    in H-chain disease, 199
    in idiopathic cryoglobulinemia, 144
    in macroglobulinemia (Waldenström's), 52,
        144, 192, 194
    in multiple myeloma, *See* Myeloma cell
    in paraamyloidosis, 144
    release of antibody from, 61
    role in antibody formation, 47
    in secondary adult Fanconi syndrome, 144
    volume in body, 48
Plasma cell hepatitis, *See* Lupoid hepatitis
Plasma cell leukemia, *See* Leukemia, plasma
    cell
Plasmacytoma, extramedullary, *See* Extramed-
    ullary plasmacytoma
Plasmacytoma, solitary, *See* Solitary plasmacy-
    toma
Plasmacytomas, multiple, *See* Multiple plas-
    macytomas
Plasmacytosis, reactive, marrow in, 145
Plasmapheresis
    in treatment of macroglobulinemia (Wal-
        denström's), 197
    in treatment of multiple myeloma, 187
Plasmoma, conjunctival, *See* Conjunctival plas-
    moma
Platelets, role in bleeding manifestations, para-
    immunoglobulinopathies, 136
Pneumocystis carinii pneumonia
    in congenital sex-linked agammaglobulin-
        emia, 73

Pneumocystis carinii pneumonia (*Continued*)
in generalized adult hypoimmunoglobulinemia, 79
in Swiss-type agammaglobulinemia with
lymphopenia, 69, 100
treatment of, 107
Polyarteritis nodosa
cryoglobulins in, 134
hyperimmunoglobulinemia in, 120
Polycythemia vera associated with multiple
myeloma, 167
Polymorphonuclear leukocytes, amyloid in, 215
Polyribosomes in antibody synthesis, 47
Precipitin reaction, 42
Pregnancy in multiple myeloma, 183
Premyeloma, 203
bone pain in, 149
Primary acquired hypogammaglobulinemia (s) ,
*See* Hypoimmunoglobulinemias of late
onset
Primary hyperimmunoglobulinemia (s) , 112–
114
Primary response
immunocytes in, 52–54
in lymphoid follicles, 54
relation to lymphoid follicles, 54
Primary adult hypogammaglobulinemia (s) ,
*See* Hypoimmunoglobulinemias of late
onset
Primary hypoimmunoglobulinemia (s) , 67–90
Properdin in hypo-IgA and M-immunoglobu-
linemia, 107
Protein (s) , serum
in macroglobulinemia (Waldenström's) , 195
in multiple myeloma, 171–178
Protein-losing enteropathy with secondary hypoimmunoglobulinemia associated with
hypoalbuminemia, 90
Prothrombin, role in bleeding manifestations,
paraimmunoglobulinopathies, 135, 194
Pseudofracture in multiple myeloma, 150, 157,
165
Pulmonary fibrosis, serum immunoglobulin
concentration in, 112
Punched-out lesions of bone
in macroglobulinemia (Waldenström's) , 194
in multiple myeloma, 161–165
Pyelonephritis in multiple myeloma, 157
Pyroglobulinemia, 135
idiopathic, *See* Idiopathic pyroglobulinemia
Pyrrolidone carboxylic acid as N-terminal residue, 34

**Q**

Queyrat, benign primary, erythroplasia of, 153

**R**

Race, effect on immunoglobulins, 112
Radiologic manifestations, multiple myeloma,
161–165
Radiotherapy
in H-chain disease, 200
in multiple myeloma, 188
Random errors in DNA, 57
Rat, paraimmunoglobulinopathies of, 131
Raynaud's phenomenon
in cryoglobulinemia, 134, 160, 194
treatment of, 197
Reactive plasmacytosis, marrow in, 145
Reagins, 43
role in diagnosis, 106
Rectal biopsy
in paraamyloidosis, 216–217
role in diagnosis, 107
Regional enteritis with secondary hypoimmunoglobulinemia associated with hypoalbuminemia, 90, 101
Renal biopsy
in multiple myeloma, 181
in paraamyloidosis, 181, 216–217
Renal involvement in paraamyloidosis, 213
Renal lesions
in multiple myeloma, 147–148
in paraimmunoglobulinopathies, pathogenesis of, 137–138
Renal manifestations of multiple myeloma,
156–158, 181, 183
Renal tubular acidosis in multiple myeloma,
157
Respiratory tract involvement
in multiple myeloma, 154, 183
in paraamyloidosis, 213
Reticular dysgenesis, 67–68
infections in, 67–68, 100
mode of inheritance, 68
organ involvement in, 68
pathogenesis, 68, 96–97
white blood cells in, 67
Reticuloendothelial system
activity of, 55, 62
formation of amyloid in, 206–207
Reticulum cell (s) , 46
in idiopathic cryoglobulinemia, 144
in multiple myeloma, 145
Reticulum cell sarcoma
in ataxia-telangiectasia, 76
in familial hyper-IgA-globulinemia, 113
hyperglobulinemic purpura in, 122
hyperimmunoglobulinemia in, 120–121
lesions in multiple myeloma, 146, 181, 200
in mouse, 131

*Index*

Reticulum cell sarcoma *(Continued)*
  relationship to paraimmunoglobulinopa-
    thies, 139–140, 200
Rheumatic fever
  cryoglobulins in, 134
  plasma cells in, 144
  with secondary hypoimmunoglobulinemia,
    92
Rheumatoid arthritis
  in congenital sex-linked agammaglobulin-
    emia, 74, 116
  cryoglobulins in, 117–118, 134
  hyperimmunoglobulinemia in, 115–117
  hyperglobulinemic purpura in, 122
  immunoglobulins in, 115–117
  macroglobulins in, 195
  associated with multiple myeloma, 141, 165–
    **166**
  associated with paraamyloidosis, 214
  paraimmunoglobulinemia in, 201
  rheumatoid factor in, 116–118
  with secondary hypo-immunoglobulinemia,
    92, 103
  serum immunoglobulin concentration in,
    112
Rheumatoid factor
  as specific agglutinator, 20–21
  cryoglobulin activity of, 118–119
  determination of, 116–117
  in families of patients with acquired hypo-
    immunoglobulinemia of late onset, 104
  in hyperglobulinemic purpura, benign (Wal-
    denström's), 123
  incidence of, 117
  in infectious mononucleosis, 121
  properties of, 116
  in rheumatoid arthritis, 116–118
  in Sjögren's syndrome, 118
  in thyroiditis, 118
"Rheumatoid factor" hyperglobulinemias, 118–
  119
RNA, defective synthesis of, 99
Rouleaux formation
  in macroglobulinemia (Waldenström's), 194
  in multiple myeloma, 169–170
Rubella
  gamma globulin in prevention of, 108
  immunoglobulins in, 114
Russell bodies
  in conjunctival plasmoma, 146
  electron micrograph of, 52
  in myeloma cells, 144, 170

**S**

Salmonellosis, immunoglobulins in, 114
Sarcoidosis

Sarcoidosis *(Continued)*
  cryoglobulins in, 119
  hyperglobulinemic purpura in, 122
  hyperimmunoglobulinemia in, 122
  immunoglobulins in, 122
  infections in, 44
  paraimmunoglobulinemia in, 201
  rheumatoid factor in, 117
  with secondary hypoimmunoglobulinemia,
    92, 93
Sarcolysin in treatment of multiple myeloma,
  190–191
Schick test, role in diagnosis, 106
Schultz-Dale reaction, 43
Scleroderma
  associated with hypoimmunoglobulinemia,
    103
  hyperglobulinemia in, 112
  hyperimmunoglobulinemia in, 120
Secondary acquired hypoimmunoglobulinemia (s), *See* Secondary hypoimmunoglobulinemia (s)
Secondary hyperimmunoglobulinemia (s), 114–
  125
Secondary hypoimmunoglobulinemia (s), 90–93
  associated with autoimmune diseases, 92
    infections in, 101
    pathology of, 97, 99
  associated with chronic infections, 92–93
  associated with hypoalbuminemia, 90–91
    infections in, 101
  associated with malignancies of the reticulo-
    endothelial system, 91–92, 106
    infections in, 101
    pathogenesis of, 96–98
  associated with pernicious anemia, 92
Secondary response, immunocytes in, 52–54
Selective adult hypoimmunoglobulinemia (s),
  80–89
  infections in, 101
  intestinal lesions in, 101
Selective hypo-IgA-globulinemia, 80–84
Selective hypo-IgA and G-globulinemia with
  increased IgM, 84–88
  cellular changes in, 84–87
  mode of inheritance, 86
  pathogenesis of, 87–88
  splenectomy in, 110
Selective hypo-IgA and M-globulinemia with
  normal IgG, 8
  mode of inheritance of, 88
  properties of, 107
Selective hypo-IgA and M-globulinemia with
  slight decrease in IgG, 88–89
Selective hypo-IgD-globulinemia, 89
Selective hypo-IgG-globulinemia, 84

Selective hypo-IgM-globulinemia, 89
Selective theories, 55, 59
Serum hepatitis
  gamma globulin in attenuation of, 108
  immunoglobulins in, 125
Serum levels, immunoglobulins
  in clinical disorders, 112
  normal, 13, 61, 63–65
Serum sickness, 43
  Forssman antibodies in, 121
Sex-linked agammaglobulinemia, congenital,
    *See* Congenital sex-linked agammaglobu-
    linemia
Sia euglobulin test
  in macroglobulinemia (Waldenström's) , 181,
    195
  in multiple myeloma, 181
Sjögren's syndrome
  cryoglobulins in, 118, 134
  hyperglobulinemic purpura in, 122
  rheumatoid factor in, 118
  serum immunoglobulin concentration in,
    112
Skin attachment, 20
Skin biopsy in paraamyloidosis, 181, 216–217
Skin manifestations
  in multiple myeloma, 160, 161
  in paraamyloidosis, 208–209
Sodium fluoride in treatment of multiple mye-
    loma, 187–188
Solitary myeloma, *See* Solitary plasmacytoma
Solitary plasmacytoma, 146, 151–152
  prognosis of, 182–183
Somatic crossing over, 56–57
Somatic mutation, 127, 129, 132, 141, 204
Somatic recombination, 57
Spleen
  antibody production in, 54
  immunocytes in, 52
  transplantation of, 110
Splenectomy in treatment of selective hypo-IgA-
    and G-immunoglobulinemia with in-
    creased IgM, 110
Splenic puncture in multiple myeloma, 170,
    181
Splenomegaly
  in multiple myeloma, 158
  in paraamyloidosis, 212
  in paraimmunoglobulinopathies, pathogen-
    esis of, 132
Sprue, nontropical with secondary hypoim-
    munoglobulinemia associated with hypo-
    albuminemia, 90, 101
Spurious macroglobulinemia, *See* "Rheumatoid
    factor" hyperglobulinemia, 118–119
sRNAs, 57

Steric relationships, 58
Steroids, anabolic, in treatment of multiple
    myeloma, 186
Stilbamidine in treatment of multiple mye-
    loma, 189
Subacute bacterial endocarditis
  cryoglobulins in, 134
  immunoglobulins in, 114
  rheumatoid factor in, 117
Swiss-type agammaglobulinemia with lympho-
    penia, 68–72
  cellular changes in, 68–71
  contraindication to immunization, 72
  definition of, 68–69
  immunoglobulins in, 69
  infections in, 69, 100
  intestinal lesions in, 101
  lymph node biopsy in, 107
  mode of inheritance, 71–72
  organ involvement in, 69–71
  pathogenesis of, 96–97
  Pneumocystis carinii pneumonia in, 69
  rectal biopsy in, 107
  treatment of, 72
Synthesis rate, immunoglobulins, 61
Syphilis
  cryoglobulins in, 134
  immunoglobulins in, 115
  rheumatoid factor in, 117
Systemic lupus erythematosus, *See* Lupus ery-
    thematosus
Systemic manifestations of multiple myeloma,
    161

**T**

Theories of antibody production, 55–60
Thesaurocytes in multiple myeloma, 144–145
Thioflavin T stain for amyloid, 205
Thioguanine, suppression of immune response
    by, 55
Thrombocytopenia in paraimmunoglobulin-
    opathies
  pathogenesis of, 132
Thymectomized animals, 52–53, 69–71
Thymocytes, nonstimulation by phytohemag-
    glutinin, 52
Thymoma
  associated with multiple myeloma, 136
  in generalized adult hypoimmunoglobu-
    linemia, 79, 104
  hyperglobulinemic purpura in, 122
  in hypoimmunoglobulinopathies, 104–106
  paraimmunoglobulinemia in, 201
  in selective hypo-IgA and G-globulinemia
    with increased IgM, 86
  in selective hypo-IgA and M-globulinemia

Thymoma (*Continued*)
    with slight decrease in IgG, 89
    pathogenesis of, 97
Thymus
    activity of, 52–53
    embryology of, 95–96
    immunocytes in, 52
    transplantation of, 110
Thymus-dependent lymphoid tissue, 95–96
Thyroiditis
    cryoglobulins in, 118
    rheumatoid factor in, 118
Tolerance, immunologic, 54, 60
Tongue biopsy in paraamyloidosis, 216
"Toxic polyneuritis" in multiple myeloma, 155
Toxoplasmosis
    immunoglobulins in, 114
    in multiple myeloma, 156
Transferrin in urine, 179
Transformation, 56
Transplantation immunity, antibody levels in, 43
Transplantation of organs in treatment of hypoimmunoglobulinopathies, 110
Transport piece, 42
Triethylene melamine in treatment of macroglobulinemia, 198
Trypanosomiasis, immunoglobulins in, 115
Tuberculosis
    hyperglobulinemic purpura in, 122
    immunoglobulins in, 115
    rheumatoid factor in, 117
Tumor cells, myeloma, distribution of, 146–147
Tumor formation in multiple myeloma, 150–153
Typhoid fever, immunoglobulins in, 114
Typhus, immunoglobulins in, 115

U

Ulcerative colitis
    with secondary hypoimmunoglobulinemia associated with hypoalbuminemia, 90, 101
    serum immunoglobulin concentration in, 112
Urethan in treatment of multiple myeloma, 188–189
Urethan-gel reaction in multiple myeloma, 181
Uric acid
    in H-chain disease, 199

Uric acid (*Continued*)
    in multiple myeloma, 180–181
    in myeloma kidney, 138, 148, 157
    in paraamyloidosis, 215
    in paraimmunoglobulinopathies, 138
Urinalysis
    in H-chain disease, 199
    in macroglobulinemia (Waldenström's), 194
    in multiple myeloma, 178–179
Urine, immunoglobulin loss in, 62

V

Vaccinia, progressive
    in congenital sex-linked agammaglobulinemia, 73
    gamma globulin in therapy of, 108
    in Swiss-type agammaglobulinemia with lymphopenia, 69
van Gieson stain for amyloid, 205
Varicella, gamma globulin in modification of, 108
Vertebral collapse
    in multiple myeloma, 146
    pathogenesis of, 132
Vinblastine in treatment of multiple myeloma, 189
Viruses as etiologic agent of paraimmunoglobulinopathy, 127–128

W

Waldenström's hyperglobulinemic purpura, *See* Hyperglobulinemic purpura, benign
Waldenström's macroglobulinemia, *See* Macroglobulinemia (Waldenström's)
Wassermann reaction
    in infectious mononucleosis, 121
    in lupus erythematosus, 119–120
    in multiple myeloma, 181
    in rheumatoid arthritis, 117
Weight loss
    in multiple myeloma, 158
    in paraamyloidosis, 214

X

X chromosome, 99
    in familial hyper-IgA-globulinemia, 114
Xanthelasma in multiple myeloma, 160
X-ray, *See* Radiologic and Radiotherapy